Recent Innovations in Surgical Procedures of Pancreatic Neoplasms

Juan Bellido Luque
Angel Nogales Muñoz

Editors

Recent Innovations in Surgical Procedures of Pancreatic Neoplasms

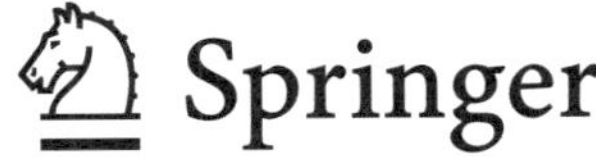

Editors
Juan Bellido Luque
Biliopancreatic Surgical Division
Hospital Universitario Virgen Macarena
Sevilla, Spain

Angel Nogales Muñoz
Biliopancreatic Surgical Division
Hospital Universitario Virgen Macarena
Sevilla, Spain

ISBN 978-3-031-21353-3   ISBN 978-3-031-21351-9   (eBook)
https://doi.org/10.1007/978-3-031-21351-9

This Springer imprint is published by the registered company Springer Nature Switzerland AG
The registered company address is: Gewerbestrasse 11, 6330 Cham, Switzerland

Foreword

In the twentieth century, the development of surgery was decisive in increasing the survival of surgical patients with the introduction of resective techniques, especially in oncologic pathology.

The improvement of anesthesia and resuscitation units have facilitated the better recovery of patients and the subsequent implantation of specific units within the surgical departments, where significant growth was experienced with a significant improvement in results.

In the second half of the last century, surgical techniques were fundamentally performed using open approaches, with extensive abdominal resections, which developed significant rate of sequelae after surgery in order to achieve optimal oncological results.

Subsequently, it was found that less invasive techniques, with limited excision, good oncological results were achieved. The development of action protocols (such as sentinel node determination in breast tumor pathology and biopsies directed by harpoons) contributed to those oncological results.

The quality-of-life tests after surgery were decisive to analyze the implanted surgical techniques and their viability. There are multiple therapeutic options, independent of the surgical interventions and where the opinions of the patients begin to be important in the surgical decision-making process. Endoluminal endoscopic techniques led an advance in the second half of the twentieth century that facilitated earlier diagnoses that facilitated better results after surgery, as well as the resolution of different issues in the area of the common bile duct, Endoscopic Retrograde Cholangiopancreatography (ERCP), and esophagus. They forced more aggressive surgeries and with worse long-term results.

In the last decade of the twentieth century, the development of laparoscopy began with quick implementation in developed countries. Firstly, cholecystectomy was disseminated as a standard technique achieving excellent results in terms of lower associated costs and rapid patients' recovery compared to open techniques. With dizzying speed and the support of the advancement of industrial technology, in optics and instrumentation, advanced laparoscopy was launched in areas of coloproctology with essentially the approach to oncological resections, obtaining good results with less morbidity and mortality and greater efficiency.

In the hepatobiliary and pancreas areas, the development has become widespread in the last decade of the twenty-first century, taking into account that its implantation has been conditioned due to the high complexity of the techniques and the need to find adequate development platforms such as robotics and 3D. It began with hand-assisted techniques in liver surgery; until today, the interventions are reproduced before open surgery and currently by full minimally invasive approach.

The improvement of other areas such as the "fastrack" protocols (multimodal rehabilitation) and lately the RICA route together with the optimization of the nutritional status in surgical patients achieve a decrease in response to surgical stress and a more comfortable and earlier recovery. Better results, less associated morbidity, and more efficiency are achieved, with the consequent reduction in healthcare costs and improved health outcomes. In addition, it has achieved a satisfactory view of the resources receiver, which is the surgical patient.

Surgical Department   Fernando Oliva Mompeán
Virgen Macarena Hospital,
Sevilla, Spain

Preface

Pancreatic cancer is the seventh most common cause of cancer-related death across the world. It has the lowest survival rate of all cancers, just 2–10% of those diagnosed survive for 5 years. Survival has improved for most cancers over the last 40 years but not for pancreatic cancer. Pancreatic cancer is nearly always diagnosed too late making the overall median survival for a person diagnosed with metastatic pancreatic cancer for 4.6 months.

The most important key to improve those statistics is the early diagnosis: patients who are diagnosed in time for surgery have a much higher likelihood of surviving for 5 years.

Only 20–30% of patients at the time of pancreatic cancer diagnosis are considered candidates for surgery, while 70–80% of patients eventually fail to receive curative treatment mainly due to systemic metastasis.

Pancreatectomy is a complex surgical procedure requiring multiple anastomoses. This is reason of high postoperative morbidity rates (pancreatic leakage, bleeding, delayed gastric emptying), high late operative morbidity rates (exocrine and endocrine pancreatic insufficiency).

The previous results in survival, prognosis, and poor survival outcomes after curative resection have been the reason that pancreatic surgeons have doubts about the role of surgery as the definitive treatment for pancreatic cancer. There is a lack of high-level evidence in the field of pancreatic surgery. Current issues in pancreatic surgery could be:

- standard pancreaticoduodenectomy vs. pylorus preservation
- standard vs. extended lymphadenectomy
- role of major vessel resections
- best reconstruction method:
    - pancreaticojejunostomy vs. pancreaticogastrostomy
    - dunking/invaginating method vs. duct-to-mucosa anastomosis
    - role of internal vs. external vs. no stent
- pancreatic transection in distal pancreatectomy
    - mechanical transection vs. transection with sealing devices
    - role of reinforced cartridges
- resectability criteria
- timing of surgery: upfront surgery, surgery after neoadjuvant therapy

The main objective of this book is to clarify these issues related to pancreatic cancer surgery, contributing to solve this lack of evidence. For this

"

proposes, the highest level of evidence (meta-analysis and systematic reviews) is used to answer the main questions related to this topic.

Writing a book is hard but more rewarding than I could have ever imagined. None of this would have been possible without my colleagues and friends in Biliopancreatic Surgical Division, Gastrointestinal Surgical Department, Virgen de la Macarena Hospital, Seville, Spain (Angel Nogales Muñoz and Inmaculada Sanchez-Matamoros Martin). They have always given me the time and support to achieve the goals in my surgical career.

A very special thanks to all authors who have contributed to the chapters of this book. Their dedication and interest on this project have been extremely important for this idea to come true.

I'm eternally grateful to my parents. They taught me discipline, tough love, manners, respect, and so much more that has helped me succeed in life. I truly have no idea where I'd be if they haven't given me a roof over my head.

To my wife Loli: Thanks for always being the person who gives me shine during the dark days. She sustained me in ways that I never knew that I needed. She never stopped me and only encouraged me to achieve my goal.

To my son Juan: Thanks for waiting for me awake every night when I come home after a hard day to play with him. Thanks for letting me spend time in this achievement. Without your smile we could not exist.

To my sisters, Chely and Silvia: Thank you for your understanding and support during all these years.

Finally, to all those who have been a part of my getting there: Aruna R Sharma (Book project coordinator) and Donatella riza (Executive editor).

Seville, Spain   Juan Bellido Luque

Contents

Introduction to Diagnosis and Treatment in Pancreatic Neoplasms

Javier Padillo-Ruiz

1.1 The Environment for Nihilism in Pancreatic Cancer

If we adapt the concept of nihilism to our medical field, we could consider it as the approach to knowledge from a fatalistic point of view: in the end, everything is reduced to nothing and, therefore, nothing makes sense. The first World Pancreatic Cancer Day, held in Spain in 2014, had the following headline in the media: "Nihilism is the usual tendency in pancreatic cancer" [1]. It is certainly difficult to find scientific articles that do not begin by describing pancreatic cancer as an intractable malignant tumor with a very poor prognosis. Unfortunately, its incidence is increasing and according to GLOBOCAN 2020 [2], it is the twelfth most common cancer in the world, with 495,773 new cases. However, it is the 7th leading cause of cancer-related deaths, causing 466,003 deceases (4.5% of all cancer deaths). While mortality is declining in other types of cancers, it is increasing in pancreatic cancers. Generally, after diagnosis, only 24% of people survive 1 year and 9% live for 5 years [3]. This situation is not new and, unfortunately, there have not been great advances with enough impact on the results. The keys to this situation that causes nihilism are:

- Pancreatic cancer is mainly diagnosed at an advanced stage. Regrettably, 80–90% of patients present unresectable tumors at the time of diagnosis [4].
- Surgery is the only curative therapeutic option. However, even when resection is performed successfully, the overall survival as well as the disease-free survival rates remain very low due to local recurrence or distant spread [5].

Beyond the epidemiological and screening aspects, this chapter will address the most relevant general aspects of the diagnostic and therapeutic approach and the possible future approaches to improve results.

1.2 Key Points in the Diagnosis of Pancreatic Cancer

1.2.1 Molecular Diagnosis: Toward the Early Diagnosis in Pancreatic Cancer

When the patient presents symptoms of pancreatic cancer, both body and head, the tumor is, in a high percentage of cases, advanced. This makes it necessary to look for other signs that facilitate the diagnosis in earlier stages, for

J. Padillo-Ruiz (✉)
Department of General Surgery, Virgen del Rocio Hospital, Seville, Spain

Seville, Spain

instance, germline mutations which are involved in pancreatic cancer development [6, 7]. According to the National Comprehensive Cancer Network guideline, germline testing must be done for any patient with confirmed pancreatic cancer [8].

Ductal intraepithelial neoplasia (PanIN) is considered the most common type of pancreatic adenocarcinoma precursor. There are complex mutational steps from this event until cancer dissemination that include Kras, Ckn2a, Tp53, or Smad4 mutations. From them, Kras gene is mutated in more than 90% of cases [9] and G12D mutation is the most commonly observed [10]. The severity of the cancer evolution is associated with the number of mutant genes. Recently, in a meta-analysis carried out by Zhao et al. [11], it was assessed that the detection of microRNAs was related to not only the prognosis of pancreatic cancer, but also the identification of therapeutic targets [12]. Similarly, promising advances have been developed under the name of "omics". The "omics" concept includes the evaluation of circulating biomarkers, exosomes, or cell-free DNA (cfDNA) through different sequencing techniques, including transcriptomic [13].

An important key is where these markers can be more expressive, either in peripheral blood or in portal blood, where pancreatic cancer drains directly. In theory, the detection of circulating tumor cells (CTCs) in portal blood should be more accurate and it might be associated with a higher probability of liver metastases [14] (Fig. 1.1).

Earl et al. [15] evaluated CTC and DNA circulating in peripheral blood obtaining good results when they were correlated with the existence of pancreatic cancer. However, in a preliminary study carried out by Padillo et al. [16], we detected that CTCs in portal blood correlate better with tumor size and neural infiltration than in peripheral blood.

The fact of discovering a CTC would absolutely not imply the appearance of distant metastases since clusters of cells would be needed for them to occur. It remains to be defined which is the cut-off point for the number of CTCs from which the existence of a high risk of distant disease could be considered. This type of information is relevant to plan the actions to undertake.

In summary, the in-depth study of mutations and their early detection, as well as markers such as microRNA, CTC, cfDNA, or exosomes could allow new therapeutic targets. Due to the fact that a large number of biomarkers are proposed, a platform for the validation of the biomarkers used to detect early stages of pancreatic cancer has been proposed [17].

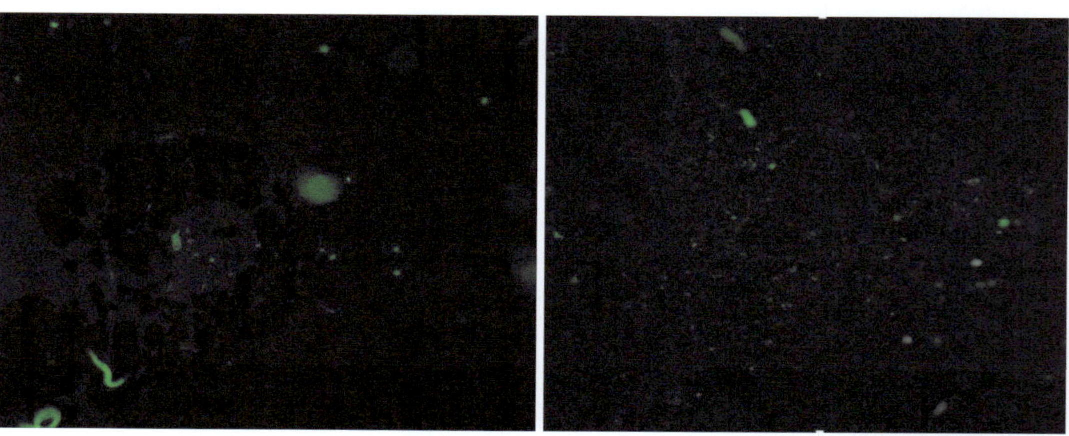

Fig. 1.1 Portal vein vs. peripheral CTCs assessment. Samples from the same patient; Portal blood: 2.170 CTCs and 15 cluster. Peripheral blood: 114 CTCs and 2 cluster

1.2.2   Radiomics: Diagnostic Imaging as a Tool for Pathological Specification and Prognosis in Pancreatic Cancer

When a patient is diagnosed with pancreatic cancer, computerized tomography (CT) scan with vascular contrast is the test of choice to assess the location, size, local extension and possible existence of distant metastases. Today, 3D reconstructions allow to obtain magnificent images that are very useful in diagnosis and treatment planning. However, as mentioned above, it is difficult to reach a diagnosis in the early stages of tumor development. Like other disciplines, radiology is working to image early lesions. Another frequent problem is to obtain a sample significant enough to have a histological diagnosis after biopsy in order to clearly guide the treatment.

Currently, radiology is generating very relevant advancements aimed at providing key preoperative information in relation to both the possible malignancy of the pancreatic lesion and the prediction of results after treatments. In this sense, the "radiomics" described by Lambin et al. [18] uses artificial intelligence and machine learning procedures in the processing of the images that are allowing to make approximations not only to the location and extension but also to the type of tumor and possible vascular or neural infiltration. Radiomics uses artificial intelligence and a machine learning approach to analyze a large amount of radiological images and extracting information from them [18], taking into account the pathology, biomarkers, and tumor phenotypes [19]. Machine learning and artificial intelligence applications allow radiomic findings to be properly correlated with overall survival as well as with the potential response to selected chemotherapy [20–22].

The decision to offer either surgery or neoadjuvant chemotherapy as the first option generates debates within the multidisciplinary committees that evaluate patients with pancreatic cancer. The developments of CT-based radiomic features have proven to be able to provide sufficiently relevant tumor information to establish the prognosis in resectable patients with pancreatic cancer. These features may be really useful to stratify patients for neoadjuvant or alternative therapies [23, 24]. Clinically, there are often doubts about the malignancy of certain types of cystic lesions, especially mucinous ones, and finally, after surgery, there might be up to a 30% of discrepancy between the pre- and postoperative diagnoses. Using multiphase CT radiomics and accepted parameters from international guidelines, Polk and colleagues [25] analyzed mucinous intraductal papillary lesions (IPMNs) to assess the degree of malignancy. The authors compared the nomogram created using only the diagnostic parameters of the International Consensus Guidelines to the one resulted from using both the guidelines and radiomic images. When both tools (radiomics and guidelines) were used, the results in predicting the malignancy of the pathology were far better. Radiomics has also been carried out to assess recurrence and prognosis with other techniques. In fact, in a recent study, a CT radiomic evaluation using clinical data and textural features done in patients with advanced pancreatic cancer, the authors developed a predictive model not only for local recurrence but also for overall survival after Stereotactic Body Radiotherapy application [26, 27]. Another recent study by Tang et al. [28] developed a multiparametric nomogram for the preoperative assessment of local recurrence including clinical stage, and artificial intelligence applied to magnetic resonance imaging (MRI).

In summary, undoubtedly, radiomic tools will allow more precise decisions to be made, generating confidence in both patients and professionals.

1.3   Key Points in the Treatment of Pancreatic Cancer

1.3.1   Medical Treatment: Personalized and Precision Therapy in Pancreatic Cancer

Nowadays, chemotherapy is recommended as a palliative treatment and as an adjuvant therapy in almost all patients after surgery. As adjuvant therapy, in general, it is recommended not to delay the start of chemotherapy excessively, which is why most protocols start it in the first 3 months after surgery [29, 30]. At present, from the PRODIGE study 24, the treatment of choice in Western countries is the combination of modified FOLFIRINOX (m FOLFIRINOX) [31]. In the study carried out in resected patients, the results showed significant differences in favor of FOLFIRINOX versus Gemcitabine in both pancreatic cancer disease-free survival (21.6 vs. 12.8 months, respectively) and overall patient survival (54.4 vs. 35 months, respectively).

Regarding neoadjuvant chemotherapy, currently there is no doubt about the use of neoadjuvant therapy in locally advanced pancreatic carcinoma. Some meta-analyses performed to evaluate FOLFIRINOX as neoadjuvant chemotherapy, reported a 67.8% resection rate and an 83.9% R0 resection rate [32]. However, since no well-designed studies are included in this meta-analysis, prospective randomized trials are necessary to evaluate properly the role of neoadjuvant therapy. The role of FOLFIRINOX as neoadjuvant therapy in resectable pancreatic cancer is under several studies (NCT02172976, NCT02562716, NCT02243007, NCT02345460). Although current clinical guidelines used routinely in pancreatic adenocarcinoma support the use of neoadjuvant chemotherapy, more prospective trials and meta-analysis including not only chemotherapy but also stereotactic radiotherapy as neoadjuvant therapy are needed to evaluate perioperative strategies in patients with both unresectable and resectable pancreatic cancer. However, as previously shown, despite significantly improving the result over the established standard, the results are still not comparable to those of other tumors. Current guidelines will probably change, mainly those related to the progress in the knowledge of the tumor biology, which could help define the best choice of chemotherapy. According to our research, in pancreatic cancer, better results are obtained when combinations of drugs are used [33, 34].

In the evaluation of medical treatment of pancreatic cancer, the biomarkers that provide relevant diagnostic and prognostic information will have to be taken into account. From the different biomarkers currently being analyzed to assess therapeutics, possibly the most developed one is Circulating Tumor DNA (ctDNA) [29]. Detectable ctDNA before surgery has been associated with a worse prognosis, and when detected after, it has been connected to local recurrence and a significant decrease in survival. The next steps to be evaluated in prospective studies would be whether once this measurement technique is established, the detection of ctDNA could be a systematic indication of the administration of neoadjuvant. One might even wonder whether in patients who continue to present ctDNA after neoadjuvant treatment the surgery is suitable or not. Possibly, the answer is not only in the ctDNA, but in the joint evaluation with other biomarkers such as the measurement of Circulating Tumor Cells (CTCs) as previously mentioned [16], and the measurement of systemic inflammatory markers such as neutrophil-to-lymphocyte ratio (NLR) [35]. In these cases, it would be necessary to determine the cut-off points from which its detection is associated with metastases not yet visualized in CT scan images and with the indication of one therapy or another.

But in addition to using biomarkers that help us determine whether a patient would receive surgery or chemotherapy, it is key to personalize cancer therapies including the predictive pathological biomarkers related to the effectiveness of chemotherapy. This line has been specially worked on with Gemcitabine and 2 markers: the equilibrative nucleoside transporter 1 (hENT1) [36] and the phosphorylation by deoxycytidine kinase (dCK) [37]. First is the main transporter that allows the absorption of Gemcitabine into the cell, and the second facilitates the conversion of Gemcitabine into active metabolites. When an increase in the expression of hENT1 or dCK is detected, the permeation to Gemcitabine will be greater and therefore better oncological results could be obtained. These results must be confirmed in long prospective series to be incorporated into the decision algorithms in the clinical guidelines.

On the other hand, pancreatic adenocarcinoma presents different histopathological structures (angiogenesis, stroma, stellate cells, immune cells, etc.) that must be approached individually, since pancreatic adenocarcinoma does not express them equally in all patients. This would lead us to wonder whether the same group of drugs should be applied to all patients or not, when to do it, the doses, etc.

Indeed, at present, transcriptomics and bioinformatics are modifying the approach to these tumors. Based on transcriptomic profiles after bioinformatics analysis, five subtypes of adenocarcinomas have been described: "pure basal-like," "stroma-activated," "desmoplastic," "immune classical," and "pure classical" [38]. As observed in the preliminary results of the COMPASS study in which the effectiveness of FOLFIRINOX was assessed according to the histological subtype of pancreatic adenocarcinoma [39], this classification allowed to determine the best chemotherapy treatment, identifying the specific target in each case. Although more prospective studies that include the different options are needed, work is being done with immunomodulatory, antistromal, and cytotoxic drugs with personalized programming based on the predominant molecular subtypes.

The culmination of all the above is the incorporation of artificial intelligence and radiomic machine learning together with the rest of the biomarkers in order to select the drug which will enable us to obtain the best response to chemotherapy treatment. In a study by Kaississ et al. [40], artificial intelligence and machine learning associated with radiomics made it possible to identify the subtypes of adenocarcinoma of pancreas which were correlated with disease-free survival and overall survival according to the predicted response to Gemcitabine or FOLFIRINOX.

In summary, although the implementation of FOLFIRINOX has improved the results obtained with monotherapy, they are still substantially inferior to other tumors. Hence, the lines of work are focused on personalized therapies to the molecular structure of the tumor through transcriptomic studies, identifying the ideal drug combination for the molecular composition of the tumor. To achieve the greatest therapeutic effectiveness on these molecular structures, it is essential to identify drug effectiveness markers that ensure a high level of permeation in the neoplastic tissue. Finally, in all this algorithm, we will have to take into account biological markers such as ctDNA that will help us define which patients can benefit from one type of therapy or another and their results.

1.3.2 The Surgical Approach as a Guarantor of the Locoregional Eradication of Pancreatic Cancer

As with chemotherapy, the surgical approach does not offer the results that are obtained from oncological surgery in other locations. In pancreatic cancer, the follow-up of the patients has revealed a poor survival rate due to high cancer recurrence. Unfortunately, the rate of surgical margin affected (R1) remains too high, especially in the increasingly frequent cases of locally advanced tumors with prior neoadjuvant treatment [41]. The technique of approaching the superior mesenteric artery initially ("artery-first" approach) has been proposed to try to reduce the rate of R1 [42] (Fig. 1.2). However, in the multicenter randomized study carried out by the pancreas surgery groups in Spain, it has not shown superiority compared to the classical technique of approaching the hilum and portal vein in the first place in duodenopancreatectomy [43]. Regardless of the approach route, to achieve a complete excision of pancreatic cancer, especially in locally advanced tumors, it is necessary to perform a complete vascular approach with dissection of the spleno-porto-meseraic venous axis, mesenteric artery and hepatic artery-celiac trunk (Fig. 1.3). A complete dissection of all these structures is essential to be able to carry out vascular resections when the tumor requires it. These resections may be more localized and be reconstructed with end-to-end venous suture (Fig. 1.4), or more extensive when it affects the confluence of the ileo-ceo-colic and jejunal

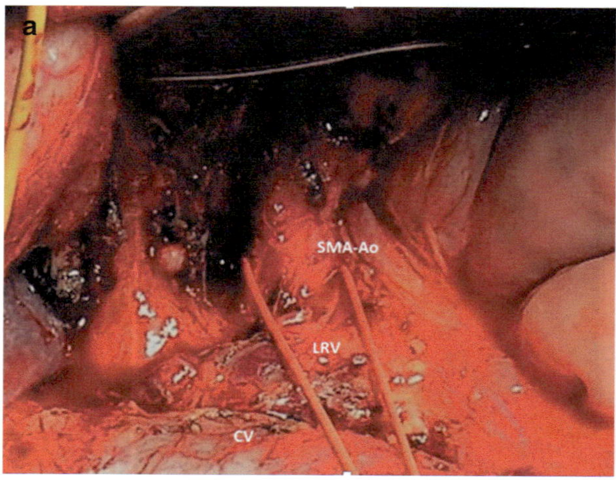

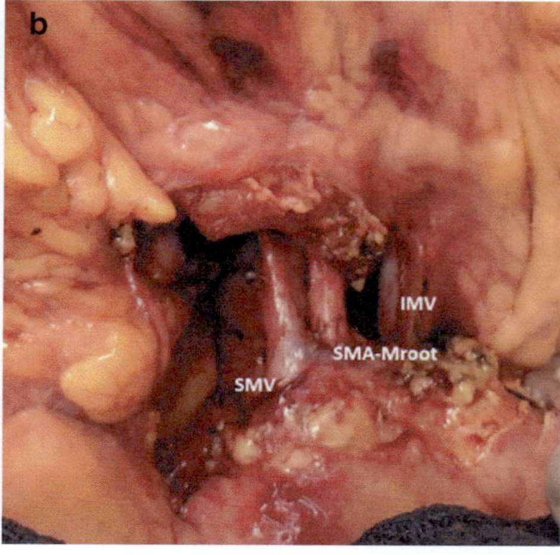

Fig. 1.2 Artery-first approach. (**a**) Proximal approach; *SMA-Ao* superior mesenteric artery at the bifurcation of aorta, *LRV* left renal vein, *CV* cava vein. (**b**) Distal approach; *SMV* superior mesenteric vein, *SMA-Mroot* superior mesenteric artery at mesenteric root, *IMV* inferior mesenteric vein

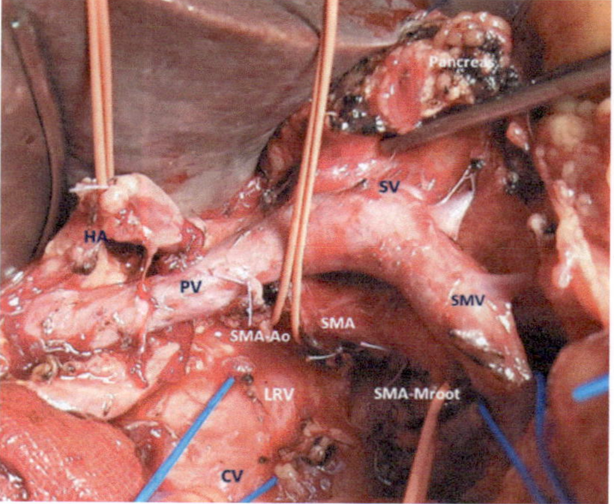

Fig. 1.3 Vascular dissection in duodenopancreatectomy. *HA* hepatic artery, *PV* portal vein, *SV* splenic vein, *SMV* superior mesenteric vein, *SMA* superior mesenteric artery, *SMA-Ao* superior mesenteric artery at the bifurcation of aorta, *SMA-Mroot* superior mesenteric artery at mesenteric root, *LRV* left renal vein, *CV* cava vein

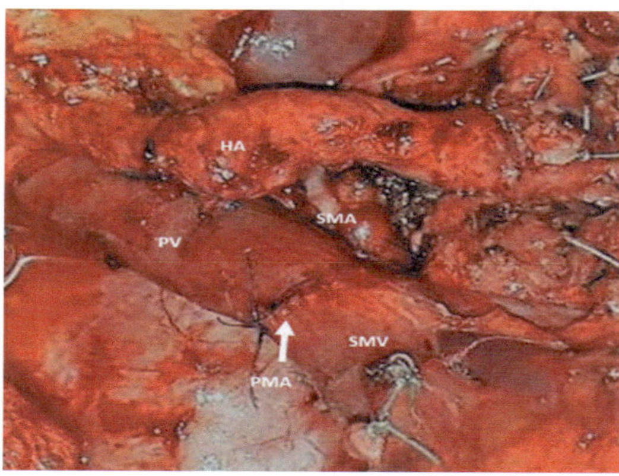

Fig. 1.4 End-to-end venous reconstruction. *HA* hepatic artery, *PV* portal vein, *SMV* superior mesenteric vein, *SMA* superior mesenteric artery, *PMA* porto-mesenteric anastomosis

venous branches in the superior mesenteric vein, requiring a Y prosthesis (Fig. 1.5). The relevance of the experience of the surgeons and the volume of activity of the units for this type of intervention and its impact on surgical and oncological results have been widely discussed. In a study carried out in hospitals in Germany and the Netherlands, they observed that centers with smaller volumes had higher mortality in pancreatic cancer interventions [44]. On the other hand, regarding oncologic approach, less delay in chemotherapy was also found in hospitals with a higher volume of cases [45].

In all this debate on how to optimize oncologic-surgical results, and even without reaching a clear global strategy, the minimally invasive surgery appears. The general benefits of laparoscopic surgery are indisputable, but it is necessary to assess them in each type of intervention. According to the aforementioned, it is obvious that it must ensure an oncological

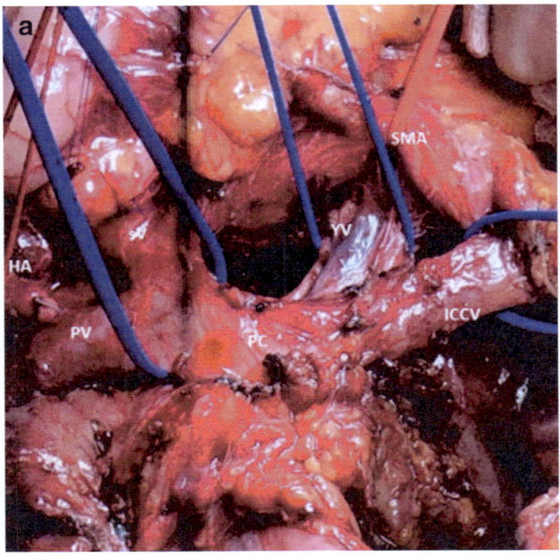

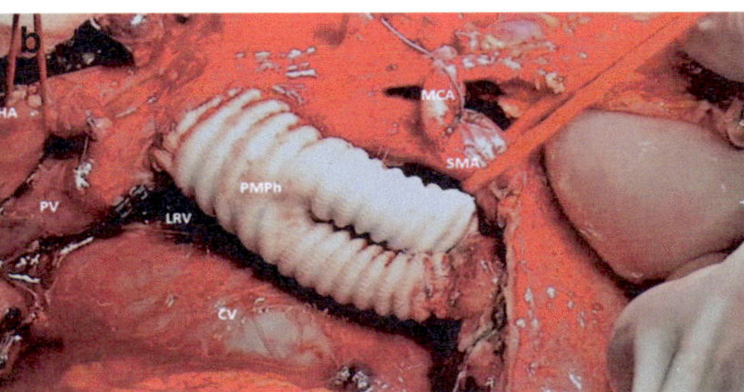

Fig. 1.5 Tumoral invasion of confluence of the ileo-ceo-colic and jejunal venous branches in the superior mesenteric vein, requiring a Y prosthesis. (**a**) *HA* hepatic artery, *PV* portal vein, *SV* splenic vein, *YV* jejunal vein, *ICCV* ileo-ceco-colic vein, *SMA* superior mesenteric artery, *PC* pancreatic cancer. (**b**) *HA* hepatic artery, *PV* portal vein, *SMA* superior mesenteric artery, *MCA* middle colic artery, *LRV* left renal vein, *CV* cava vein, *PMph* porto-mesenteric prosthesis

result at least equal to open surgery and maintain morbidity and mortality standards. Bearing in mind that laparoscopic surgery requires a specific learning curve, one might wonder if it is reasonable to assume even worse results in a pathology with surgical results still to be improved. In body and tail tumors, in which a distal pancreatectomy with lymph node cleansing must be performed, there are different experiences supporting the feasibility and safety of laparoscopic surgery [46]. Nevertheless, because of the reported excess mortality in the randomized LEOPARD-2 trial (10 vs. 2%), currently there is no consensus to recommend a laparoscopy approach for pancreaticoduodenectomy, despite an equivalent quality of exeresis [47]. A recent meta-analysis [48] concluded that, according to the level of evidence, laparoscopic duodenopancreatectomy has no advantage when compared to open surgery. However, nowadays, the quality of evidence is very low regarding the learning curve results in this type of surgery. In this sense, it could be interesting to evaluate the learning curve with a robotic approach to duodenopancreatectomy that, in general, seems to be quite less steep than with the standard laparoscopic approach [49]. As a positive aspect of the laparoscopic approach in patients without severe complications, laparoscopic surgery allows to increase the adjuvant chemotherapy rate as well as to reduce the delay in chemotherapy, due to a prompt recovery [45]. In these cases, in which the same surgical oncological (R0) and morbidity and mortality results can be assured, these considerations may be important.

One aspect that will have to be evaluated is the impact that minimally invasive surgery could have on the intraoperative spread of neoplastic disease. In patients with pancreatic cancer, the pancreas manipulation during open surgery may increase the tumor cell spread via the portal vein and thus increase the risk of liver metastasis. Theoretically, a non-touch isolation technique might reduce the circulating tumor cell (CTC) spread. Thus, we have designed a prospective multicenter randomized study to monitor the CTC level during open pancreaticoduodenectomy in patients with carcinoma of the head of the pancreas [50]. In this study, non-touch and

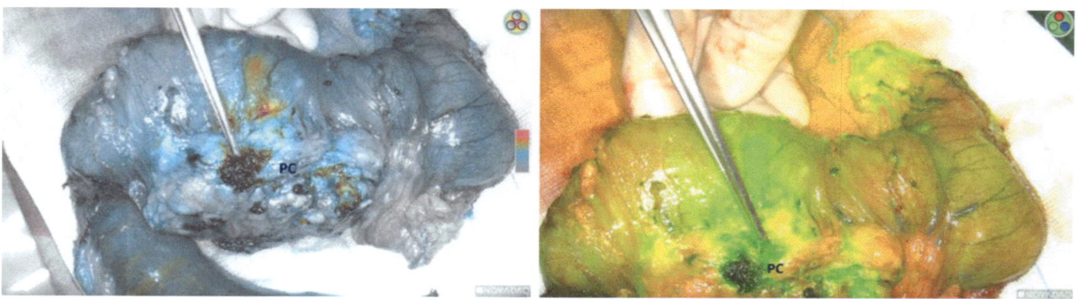

Fig. 1.6 Intraoperative use of indocyanine green. *PC* pancreatic cancer

artery-first approaches are compared and long-term follow-up results will be evaluated according to intraoperative CTC levels. It might as well be interesting to develop this study including a laparoscopic approach that could reduce the tumor manipulation and, consequently, the CTC spread.

Regardless of the approach route, a very limiting aspect of pancreatic cancer surgery is the high local recurrence rate. There are currently different and novel lines of research that seek to optimize the effects of systemic treatment of pancreatic cancer by implementing the locoregional effect of chemotherapeutic agents. One of the ways is to facilitate the arrival of chemotherapeutic and/or immunotherapeutic drugs to tumor cells. For this, the use of various vehicles (lysosomes, exosomes, vectors, etc.) is proposed which, when administered systemically and loaded with drugs, lead them to tumor cells. However, these strategies often fail in their mission to get the medication to the neoplastic cell due to the dense stromal matrix that pancreatic adenocarcinomas have. This matrix is responsible for the poorly vascularized and immunosuppressive microenvironment characteristic of this type of tumor. Hence, research is currently being conducted on formulas that allow high concentrations of chemotherapy/immunotherapy and antistromal medication in the tumor itself to generate a synergistic antineoplastic effect. Based on the contributions made in the field of peritoneal carcinomatosis, using hyperthermic intraoperative intraperitoneal chemotherapy (HIPEC), our research group has developed a biodevice (TARTESSUS®) (FISEVI-19004) that releases chemotherapy drugs on a scheduled basis. Applied locally after resection, this biodevice would release chemotherapeutic agents in a delayed and controlled manner to promote local permeation and reduce recurrences. These studies are currently in the development phase.

At present, another development to reduce the incidence of R1 and ensure a good lymphadenectomy is indocyanine green-guided surgery (Fig. 1.6). Fluorescent structures showed during operation allow the surgeon not only to identify potential lymphatic dissemination but also to be sure that resected mesopancreas tissue is free of tumor [51, 52]. In our experience, it has both served to facilitate the identification of lymphadenopathy or free margin, and to detect multicentric lesions not identified in the preoperative tests that have modified the expected surgical technique, changing the cephalic duodenopancreatectomy for a total duodenopancreatectomy.

To sum up, navigation tools must be key to achieving radical goals in pancreatic cancer oncological surgery. In both open and laparoscopic or robotic surgery, they should be incorporated progressively. In the same way as in chemotherapeutic medical treatment, the application of radiomics can play a crucial role in the personalization of treatments. The intraoperative incorporation of radiomics with artificial intelligence and machine learning developments, together with the current fluorescence, should contribute to important advances to carry out the surgical approach of each patient in a personalized way.

Acknowledgments To my colleagues of the University Hospital Virgen del Rocio HPB Unit and IBIS Pancreas Cancer Research Team: Gomez- Bravo MA, Suarez G, Alamo JM, Marin LM, Bernal C, Cepeda C, Beltran P, Calero F, Pereira S, Castillo JM, Macher H, Gallego I, Perez H, Borrero JJ.

References

1. https://www.diariomedico.com/2014/11/13/areaci-entifica/especialidades/oncologia/investigacion/nihilismo-es-tonica-actual-cancer-pancreas
2. https://gco.iarc.fr/today/data/factsheets/cancers/13-Pancreas-fact-sheet.pdf
3. World Health Organization. World cancer report 2020.
4. Rawla P, Sunkara T, Gaduputi V. Epidemiology of pancreatic cancer: global trends, etiology and risk factors. World J Oncol. 2019;10:10–27.
5. Siegel RL, Miller KD, Jemal A. Cancer statistics, 2018. CA Cancer J Clin. 2018;68:7–30.
6. Solomon S, Das S, Brand R, Whitcomb DC. Inherited pancreatic cancer syndromes. Cancer J. 2012;18:485–91.
7. Greer JB, Whitcomb DC, Brand RE. Genetic predisposition to pancreatic cancer: a brief review. Am J Gastroenterol. 2007;102:2564–9.
8. National Comprehensive Cancer Network. NCCN Guidelines for Treatment of Cancer by Site. Available online: https://www.nccn.org/professionals/physician_gls/default.aspx#site
9. Jones S, Zhang X, Parsons DW, Lin JC, Leary RJ, Angenendt P, Mankoo P, Carter H, Kamiyama H, Jimeno A, Hong SM, Fu B, Lin MT, Calhoun ES, Kamiyama M, Walter K, Nikolskaya T, Nikolsky Y, Hartigan J, Smith DR, Hidalgo M, Leach SD, Klein AP, Jaffee EM, Goggins M, Maitra A, Iacobuzio-Donahue C, Eshleman JR, Kern SE, Hruban RH, Karchin R, Papadopoulos N, Parmigiani G, Vogelstein B, Velculescu VE, Kinzler KW. Core signaling pathways in human pancreatic cancers revealed by global genomic analyses. Science. 2008;321:1801–6.
10. Morris JPT, Wang SC, Hebrok M. KRAS, Hedgehog, Wnt and the twisted developmental biology of pancreatic ductal adenocarcinoma. Nat Rev Cancer. 2010;10:683–95.
11. Zhao F, Wei C, Cui M-Y, Xia Q-Q, Wang S-B, Zhang Y. Prognostic value of microRNAs in pancreatic cancer: a meta-analysis. Aging. 2020;12:9380–404.
12. Ryan DP, Hong TS, Bardeesy N. Pancreatic adenocarcinoma. N Engl J Med. 2014;371:1039.
13. Zhang X, Shi S, Zhang B, Ni Q, Yu X, Xu J. Circulating biomarkers for early diagnosis of pancreatic cancer: facts and hopes. Am J Cancer Res. 2018;8:332–53.
14. Liu X, Li C, Li J, Yu T, Zhou G, Cheng J, Li G, Zhou Y, Lou W, Wang X, Gong G, Liu L, Che Y. Detection of CTCs in portal vein was associated with intrahepatic metastases and prognosis in patients with advanced pancreatic cáncer. J Cancer. 2018;9:2038–45.
15. Earl J, Garcia-Nieto S, Martinez-Avila JC, Montans J, Sanjuanbenito A, Rodríguez-Garrote M, Lisa E, Mendía E, Lobo E, Malats N, Carrato A, Guillen-Ponce C. Circulating tumor cells (Ctc) and kras mutant circulating free Dna (cfdna) detection in peripheral blood as biomarkers in patients diagnosed with exocrine pancreatic cáncer. BMC Cancer. 2015;15:797–807.
16. Padillo J, Pereira S, Villanueva P, Suarez G, Marin L, Bernal C, Cepeda C, Beltran P, Alamo JM, Gomez MA, Muntane J. CTSs evaluation as prognostic marker in pancreatic cancer. Portal vein versus peripheral blood sample determination. ISLB Meeting 2020.
17. Young M, Wagner P, Ghosh S, Rinaudo JA, Baker SG, Zaret KS, Goggins M, Srivastava S. Validation of biomarkers for early detection of pancreatic cáncer: summary of the Allience of Pancreatic Cancer Consortia for workshop. Pancreas. 2018;47:135–41.
18. Lambin P, Rios-Velazquez E, Leijenaar R, Carvalho S, van Stiphout R, Granton P, Zegers CML, Gillies R, Boellard R, Dekker A, Aerts HJW. Radiomics: extracting more information from medical images using advanced feature analysis. Eur J Cancer. 2012;48:441–6.
19. Kato S, Honda K. Use of biomarkers and imaging for early detection of pancreatic cancer. Cancers. 2020;12:1965.
20. Jiang Y, Yuan Q, Lv W, Xi S, Huang W, Sun Z, Chen H, Zhao L, Liu W, Hu Y, Lu L, Ma J, Li T, Yu J, Wang Q, Li G. Radiomic signature of (18)F fluorodeoxyglucose PET/CT for prediction of gastric cancer survival and chemotherapeutic benefits. Theranostics. 2018;8:5915–28.
21. Yang L, Gu D, Wei J, Yang C, Rao S, Wang W, Chen C, Ding Y, Tian J, Zeng M. A radiomics nomogram for preoperative prediction of microvascular invasion in hepatocellular carcinoma. Liver Cancer. 2019;8:373–86.
22. Ma X, Wei J, Gu D, Zhu Y, Feng B, Liang M, Wang S, Zhao X, Tian J. Preoperative radiomics nomogram for microvascular invasion prediction in hepatocellular carcinoma using contrast-enhanced CT. Eur Radiol. 2019;29:3595–605.
23. Khalvati F, Zhang Y, Baig S, Lobo-Mueller EM, Karanicolas P, Gallinger S, Masoom A. Haider prognostic value of CT radiomic features in resectable pancreatic ductal adenocarcinoma. Sci Rep. 2019;9:5449.
24. Permuth JB, Choi J, Balarunathan Y, Kim J, Chen D-T, Chen L, Orcutt S, Doepker MP, Gage K, Zhang G, Latifi K, Hoffe S, Jiang K, Coppola D, Centeno BA, Magliocco A, Li Q, Trevino J, Merchant N, Gillies R, Malafa M, Florida Pancreas Collaborative. Combining radiomic features with a miRNA classifier may improve prediction of malignant pathology for pancreatic intraductal papillary mucinous neoplasms. Oncotarget. 2016;7:85785–97.
25. Polk SL, Choi JW, McGettigan MJ, Rose T, Ahmed A, Kim J, Jiang K, Balagurunathan Y, Qi J, Farah PT, Rathi A, Permuth JB, Jeong D. Multiphase computed tomography radiomics of pancreatic intraductal pap-

illary mucinous neoplasms to predict malignancy. World J Gastroenterol. 2020;26:3458–71.

26. Cozzi L, Comito T, Fogliata A, Franzese C, Franceschini D, Bonifacio C, Tozzi A, Di Brina L, Clerici E, Tomatis S, Reggiori G, Lobefalo F, Stravato A, Mancosu A, Zerbi A, Sollini M, Kirienko M, Chiti A, Scorsetti M. Computed tomography based radiomic signature as predictive of survival and local control after stereotactic body radiation therapy in pancreatic carcinoma. PLoS One. 2019;14(1):e0210758. https://doi.org/10.1371/journal.pone.0210758.

27. Parr E, Du Q, Zhang C, Lin C, Kamal A, McAlister J, Liang X, Bavitz K, Rux G, Hollingsworth M, Baine M, Zheng D. Radiomics-based outcome prediction for pancreatic cancer following stereotactic body radiotherapy. Cancers. 2020;12:1051.

28. Tang T-Y, Li X, Zhang Q, Guo C-X, Zhang X-Z, Lao M-Y, Shen Y-N, Xiao W-B, Ying S-H, Sun K, Yu R-S, Gao S-L, Que R-S, Chen W, Huang D-B, Pang P-P, Bai X-L, Liang T-B. Development of a novel multiparametric MRI radiomic nomogram for preoperative evaluation of early recurrence in resectable pancreatic cancer. J Magn Reson Imaging. 2020;52:231–45.

29. Turpin A, el Amrani M, Bachet JB, Pietrasz D, Schwarz L, Hammel P. Adjuvant pancreatic cancer management: towards new perspectives in 2021. Cancers. 2020;12:3866.

30. Valle JW, Palmer D, Jackson R, Cox T, Neoptolemos JP, Ghaneh P, Rawcli E, Bassi C, Stocken DD, Cunningham D, O'Reilly D, Goldstein D, Robinson BA, Karapetis C, Scarfe A, Lacaine F, Sand J, Izbicki J, Mayerle J, Dervenis C, Oláh A, Butturini G, Lind PA, Middleton MR, Anthoney A, Sumpter K, Carter R, Büchle MK. Optimal duration and timing of adjuvant chemotherapy after definitive surgery for ductal adenocarcinoma of the pancreas: ongoing lessons from the ESPAC-3 study. J Clin Oncol. 2014;32:504–12.

31. Conroy T, Hammel P, Hebbar M, Ben Abdelghani M, Wei AC, Raoul JL, Choné L, Francois E, Artru P, Biagi JJ, Lecomte T, Assenat E, Faroux R, Ychou M, Volet J, Sauvanet A, Breysacher G, Di Fiore F, Cripps C, Kavan P, Texereau P, Bouhier-Leporrier K, Khemissa-Akouz F, Legoux JL, Juzyna B, Gourgou S, O'Callaghan CJ, Jouffroy-Zeller C, Rat P, Malka D, Castan F, Bachet JB, Canadian Cancer Trials Group and the Unicancer-GI-PRODIGE Group. FOLFIRINOX or Gemcitabine as adjuvant therapy for pancreatic cancer. N Engl J Med. 2018;379:2395–406.

32. Janssen QP, Buettner S, Suker M, Beumer BR, Addeo P, Bachellier P, Bahary N, Bekaii-Saab T, Bali MA, Besselink MG, Boone BA, Chau I, Clarke S, Dillhoff M, El-Rayes BF, Frakes JM, Grose D, Hosein PJ, Jamieson NB, Javed AA, Khan K, Kim KP, Kim SC, Kim SS, Ko AH, Lacy J, Margonis GA, McCarter MD, McKay CJ, Mellon EA, Moorcraft SY, Okada KI, Paniccia A, Parikh PJ, Peters NA, Rabl H, Samra J, Tinchon C, van Tienhoven G, van Veldhuisen E, Wang-Gillam A, Weiss MJ, Wilmink JW, Yamaue H, Homs MYV, van Eijck CHJ, Katz MHG, Groot KB. Neoadjuvant FOLFIRINOX in patients with borderline resectable pancreatic cancer: a systematic review and patient-level meta-analysis. Natl Cancer Inst. 2019;111:782–94.

33. Padillo FJ, Ruiz-Rabelo JF, Cruz A, Perea MD, Tasset I, Montilla P, Tunez I, Muntane J. Melatonin and celecoxib improve the outcomes in hamsters with experimental pancreatic cancer. J Pineal Res. 2010;49:264–70.

34. Ruiz-Rabelo J, Vázquez R, Arjona A, Perea D, Montilla P, Túnez I, Muntané J, Padillo J. Improvement of capecitabine antitumoral activity by melatonin in pancreatic cancer. 2011;40:410–4.

35. Bhatti I, Peacock O, Lloyd G, Larvin M, Hall RI. Preoperative hematologic markers as independent predictors of prognosis in resected pancreatic ductal adenocarcinoma: neutrophil-lymphocyte versus platelet-lymphocyte ratio. Am J Surg. 2010;200:197–203.

36. Conroy T, Ducreux M. Adjuvant treatment of pancreatic cancer. Curr Opin Oncol. 2019;31:346–53.

37. Maréchal R, Bachet J-B, Mackey JR, Dalban C, Demetter P, Graham K, Couvelard A, Svrcek M, Bardier-Dupas A, Hammel P, et al. Levels of gemcitabine transport and metabolism proteins predict survival times of patients treated with gemcitabine for pancreatic adenocarcinoma. Gastroenterology. 2012;143:664–74.

38. Puleo F, Nicolle R, Blum Y, Cros J, Marisa L, Demetter P, Quertinmont E, Svrcek M, Elarouci N, Iovanna J, Franchimont D, Verset L, Galdon MG, Devière J, de Reyniès A, Laurent-Puig P, Van Laethem JL, Bachet JB, Maréchal R. Stratification of pancreatic ductal adenocarcinomas based on tumor and microenvironment features. Gastroenterology. 2018;155:1999–2013.

39. Aung KL, Fischer SE, Denroche RE, Jang GH, Dodd A, Creighton S, Southwood B, Liang SB, Chadwick D, Zhang A, O'Kane GM, Albaba H, Moura S, Grant RC, Miller JK, Mbabaali F, Pasternack D, Lungu IM, Bartlett JMS, Ghai S, Lemire M, Holter S, Connor AA, Moffitt RA, Yeh JJ, Timms L, Krzyzanowski PM, Dhani N, Hedley D, Notta F, Wilson JM, Moore MJ, Gallinger S, Knox JJ. Genomics-driven precision medicine for advanced pancreatic cancer: early results from the COMPASS trial. Clin Cancer Res. 2018;24:1344–54.

40. Kaissis G, Ziegelmayer S, Lohöfer F, Steiger K, Algül H, Muckenhuber A, Yen HY, Rummeny E, Friess H, Schmid R, Weichert W, Siveke JT, Braren R. A machine learning algorithm predicts molecular subtypes in pancreatic ductal adenocarcinoma with differential response to gemcitabine-based versus FOLFIRINOX chemotherapy. PLoS One. 2019;14(10):e0218642. https://doi.org/10.1371/journal.pone.0218642.

41. Hackert T. Surgery for pancreatic cancer after neoadjuvant treatment. Ann Gastroenterol Surg. 2018;2:413–8.

42. Inoue Y, Saiura A, Yoshioka R, Ono Y, Takahashi M, Arita J, Takahashi Y, Koga R. Pancreatoduodenectomy with systematic mesopancreas dissection using a supracolic anterior artery-first approach. Ann Surg. 2015;262:1092–101.

43. Sabater L, Cugat E, Serrablo A, Suarez-Artacho G, Diez-Valladares L, Santoyo-Santoyo J, Martín-Pérez E, Ausania F, Lopez-Ben S, Jover-Navalon JM, Garcés-Albir M, Garcia-Domingo MI, Serradilla M, Pérez-Aguirre E, Sánchez-Pérez B, Di Martino M, Senra-Del-Rio P, Falgueras-Verdaguer L, Carabias A, Gómez-Mateo MC, Ferrandez A, Dorcaratto D, Muñoz-Forner E, Fondevila C, Padillo J. Does the artery-first approach improve the rate of R0 resection in pancreatoduodenectomy? A multicenter, randomized, controlled trial. Ann Surg. 2019;270:738–46.

44. Mackay TM, Wellner UF, van Rijssen LB, Stoop TF, Busch OR, Groot Koerkamp B, Bausch D, Petrova E, Besselink MG, Keck T, Dutch Pancreatic Cancer Group and DGAV StuDoQ|Pancreas. Variation in pancreatoduodenectomy as delivered in two national audits. Br J Surg. 2019;106:747–55.

45. Kutlu OC, Vega EA, Salehi O, Lathan C, Kim S, Krishnan S, Stallwood C, Kozyreva O, Conrad C. Laparoscopic pancreatectomy for cancer in high volume centers is associated with an increased use and fewer delays of adjuvant chemotherapy. HPB (Oxford). 2020;25:S1365-182X(20)31146-1.

46. Kawabata Y, Hayashi H, Kaji S, Fujii Y, Nishi T, Tajima Y. Laparoscopic versus open radical antegrade modular pancreatosplenectomy with artery-first approach in pancreatic cáncer. Langenbecks Arch Surg. 2020;405:647–56.

47. van Hilst J, de Rooij T, Bosscha K, Brinkman DJ, van Dieren S, Dijkgraaf MG, Gerhards MF, de Hingh IH, Karsten TM, Lips DJ, Luyer MD, Busch OR, Festen S, Besselink MG, Dutch Pancreatic Cancer Group. Laparoscopic versus open pancreatoduodenectomy for pancreatic or periampullary tumours (LEOPARD-2): a multicentre, patient-blinded, randomised controlled phase 2/3 trial. Lancet Gastroenterol Hepatol. 2019;4:199–207.

48. Nickel F, Haney CM, Kowalewski KF, Probst P, Limen EF, Kalkum E, Diener MK, Strobel O, Müller-Stich BP, Hackert T. Laparoscopic versus open pancreaticoduodenectomy: a systematic review and meta-analysis of randomized controlled trials. Ann Surg. 2020;271:54–66.

49. Shyr B-U, Chen S-C, Shyr Y-M, Wang S-E. Learning curves for robotic pancreatic surgery-from distal pancreatectomy to pancreaticoduodenectomy. Medicine (Baltimore). 2018;97:e13000.

50. Padillo J (Principal Investigator). Role of CTC's spread during pancreaticoduodenectomy in patients with pancreatic and periampullary tumors (CETUPANC). ClinicalTrials.gov Identifier: NCT03340844.

51. Qi B, Crawford AJ, Wojtynek NE, Holmes MB, Souchek JJ, Almeida-Porada G, Ly QP, Cohen SM, Hollingsworth MA, Mohs AM. Indocyanine green loaded hyaluronan-derived nanoparticles for fluorescence-enhanced surgical imaging of pancreatic cáncer. Nanomedicine. 2018;14:769–80.

52. Baiocchi GL, Diana M, Boni L. Indocyanine green-based fluorescence imaging in visceral and hepatobiliary and pancreatic surgery: state of the art and future directions. World J Gastroenterol. 2018;24:2921–30.

Pancreatic Cystic Neoplasms: Serous Cystadenoma, Mucinous Cystadenoma

2

Inmaculada Sanchez-Matamoros Martin,
Juan Bellido-Luque, Juan Manuel Castillo Tuñón,
and Angel Nogales Muñoz

Pancreatic cystic neoplasms (PCNs) are classified depending on their histology.

Due to the well-known low survival rate of pancreatic cancer and the increase in the prevalence of pancreatic cystic lesions, some of them precursors of it, there is a great need to improve the characterization of premalignant cystic lesions, performing surgery on those who need it and avoiding surveillance and unnecessary interventions, since this surgery has not negligible morbidity and mortality rates.

When a patient is identified with a pancreatic cystic lesion, the first thing to determine is their malignant potential; in general, they can be divided as shown in the classification (Table 2.1) into benign, malignant, and precursors, although in general pancreatic cysts can be classified into mucinous or non-mucinous, the latter will rarely undergo a malignant transformation unlike the former [1].

Pancreatic cystic neoplasms were considered a rare entity but are now becoming more common, accounting for 10–15% of all pancreatic cystic lesions and 1% of all pancreatic lesions [2], with variable malignant potential. In general,

intraductal papillary mucinous neoplasia (IPMN), mucinous cystic neoplasia (MCN), and serous cystadenoma (SCA) are the most common cystic neoplasms of the pancreas. IPMN and MCN are thought to potentially lead to pancreatic ductal adenocarcinoma, while SCA is largely benign [3].

Due to increasing growth in the aging population and the advancement of imaging techniques that improve the sensitivity of detection rates and shrinking lesions, the prevalence of pancreatic cystic lesions worldwide has increased dramatically over the past two decades [4]. If the prevalence is adjusted by age and gender, we will have in the general population approximately 2%, although it would increase exponentially with age, being able to reach older people up to 45%.

The most frequent way to diagnose them is incidental, in patients who have performed imaging tests for other reasons, so they can be called incidentalomas, although many are diagnosed in symptomatic patients. Depending on the technique used, the incidence rate varies, so in magnetic resonance imaging (MRI) it can reach up to 19.6% [4].

Pancreatic cystic neoplasms, although they are generally asymptomatic, in case of presenting symptoms they are usually nonspecific, such as asthenia, nausea and vomiting, abdominal or back pain, jaundice, steatorrhea, pancreatitis, or

I. Sanchez-Matamoros Martin (✉) · J. Bellido-Luque
J. M. C. Tuñón · A. Nogales Muñoz
Hepatobiliopancreatic Unit Surgical Department,
Virgen Macarena University Hospital, Seville, Spain
e-mail: anogal@telefonica.net

Table 2.1 Histological classification of pancreatic cyst tumors

Benign tumors
1. Serous cystoadenoma
(a) Microcystic
(b) Macrocystic
(c) Solid
(d) Von-hippel lindau syndrome associated
(e) Mixed serous-neuroendocrine neoplasm
2. Seorus cystadenocarcinoma
3. Low grade Glandular intraepithelial neoplasia
4. High grade Glandular intraepithelial neoplasia
5. Intraductal papillary mucinous neoplasm with low grade intraepithelial neoplasia
6. Intraductal papillary mucinous neoplasm with high grade intraepithelial neoplasia
7. Intraductal papillary mucinous neoplasm with associated invasive carcinoma
8. Intraductal oncocytic papillary neoplasm
9. Intraductal oncocytic papillary neoplasm with associated invasive carcinoma
10. Intraductal tubulopapillary neoplasm
11. Intraductal tubulopapillary neoplasm with associated invasive carcinoma
12. Mucinous cystic neoplasm with low grade intraepithelial neoplasia
13. Mucinous cystic neoplasm with high grade intraepithelial neoplasia
14. Mucinous cystic neoplasm with associated invasive carcinoma
Malign tumors
1. Duct adenocarcinoma
(a) Colloide carcinoma
(b) Poorly cohesive carcinoma
(c) Signet rign cell carcinoma
(d) Medullary carcinoma
(e) Adenosquamous carcinoma
(f) Epidermoid carcinoma
(g) Larg cell carcinoma with rhabdoid phenotype
(h) Carcinoma undifferenciated
(i) Undifferenciated carcinoma with osteoclast-like giant cell
2. Acinar cell carcinoma
(a) Acinar cell cystadenocarcinoma
(b) Mixed acinar-neuroendocrine carcinoma
(c) Mixed acinar-endocrine-ductal carcinoma
(d) Mixed acinar-ductal carcinoma
3. Pancreatoblastoma
4. Solid pseudopapillary neoplasm with high grade dysplasia

palpable mass. Clinical symptoms, especially weight loss, jaundice, and pain, are associated with a high risk of malignancy [5].

Currently, three guidelines are used to guide the follow-up and surgical referral of patients presenting with asymptomatic pancreatic cystic lesions: The 2017 International Pancreatology Association's Fukuoka Guidelines [6], the 2015 American Gastroenterological Association (AGA) Guidelines [7], and the 2018 European Evidence-Based Guidelines (EEG) [8]. The fact that there are different consensus guidelines in use indicates the imperfect state of knowledge about pancreatic cystic lesions and pancreatic cancer and the urgent need for better biological characterization of these lesions.

The most commonly used diagnostic tools for pancreatic cystic lesions include computed tomography (CT), MRI, and endoscopic ultrasound (EUS) ± fine needle aspiration, all of them have low sensitivity and specificity for identifying high- and low-risk patients [7].

The differential diagnosis of a pancreatic cyst by USE will depend on the morphology and size of the cyst, the number of cysts present, the characteristics of the wall and internal structures, calcification, position in relation to the main pancreatic duct, and the presence of background lesions; these descriptors are highly dependent on the operator and the characterization of the cyst without cystic fluid analysis is limited.

Because imaging alone has limitations with respect to a definitive diagnosis, fine needle aspiration (FNA) puncture, and cystic fluid examination by cytology and biochemical analysis, they have been extensively studied and demonstrated clinical utility in the diagnosis of pancreatic cystic neoplasms.

Although FNA can be performed percutaneously guided by CT or ultrasonography (US), it is usually radioguided by EUS, because it has better image resolution (the tumor is closer to the transducer) and has fewer complications. Even so, it has an associated morbidity, so it should be justified and performed if the results of it will influence the therapeutic plan.

FNA should not be performed when:

- The characteristics of the image of the cystic lesion are diagnostics, and performing the appropriate treatment of it.
- If the lesion is symptomatic since it has indication of resection.

Macroscopically, the fluid aspirated in SCA is usually transparent, thin, and mucin-free, unlike MCNs where the fluid is thick, viscous, and mucinous. If the biochemistry of the same is analyzed, other differences are found for mucin, for amylase and tumor markers (Table 2.2).

Amylase in the cystic fluid, if >5 times serum levels, indicates that there is a communication of the pancreatic duct with the cyst, so it serves to exclude serous cystic neoplasms and mucinoses [9].

The Carcinoembrionary Antigen (CEA) level of the cyst fluid is the most accurate test to determine whether the cyst is mucinous and to differentiate a mucinous neoplasm from an SCA with reasonable reliability [10]; however, cystic CEA levels are not a reliable marker for differentiating benign mucinous cystic neoplasms from malignant one, as it is increased in all mucinous cysts [11].

Cystic fluid cytology has a high specificity for malignancy or high-grade dysplasia, but low sensitivity due to the low cellularity of the samples [12]; as a result, cytological examination of cystic fluid is often undiagnosed. It may be useful in differentiating mucinous from non-mucinous cysts by identifying mucin-producing cells.

Endoscopic retrograde cholecistopancreatography (ERCP) has a higher risk of adverse events and a lower sensitivity and specificity in identifying the type of PCNs than conventional radiology and USE, so it should not be used for this indication [13].

To date, for pancreatic cystic neoplasms, there are no blood biomarkers for clinical use available to differentiate the type of pancreatic cyst, identify high-grade dysplasias or cancer, as well as for monitoring them in daily clinical practice.

Each type of pancreatic cystic neoplasm will have an algorithm for its treatment depending on the type it is and that will be seen in its corresponding sections and in the case of being faced with a cyst of unclear etiology of <15 mm and without risk factors of malignancy, it will be reevaluated from year to year for 3 years, if during this time it remains stable it will be followed every 2 years. If the cyst is >15 mm it will be followed every 6 months in the first year and then annually [14].

Because PCNs present a greater risk of malignancy the larger they are in size and knowing that any indefinite cyst can be mucinous in nature, it is why surveillance is recommended in both [15].

The long-term evolution of PCN as well as indefinite pancreatic cysts are unknown; therefore, follow-up should be lifelong, unless the patient refuses or is not a candidate for surgery [8].

Table 2.2 Analysis of cyst fluid aspirate

	Serous cystic neoplasms	Mucinous cystic neoplasm
Sex ratio (M/F)	1:3–4	1:9
Age range (year)	60–80	30–50
Location in pancreas	Variable	Body/tail (90%) >> head
Characteristics of lesions	Multiple, small (<2 cm) microcysts, honeycombed; rarely a unilocular microcyst; characteristic central stellate calcification (30%) Rarely macrocystic	Unilocular or multiloculated macrocysts >2 cm, smooth external contour
Findings suggestive of malignancy	Rare <1% serous cystadenocarcinoma, invasive and/or metastatic lesions	10–17% Eggshell calcification, solid component or mural nodule
Communication of cystic area with pancreatic duct	Absent	Absent

2.1 Serous Cystadenoma

Benign neoplasm of the pancreas of presumed ductal origin but of a non-mucinous nature. It is a benign tumor and more frequent in women (75%) with an average age in resected patients of 60 years (Table 2.3).

They represent more than 30% of pancreatic cystic neoplasms, 1% of non-endocrine pancreatic neoplasms, and about 16% of resected cystic tumors of the pancreas, and can be located anywhere in the pancreas [16, 17].

Very few cases of malignancy have been reported (less than 1%), approximately 30 cases have been reported in the world literature, and they are typically locally invasive lesions rather than metastatic diseases [18].

Several morphological variants have been described including microcystic serous cystadenomas, macrocystic (oligocystic), solid serous adenoma, and serosa cystic neoplasm associated with Von Hippel-Lindau (VHL) [19]. Often the term serous cystadenoma refers indistinctly to both the micro and macrocystic variants.

The *microcystic* (multilocular) form consists of innumerable small tubular structures, of different shapes and with irregular contours, most subcentimetric. It is the typical and most commonly described form of serous cystadenoma, also called "honeycomb" (Table 2.3), creating a unique configuration diagnosis of this type of tumor, similar to a sponge. It is formed by multiple cysts of small size, with characteristic septums and a thick fibrous wall, the cysts are lined with a glycogen-rich cuboidal epithelium, with uniform round nuclei with homogeneous dense chromatin and a prominent microvascular network that hugs the epithelium (Fig. 2.1).

The classic radiological image in CT or MRI is a "spongy" or "honeycomb" multilobular mass and in 30% of cases with a central scar that may or may not be calcified and is pathognomonic of the microcystic variant (Fig. 2.2).

Sometimes radiological imaging can be confused with an endocrine solid pancreatic neoplasm [20], in which case USE with biopsy and fluid sampling may be necessary to support the diagnosis.

Table 2.3 Features of SCA and MCN

	Cytologic	Viscosity	CEA level (ng/ml)	Ca 19.9	Amylase	Mucin
Serous cystic neoplasms	Negative or celular sheets of glycogen-containing, cuboidal cells	Low	Low, <5	Normal	Low <250 U/l	None
Mucinous cystic neoplasm	Mucin- containing columnar cells	High	High, >5	↑	Low <250 U/l	Present

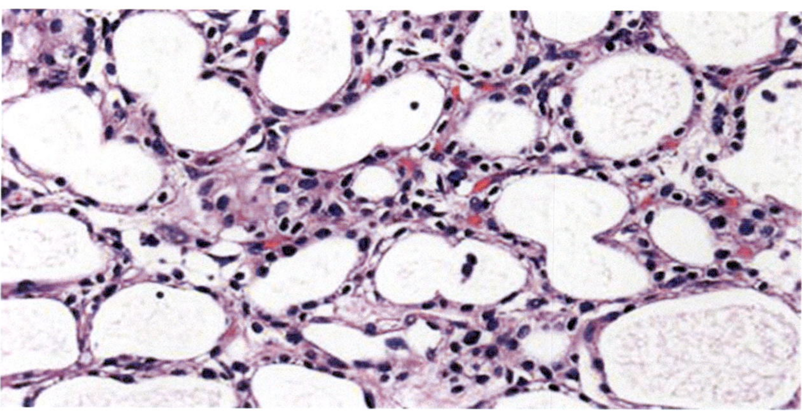

Fig. 2.1 Serous cystadenoma, microcystic type

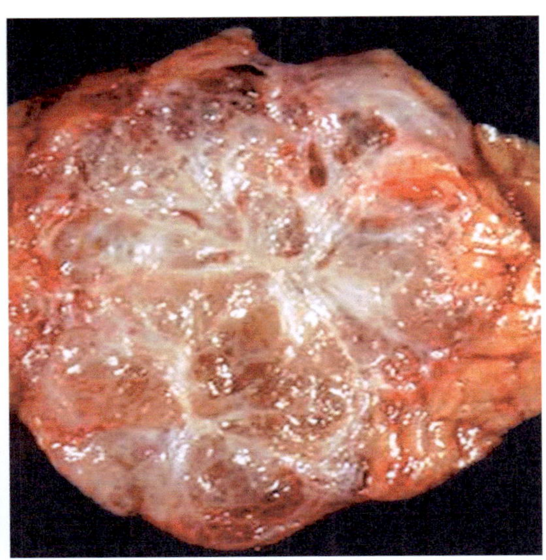

Fig. 2.2 Serous cystadenoma, central stellate calcification

Macrocystics or oligocystics (uniloculars) forms have much larger cysts (centimeters), in smaller numbers (typically less than 10) [19] and are devoid of central fibrosis or calcification. They account for approximately 10% of serous cystadenomas. It can radiographically simulate intraductal papillary mucinous neoplasms, mucinous cystic neoplasms, and pseudocysts, especially if only one cyst is evident, so this variant can be much more difficult to diagnose.

The presence of small peripheral cysts on imaging such as USE, and the low level of CEA, support the diagnosis of an oligocystic serous cystadenoma.

Rarely, the lesions are multiple, specifically when associated with VHL [19].

They can cause nonspecific symptoms, such as epigastric abdominal pain and weight loss; currently, most of them are diagnosed by chance and are asymptomatic, except in cases located in the pancreatic head and/or with large tumor size, where they present a more aggressive behavior due to their mass effect, or by direct invasion to adjacent organs or blood vessels or metastases to lymph nodes or other organs. Most cases are treated conservatively and can be followed up with serial imaging tests to ensure that it does not have rapid growth.

Serous cystadenoma has a very slow growth (<5 mm/year) [21], with an estimated doubling time of 12 years [22]. Approximately 60% of SCAs remain stable in size and only 40% of them increase in size is observed [8]. All this means that having a definitive diagnosis and in small tumors, the treatment is surveillance and in case of symptomatic or large lesions, the option of elective treatment is surgery.

FNA diagnosis of serous neoplasms has proven to be challenging due to the very low aspiration cellularity, probably due to the cohesion and adhesion of cells to tissue. Tumor cells are soft, cubic, and arranged in loose groups or monolayers and the cytoplasm is usually vacuolized; however, the cells are usually stripped of the cytoplasm, showing only small, round nuclei with fine but dense and homogeneous nuclear chromatin [23].

Presurgical diagnosis of pancreatic cysts has traditionally been based on the measurement of cyst fluid amylase, as well as tumor markers CA19-9 and CEA to identify and distinguish mucinous neoplasms from non-mucinous lesions such as serous ones. However, the sensitivity and specificity of these markers are relatively low.

Amylase may exclude pancreatic pseudocysts, values <250 U/l have a sensitivity of 0.44 and specificity of 0.98; but no difference between other mucinous and non-mucinous cysts [8] (Table 2.2).

There is a published study showing in an ELISA analysis of cystic fluid and tumor tissue, that vascular endothelial growth factor A (VEGF-A) was markedly elevated in serous cystic neoplasms compared to pseudocysts, papillary intraductal mucinous neoplasms, mucinous cystic neoplasms, and pancreatic ductal adenocarcinoma [24]; reaching a sensitivity of 100% and a specificity of 97% as a marker of serous cystic neoplasms, which makes it a very promising biomarker for the diagnosis and distinction of serous cystic neoplasms from other pancreatic cysts, especially when used in conjunction with CEA [24].

The identification of cyst-specific somatic mutations (involving the KRAS, GNAS, RNF43, CTNNB1, and VHL genes) offers great promise in the presurgical diagnosis of pancreatic cysts. KRAS and GNAS mutations have been shown to have 96% sensitivity and 100% specificity to differentiate intraductal papillary mucinous neoplasia from serous cystic neoplasia [25].

The fluid of the serous cystadenoma is transparent and watery, colorless, yellow, or blood-stained appearance, they may even have foci of hemorrhage [26] (Table 2.2). It presents very low levels of CEA, typically <5 ng/ml, but in the microcystic variant (the most frequent found), it may be difficult to obtain; however, the oligo-quistic variant, more infrequent in its finding, but more difficult in its diagnosis (radiologically with characteristics superimposable to mucinous cystic neoplasia and intraductal papillary muci-nous neoplasia of secondary branch), the pres-ence of peripheral small cysts in echoendoscopy and low levels of CEA support the diagnosis of oligocystic serous cystadenoma.

If we have a clear diagnosis of serous cystic neoplasia, with radiological evidence of it and asymptomatic, they should be followed for 1 year; subsequently, follow-up based on symp-toms is recommended. In case of having an uncertain diagnosis, follow-up is required [8].

Only if there is a clear diagnosis of serous cys-tic neoplasia and in symptomatic patients in rela-tion to compression of adjacent organs, surgery is the treatment of choice [8].

Solid *serous adenoma* is characterized by uni-form and small nests or tubules, with minimal or even no light formation. They usually lack cen-tral fibrosis and are often radiologically misinter-preted as neuroendocrine tumors. Tumor cells reveal a typical glycogen-laden clear cytoplasm and soft, round, or oval hyperchromatic nuclei [27, 28].

There are other solid neoplasms such as neu-roendocrine tumors and metastatic renal cell car-cinoma, which can have a difficult differential diagnosis with solid serous adenomas, mainly if it is in the context of VHL, since they can occur at the same time.

Serum cystic neoplasms associated with VHL usually present as a diffuse and irregular forma-tion in the pancreas, although they can do so as a localized and well-defined pancreatic mass.

Serous cystadenomas associated with VHL occur in 35–90% of patients with VHL and the most common morphological types are multiple serous cystadenoma and macrocystic variants, their course being benign.

Allelic deletions of the VHL gene (chromosome 3p) are detected in serous cystic neoplasms of patients with VHL, providing molecular evidence of their neoplastic nature; although alterations of the VHL gene can also be detected in up to 40% of sporadic cases of serous cystadenoma [19].

2.2 Mucinous Cystic Neoplasia (MCN) (Tables 2.2 and 2.3)

MCN of the pancreas is a cystic from benign to potentially low-degree malignant epithelial neo-plasm, composed of cells containing intracyto-plasmic mucin and pathologically characterized by an ovarian-type stroma. It takes the shape of spindle cells forming a compact layer under the epithelium (Fig. 2.3).

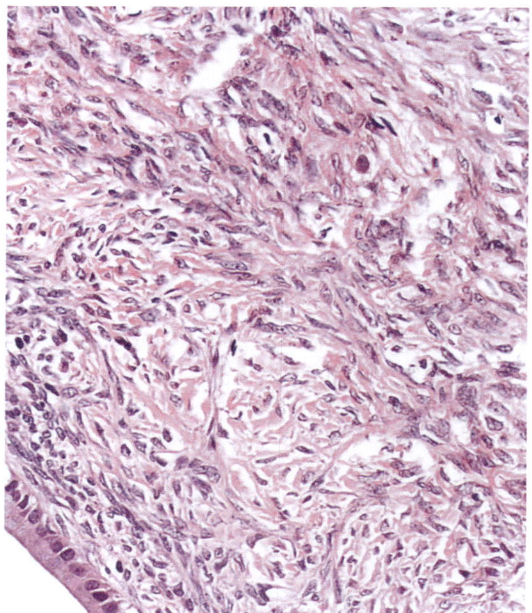

Fig. 2.3 Mucinous cystic neoplasm (ovarian-like stroma)

Spindle cells are generally positive for the estrogen receptor and progesterone receptor. As the size of the MCN increases, the characteristic stroma may become hyalinized, not being present in all the cuts, so the sampling must be sufficiently large to demonstrate this diagnostic criterion [29].

It is a rare pancreatic disease, slow growing and with a single lesion that does not communicate with the pancreatic duct although exceptions have been described [30, 31]; inside the cyst there is mucinous content, unlike serous cystic neoplasms. The size of the tumor ranges from 1 to 30 cm and they often have a complex internal structure with thin-walled lobes and variable size, although they are sometimes unilocular.

The size rate of an MCN increase should be considered. There appears to be considerably faster growth during pregnancy, which could lead to tumor rupture [32]; therefore, patients with MCN should be closely observed during pregnancy [8].

Although MCN generally is asymptomatic, unlike serous cystic neoplasms they are more commonly symptomatic, possibly due to their larger size and their more aggressive local biological behavior; so, clinical symptoms can occur as systemic manifestations, back pain, and jaundice, and should lead to suspicion of the presence of malignancy [5].

It frequently affects women (>95%) with an average age of 45 years and is usually located in the distal pancreas (>95%) [33].

It can be the origin of pancreatic adenocarcinoma and harbor invasive carcinoma, so it is classified into:

- *MCN with low-grade dysplasia (adenoma):* The epithelial lining takes the form of a single layer of cubic to columnar cells with minimal variation in the size and shape of the nucleus. It has little or no malignant potential and is called by some authors "non-mucinous cystadenoma."
- *MCN with high-grade dysplasia (carcinoma in situ).*
- *MCN with invasive carcinoma* (Less than 20% of cases) [34]. Invasion in the ovarian stroma but not beyond the capsule.

Having a large tumor size, palpable, or visible solid areas, presence of mural nodules with marked papillary projections and asymmetrically thickened walls or hypervascularization, as well as peripheral calcification in "eggshell," are known to be associated with malignancy [35].

Recurrent genetic alterations have been identified in KRAS, GNAS, and RNF43 in MCNs, although they are not specific, since they also appear in intraductal papillary mucinous neoplasms. Detection of these mutations, along with typical morphology, can facilitate diagnosis [36, 37].

Due to its malignant potential, there is an aggressive approach in clinical guidelines, considering resection as the treatment of choice, in all patients with low surgical risk.

Patients diagnosed with MCN who present [38] have a clear indication for surgery:

- Symptoms
- Size ≥ 40 mm
- Risk factors (such as the presence of wall nodules) regardless of their size

The type of surgery for these neoplasms is a standard oncological resection, that is, a distal pancreatectomy in 95% of cases, associating lymphadenectomy and splenectomy for MCNs with high-grade dysplasia or carcinoma. In cases of low risk of malignancy, a non-oncological resection, distal pancreatectomy with splenic preservation with or without preservation of splenic vessels may be performed. The approach route of this type of resection is recommended to be performed by laparoscopy, due to its demonstrated benefits over the open approach [39].

A conservative approach with surveillance in patients with low-risk MCN is currently proposed.

Patients with MCN of <40 mm asymptomatic and without risk characteristics such as wall nodules, will follow-up with MRI, EUS, or both, every 6 months in the first year and then annually if there are no changes, for life as long as they can be candidates for surgery.

For those patients with MCN between 30 and 40 mm, other factors such as age and comorbidity, as well as patient preferences, can be incorporated. For those <30 mm in size that may be difficult to have a definitive diagnosis, surveillance similar to intraductal papillary mucinous neoplasms of <3 cm is recommended.

References

1. Kromrey M-L, Bülow R, Hübner J, Paperlein C, Lerch MM, Ittermann T, Völzke H, Mayerle J, Kühn J-P. Prospective study on the incidence, prevalence and 5-year pancreatic-related mortality of pancreatic cysts in a population-based study. Gut. 2018;67:138–45.
2. Basturk O, Askan G. Benign tumors and tumor-like lesions of the pancreas. Surg Pathol Clin. 2016;9(4):619–41.
3. Sethi V, Giri B, Saluja A, Dudej V. Insights into the pathogenesis of pancreatic cystic neoplasms. Dig Dis Sci. 2017;62(7):1778–86.
4. Kane LE, Mellotte GS, Conlon KC, Ryan BM, Maher SG. Multi-omic biomarkers as potential tools for the characterisation of pancreatic cystic lesions and cancer: innovative patient data integration. Cancers. 2021 Feb;13(4):769.
5. Lennon AM, Wolfgang C. Cystic neoplasms of the pancreas. J Gastrointest Surg. 2013;17:645–53.
6. Tanaka M, Fernández-del C, Kamisawa T, Jang JY, Levy P, Ohtsuka T, Salvia R, Shimizu Y, Tada M, Wolfgang CL. Revisions of international consensus Fukuoka guidelines for the management of IPMN of the pancreas. Pancreatology. 2017;17:738–53.
7. Vege SS, Ziring B, Jain R, Moayyedi P, Adams MA, Dorn SD, Dudley-Brown SL, Flamm SL, Gellad ZF, Gruss CB. American gastroenterological association institute guideline on the diagnosis and management of asymptomatic neoplastic pancreatic cysts. Gastroenterology. 2015;148:819–22.
8. European Study Group on Cystic Tumors of the Pancreas. European evidence-based guidelines on pancreatic cystic neoplasms. Gut. 2018;67:789–804.
9. Sakorafas GH, Smyrniotis V, Reid-Lombardo KM, Sarr MG. Primary pancreatic cystic neoplasms revisited: part I: serous cystic neoplasms. Surg Oncol. 2011;20:84–92.
10. Pitman MB. Revised international consensus guidelines for the management of patients with mucinous cysts. Cancer Cytopathol. 2012;120:361–5.
11. Sherman S, et al. Fluid analysis prior to surgical resection of suspected mucinous pancreatic cysts. A single centre experience. J Gastrointest Oncol. 2011;2:208–14.
12. Maker AV, Carrara S, Jamieson NB, Pelaez-Luna M, Lennon AM, Molin MD, Scarpa A, Frulloni L, Brugge WR. Cyst fluid biomarkers for intraductal papillary mucinous neoplasms of the pancreas: a critical review from the international expert meeting on pancreatic branch-duct-intraductal papillary mucinous neoplasms. J Am Coll Surg. 2015;220:243–53.
13. Suzuki R, Thosani N, Annangi S, et al. Diagnostic yield of EUS-FNA-based cytology distinguishing malignant and benign IPMNs: a systematic review and meta-analysis. Pancreatology. 2014;14:380–4.
14. Del Chiaro M, Ateeb Z, Hansson MR, et al. Survival analysis and risk for progression of intraductal papillary mucinous neoplasia of the pancreas (IPMN) under surveillance: a single-institution experience. Ann Surg Oncol. 2017;24:1120–6.
15. Sahora K, Mino-Kenudson M, Brugge W, et al. Branch duct intraductal papillary mucinous neoplasms: does cyst size change the tip of the scale? A critical analysis of the revised international consensus guidelines in a large single-institutional series. Ann Surg. 2013;258:466–75.
16. Farrel J. Prevalence, diagnosis and management of pancreatic cystic neoplasms: current status and future directions. Gut Liver. 2015;9(5):571–89.
17. Lee LS, Clancy T, Kadiyala V, Suleiman S, Conwell DL. Interdisciplinary management of cystic neoplasms of the pancreas. Gastroenterol Res Pract. 2012;2:1–7.
18. Robinson SM, Scott J, Oppong KW, White SA. What to do for the incidental pancreatic cystic lesion? Surg Oncol. 2014;23:117–25.
19. Baskurk O, Askan G. Benign tumors and tumor-like lesions of the pancreas. Surg Pathol Clin. 2016;9(4):619–41.
20. Hayashi K, Fujimitsu R, Ida M, et al. CT differentiation of solid serous cystadenoma vs endocrine tumor of the pancreas. Eur J Radiol. 2012;81:203–8.
21. Jais B, Rebours V, Malleo G, et al. Serous cystic neoplasm of the pancreas: a multinational study of 2622 patients under the auspices of the International Association of Pancreatology and European Pancreatic Club (European Study Group on Cystic Tumors of the Pancreas). Gut. 2016;65:305–12.
22. El-Hayek KM, Brown N, O'Rourke C, et al. Rate of growth of pancreatic serous cystadenoma as an indication for resection. Surgery. 2013;154:794–800.
23. Collins BT. Serous cystadenoma of the pancreas with endoscopic ultrasound fine needle aspiration biopsy and surgical correlation. Acta Cytol. 2013;57:241–51.
24. Yip-Schneider MT, Wu H, Dumas RP, et al. Vascular endothelial growth factor, a novel and highly accurate pancreatic fluid biomarker for serous pancreatic cysts. J Am Coll Surg. 2014;218:608–17.
25. Wu J, Matthaei H, Maitra A, et al. Recurrent GNAS mutations define an unexpected pathway for pancreatic cyst development. Sci Transl Med. 2011;3:92ra66.
26. Panarelli NC, Park KJ, Hruban RH, et al. Microcystic serous cystadenoma of the pancreas with subtotal cystic degeneration: another neoplastic mimic of pancreatic pseudocyst. Am J Surg Pathol. 2012;36:726–31.
27. Lee SD, Han SS, Hong EK. Solid serous cystic neoplasm of the pancreas with invasive growth. J Hepatobiliary Pancreat Sci. 2013;20:454–6.

28. Yasuda A, Sawai H, Ochi N, et al. Solid variant of serous cystadenoma of the pancreas. Arch Med Sci. 2011;7:353–5.
29. Albores-Saavedra J, et al. Nonmucinous cystadenomas of the pancreas with pancreatobiliary phenotype and ovarian-like stroma. Am J Clin Pathol. 2013;139(5):599–604.
30. Masia R, et al. Pancreatic mucinous cystic neoplasm of the main pancreatic duct. Arch Pathol Lab Med. 2011;135(2):264–7.
31. Yamao K, et al. Clinicopathological features and prognosis of mucinous cystic neoplasm with ovarian-type stroma: a multi-institutional study of the Japan Pancreas Society. Pancreas. 2011;40(1):67–71.
32. Naganuma S, Honda K, Noriki S, et al. Ruptured mucinous cystic neoplasm with an associated invasive carcinoma of pancreatic head in a pregnant woman: report of a case and review of literature. Pathol Int. 2011;61:28–33.
33. Le Baleur Y, Couvelard A, Vullierme MP, et al. Mucinous cystic neoplasms of the pancreas: definition of preoperative imaging criteria for high-risk lesions. Pancreatology. 2011;11:495–9.
34. Farrell JJ. Prevalence, diagnosis and management of pancreatic cystic neoplasms: current status and future directions. Gut Liver. 2015;9(5):571–89.
35. Kang CM, Matsushita A, Hwang HK, et al. Experience-based surgical approach to pancreatic mucinous cystic neoplasms with ovarian-type stroma. Oncol Lett. 2018;15:2451–8.
36. Furukawa T, et al. Whole-exome sequencing uncovers frequent GNAS mutations in intraductal papillary mucinous neoplasms of the pancreas. Sci Rep. 2011;1:161.
37. Wu J, et al. Whole-exome sequencing of neoplastic cysts of the pancreas reveals recurrent mutations in components of ubiquitin-dependent pathways. Proc Natl Acad Sci U S A. 2011;108(52):21188–93.
38. Nilsson LN, Keane MG, Shamali A, et al. Nature and management of pancreatic mucinous cystic neoplasm (MCN): a systematic review of the literature. Pancreatology. 2016;16:1028–36.
39. Mehrabi A, Hafezi M, Arvin J, et al. A systematic review and meta-analysis of laparoscopic versus open distal pancreatectomy for benign and malignant lesions of the pancreas: it's time to randomize. Surgery. 2015;157:45–55.

Intraductal Papillary Mucinous Tumors Principal and Lateral Branch of IPMT: Preoperative Management, Surgical Indications, and Surgical Techniques

3

Victoria Alejandra Jiménez-García,
Ana Argüelles-Arias, Federico Argüelles-Arias,
Rafael Romero-Castro, and Marc Giovannini

3.1 Definition

IPMNs of the pancreas are PCN characterized by adenomatous proliferation of the pancreatic ductal epithelium that may affect the main duct, the branch ducts or both [1] and by neoplastic progression ranging from low-to-high grade dysplasia to invasive carcinoma.

V. A. Jiménez-García (✉) · R. Romero-Castro
Endoscopy Division and Gastroenterology Division,
Virgen Macarena University Hospital, Seville, Spain

A. Argüelles-Arias
Radiology Department, Virgen Macarena University
Hospital, Seville, Spain

F. Argüelles-Arias
Endoscopy Division and Gastroenterology Division,
Virgen Macarena University Hospital, Seville, Spain

Department of Medicine, University of Seville,
Seville, Spain
e-mail: farguelles@telefonica.net

M. Giovannini
Paoli-Calmettes Institute, Department of
Gastrointestinal Disease, Marseilles, France
e-mail: giovanninim@wanadoo.fr

3.2 Epidemiology

The first cases of IPMNs were reported in 1982 [2]. Their incidence has been increasingly reported [3] after the generalized use of noninvasive cross-sectional imaging procedures such as computed tomography (CT), magnetic resonance imaging (MRI), and magnetic resonance cholangiopancreatography (MRCP). These imaging procedures can display incidental pancreatic lesions in up to 45% of patients [4–7] being usually difficult to differentiate between their types [8]. Many incidentally pancreatic cystic lesions could be IPMNs [9]. However, the real incidence of IPMNs remains elusive because many IPMNs are asymptomatic. Probably, IPMNs account for 20–50% of pancreatic cysts and 1–3% of exocrine pancreatic tumors [10–12]. There has been observed an elevated incidence of IPMNs in patients who smoke cigarettes [13], have diabetes [14], Peutz-Jeghers syndrome [15], familial adenomatous polyposis syndrome [16], or a history of familial pancreatic adenocarcinoma [14, 17].

3.3 Classification

IPMNs could be both classified anatomically and histologically.

1. *Anatomic classification.* According to the involvement of the pancreatic duct, IPMNs could be classified into three subgroups:

   (a) Main-duct (MD)-IPMNs: The main pancreatic duct is involved and can be diffusely or segmentally dilated without stenosis with intraductal enlargement of mucin-producing ductal cells. Most of MD-IPMNs arise in the pancreatic head and can progress distally with or without affecting the side branches. MD-IPMNs require surveillance due to the risk of progression of the disease and malignancy, observed in up to 50% of MD-IPMNs [18]. Moreover, the entire pancreatic parenchyma has to be displayed during follow-up because of the increased risk of developing new-onset cancer [19, 20].

   (b) Branch-duct (BD)-IMPNs: The branch-side dilated subgroup of IPMNs are usually originated from the uncinate process, although the tail of the pancreas may be also affected. The potential for malignancy in this subgroup is lower, 10–15% [18], although, surveillance is also needed [21].

   (c) Mixed-type (MT)-IPMNs: They present features of the two former subgroups with involvement of both the main and the side branches of the pancreatic duct. Its biological behavior regarding the potential for malignancy is the same as for MD-IPMNs.

   Therefore, the anatomic classification has important practical clinical consequences in assessing the risk for malignancy. In a review of 20 studies including 3568 IPMNs, the risk of invasive carcinoma arising in association with MD-IPMNs was about 44%, while in BD-IPMNs was approximately 17% [22]. However, these figures obtained from surgical series may be higher if compared to radiological series.

2. *Histologic classification.* The epithelial lining of the papillary component of IPMNs can be classified according to morphological characteristics and immunohistochemical reaction against mucin proteins in four distinct histo-logic subtypes (intestinal, pancreatobiliary, gastric, and oncocytic type), each of them characterized by a different risk for developing dysplasia or malignancy. Invasive carcinomas arising from IPMNs have remarkably important prognostic differences being classified as tubular (ductal), colloid, and oncocyte types.

3.4 Pathogenesis

IPMNs have the potential to develop tumors with different phenotypes. So, these IPMNs present with a wide histological spectrum ranging from low, intermediate, high-grade dysplasia to invasive carcinoma.

The risk of developing malignancy is strongly related to the duct involvement [23]. Thus, a high-risk disease with high-grade dysplasia and invasive carcinoma were found after surgical resection in 61.6% of MD-IPMNs and in 18.5% of BD-IPMNs, respectively [22]. Besides, IPMNs have two peculiar, worrisome characteristics such as the frequent finding of multifocal cystic lesions and the increased risk of developing another cystic tumor or a pancreatic ductal adenocarcinoma (PDA), either synchronously or metachronously [23]. Moreover, malignant progression is not only limited to cystic lesions as flat lesions also have the potential to develop malignancy and they need to be also surveilled [24].

IPMNs follow a classic "adenoma-carcinoma sequence" being estimated the time of progression from low-grade dysplasia to invasive carcinoma around 4–6 years [25]. IPMNs are the second most common exocrine pancreatic tumor after PDA. Otherwise, invasive carcinomas arising from IPMNs have important different morphological and genetic features in comparison to the common PDA [26, 27]. So, there have been found several alterations in oncogenes such as tumor suppressor genes and epigenetic changes in hypermethylation and gene expression.

There are several main molecular features that explain the biological behavior of IPMNs and their complex progression pathways, *KRAS* and *GNAS* somatic mutations the most frequent genetic abnormalities found in IPMNs [28, 29].

Table 3.1 Adapted from Nasca et al. [30]. Rate of mutations in low and high-grade IPMN

Mutations	Low-grade IPMN (%)	High-grade IPMN (%)
KRAS	43–89	31–71
GNAS	41–77	42–72
RNF43	10	25–75
CDKN2A	<5	0–15
TP53	<5	18–20
SMAD4	<5	<5

In Table 3.1, there are expressed the rate of different mutations in low- and high-grade IPMNs according to Nasca et al. [30].

Invasive carcinomas in the pancreas with IPMNs may arise in two ways: in an associated/derived manner or in a distinct/concomitant way [31]. Associated invasive carcinomas may have a poorer prognosis than concomitant ones [32]. Anyway, the pathways of carcinogenesis by which IPMNs may progress to PDA are under study.

These comprehensive histologic and genome profile studies are needed to provide insights into the tumorigenesis of these complex lesions allowing further studies and design strategies to accurately identify both drivers and patients at risk to develop invasive carcinomas and treat them timely and properly.

3.5 Clinical Presentation

Most patients with IPMNs are asymptomatic, especially those with BD-IPMN that have been discovered after cross-sectional imaging modalities were performed for unrelated indications. In surgical series the rate of symptomatic patients is, obviously higher, about 50% in one series, being abdominal pain the most common symptom (41%), followed by weight loss (29%), acute pancreatitis 22%), and jaundice (9%) [26]. Nearly 80% of symptomatic patients have only nonspecific clinical signs such as malaise, nausea, vomiting, abdominal or back pain, or weight loss [33]. Some patients may have pancreatitis-like symptoms or acute pancreatitis attacks. In some cases, exocrine or endocrine pancreatic insufficiency as well as maldigestion may develop.

Patients with IPMNs are at risk for synchronous and metachronous pancreatic carcinoma and extrapancreatic malignancies. Therefore, the symptoms and clinical signs will depend on localization of the tumor. In a surgical series of patients with IPMNs referred for surgery, recent onset of diabetes, diagnosed 5 years before surgery, was found to be associated with a 6.9-fold increased risk of invasive carcinoma [34].

Routine laboratory tests are usually normal. In patients complaint with abdominal pain, there may be elevated levels of amylase or lipase, associated or not with increased levels of bilirubin or cholestasis enzymes. Tumor markers such as carcinoembryonic antigen (CEA) or carbohydrate antigen 19-9 (Ca 19-9) are elevated in less than 20% of noninvasive cases while if they are elevated are suggestive of malignancy [35]. In a meta-analysis, elevated serum Ca 19-9 had a sensitivity of 52% and a specificity of 88% in detecting malignancy in IPMNs [36]. Elevated serum Ca 19-9 has been included in the revised consensus of Fukuoka guidelines as a worrisome parameter [25]. However, serum elevated Ca 19-9 has not been proved useful in distinguishing high-grade dysplastic lesions and its optimal cut-off has to be determined yet [26].

3.6 Diagnostic Approach

The diagnosis work-up of IPMNs relies on high-resolution cross-sectional imaging and endoscopy techniques and has several goals [37]. Firstly, IPMNs should be differentiated from other pancreatic cystic lesions. Secondly, it has to be determined the type of IPMN. Lastly, malignancy-related findings should be identified.

Radiology To assess accurately the subtype of PCN may be difficult. Gadolinium-MRI and/or MRCP should be the first procedure indicated because it can differentiate around 40–95% of PCN in comparison to 40–81% for multidetector CT scan [21] (Fig. 3.1). So, MRI/MRCP is more sensitive than CT for identifying communication between the cysts and the main pancreatic duct, multiple cysts, nodules, and thickened walls and the size of the main pancreatic duct [21, 25, 38]. MRI also spares patients from ionizing radiation of repeated CT. Nevertheless, multimodal imaging procedures (additional CT, especially dual-phase pancreatic protocol CT) should be performed to assess calcifications, when there is a suspect of malignant PCN or a concomitant pancreatic cancer and to rule out malignant recurrence after surgery for pancreatic cancer. There are radiologic features associated with an increased risk of malignancy in IPMNs: presence of a solid component, an enhanced mural nodule (<5 mm), increasing dilation of the main pancreatic duct, 5–9.9 mm and a large cystic diameter ≥ 4 cm [21].

Endoscopy Endoscopic retrograde cholangio-pancreatography (ERCP) is increasingly less employed because of its potential associated risks and the more accurate diagnostic yield and safety profile of endoscopic ultrasound (EUS). At ERCP, a patulous "fish mouth" papilla extruding mucus could be seen with the endoscopic view in advanced cases (patognomonic of MD-IPMN) and brushing cytology and collecting pancreatic juice could be obtained. Anyway, current data do not support the routine use of ERCP [39].

EUS is the next diagnostic step in the work-up of IPMNs after MRI and CT [25]. EUS provides accurate information on localization, dimensions, and characteristic features such as septation, number of cavities, and calcifications. EUS also assesses mural nodules, the cystic wall, and the entire pancreatic parenchyma to rule out associated solid lesions. EUS has the unique capability to perform EUS-guided fine needle aspiration (EUS-FNA) for solid lesions and cystic lesions to obtain the cystic fluid content for a comprehensive study including amylase/lipase, cytology, proteins antigens, and molecular analyses.

EUS obtains high-resolution images of the entire pancreatic parenchyma and is superior to radiologic techniques, also in assessing mural nodules which are a worrisome feature and one of the stronger predictors of high-risk IPMN. However, mucin plugs could be misdiagnosed as mural nodules. Contrast-enhanced harmonic EUS (CE-EUS) can display the microvascularization of the mural nodules and parenchymal perfusion helping to differentiate them from mucin plugs (Figs. 3.2 and 3.3) with a sensitivity and specificity ranging from 89 to 96% and 64 to 88, respectively [40]. If CE-EUS displays hyperenhancement of a mural nodule, a solid mass, or septations, the concern of malignant transformation is raised and EUS-FNA should be performed according to a European guideline [21]. Besides, to make clinical management of these patients more difficult, not only cystic or mural nodules are worrisome features. Koshita et al. diagnosed with EUS 21 patients with BD-IPMNs with invasive carcinoma. They found 12 patients with mural nodules while 9 patients have flat-type invasive carcinomas with higher recurrence rates of 33 vs. 67% and a worst 5-year survival of 76 vs. 33% in those with flat-type IPMNs [24].

A prospective multicenter study has reported that needle-based confocal laser endomicroscopy (nCLE) performed during the EUS-FNA of a

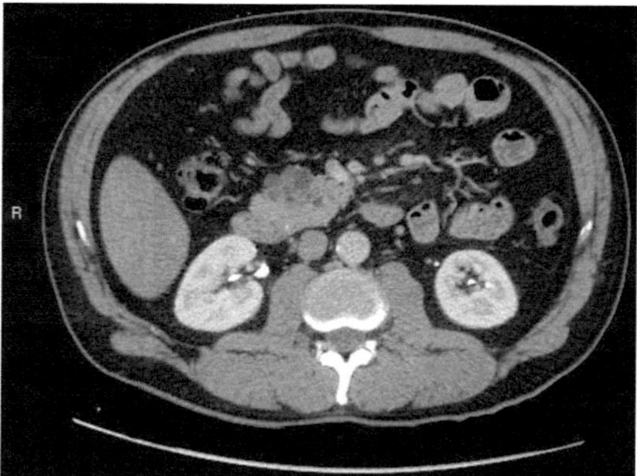

Fig. 3.1 Main duct (MD)-IPMN in the pancreatic head

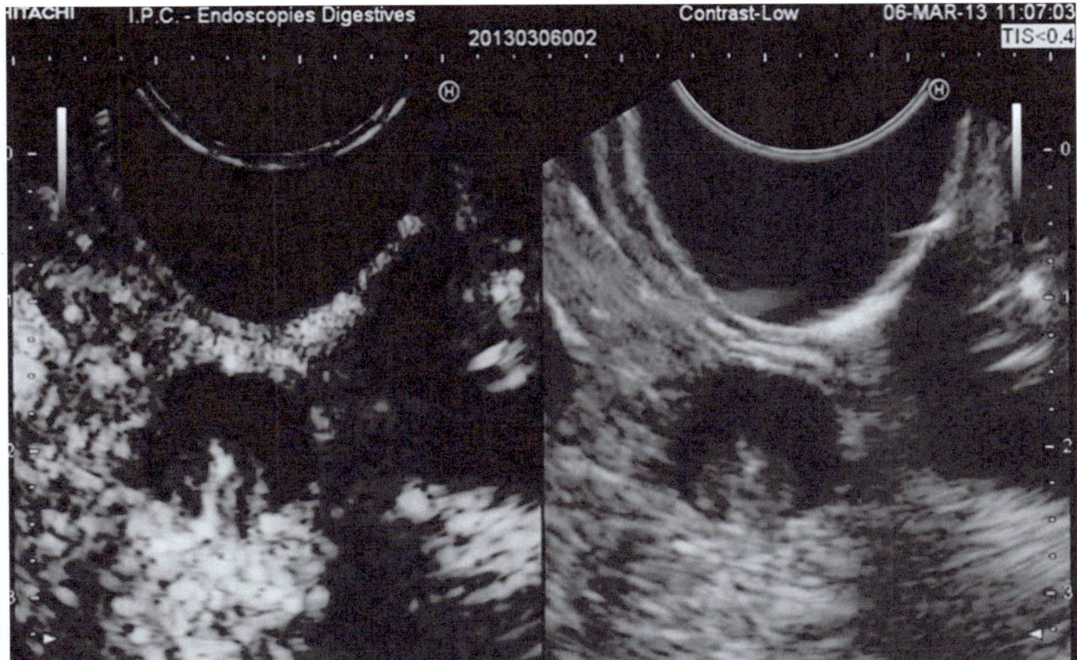

Fig. 3.2 CE-EUS showing the microvascularization of a mural nodule

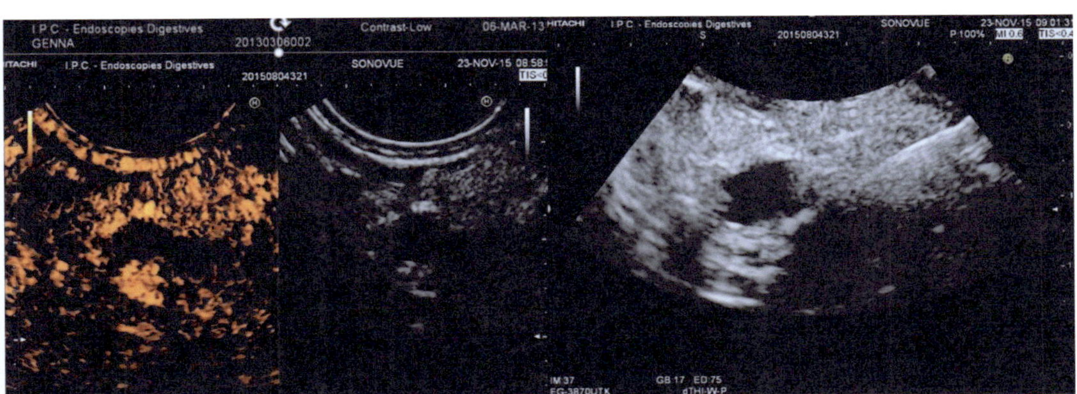

Fig. 3.3 Mural nodule enhancement after intravenous administration of Sonovue® displayed by EUS. EUS-FNA of the mural nodule. Courtesy of Professor Marc Giovannini. Institut Paoli-Calmettes, Marseilles, France

cystic lesion may be helpful in the differential diagnosis between mucinous and non-mucinous cysts [41].

Brush cytology and forceps biopsy are not yet recommended in daily clinical practice requiring these procedures further studies [21].

Finally, in patients unfit for surgery, EUS-guided radio frequency ablation would be a therapeutic option (Fig. 3.4) [42].

Cyst Fluid Analyses The study of cystic fluid obtained after EUS-FNA is evolving and remains investigational for the most part of their parameters. However, currently available data and further initiated research could help in differentiating mucinous from non-mucinous PCN and in the dire challenging clinical decision-making algorithm in detecting high-risk IPMNs. Study of the cyst fluid content encomprises cytology,

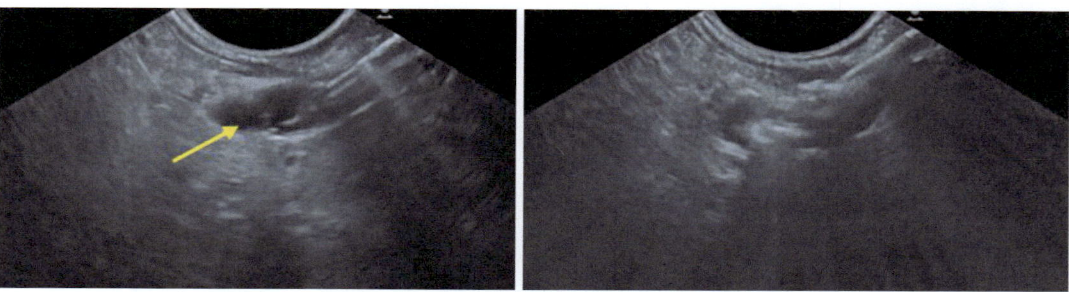

Fig. 3.4 Mural nodule (arrow) of an IPMN treated with EUS-guided RFA. Courtesy of Professor Marc Giovannini. Institut Paoli-Calmettes, Marseilles, France

biochemical analyses of CEA, Ca 19-9, viscosity, amylase/lipase and glucose, mucin stain, and proteomics and molecular analyses.

Cytology of the cystic fluid is of great value in assessing the risk of malignancy in IPMNs, although its sensitivity and specificity are hampered by the low volume, low cellular yield, and interobserver variability. The Moray micro forceps biopsy employed through a 19-gauge needle inserted into the cyst has been statistically significant superior to conventional analyses of the cystic fluid in diagnosing the specific type of the cyst [43]. However, this procedure has not been widely accepted in daily clinical practice.

CEA is the most widely employed protein marker in pancreatic cyst fluid being a valuable tool to distinguish between mucinous from non-mucinous lesions, although it cannot differentiate between benign cysts from those with high-grade dysplasia or invasive carcinoma [44]. CEA cut-off values of 109.9 and 192 ng/mL have been found to have an accuracy value of 79% and 86%, respectively, in detecting mucinous lesions [26]. The cyst fluid Ca 19-9 is not useful in distinguishing benign from malignant PCN [45]. The viscosity of IPMNs is typically thick while amylase levels will be high (>250 U/L). However, some mucinous neoplasms may have high levels of CEA and amylase also. Low levels of amylase neither rule out malignancy [46].

DNA alterations in the cyst fluid, especially mutations of *KRAS* and *GNAS* analyzed by next generation sequencing can distinguish muci-

nous from non-mucinous cysts [47], specially GNAS has been reported to have a sensitivity of 98% and a specificity of 100% in differentiated IPMNs from mucinous cystic neoplasms [48]. Different subtypes of mucin are released according to the histopathological subtype of IPMNs that also corresponds to the grade of dysplasia [49].

Interleukins levels of IL-1b, IL-5 and IL-8 have been found significantly higher in cysts with high-grade dysplasia or malignancy, being IL-1b the more accurate parameter in predicting high-risk versus low-risk with a sensitivity and specificity of 79% and 95%, respectively [50]. Prostaglandin E2 has been associated with PDA and has been found significantly higher in IPMMs compared to mucinous neoplasms ($p < 0.05$) and their levels correlated in a step-wise manner with the degree of dysplasia of the IPMN in two studies [51, 52].

MicroRNA profiling using Next Generation Sequencing displays aberrant microRNA expression in PDA and pancreatic cysts, being miR-216 the parameter most associated with dysplasia with a statistical difference in high-grade dysplasia-IPMNs and pancreatic cancer associated with IPMNs, when compared to low-grade dysplastic IPMNs [53]. Therefore, microRNA would be of great value in stratifying IPMNs [9].

Colon epithelial protein, when found in gastric and pancreatic epithelium, poses a risk of developing invasive carcinoma and react to the murine Das-1 monoclonal antibody [9, 54]. The dysplastic changes arising in the epithelial lining of the cysts may produce specific changes in the cystic fluid milieu that could be studied by several methods to investigate panels or a combination of several markers in order to better distinguish between high-risk from low-risk lesions.

To sum up, the study of cystic fluid biomarkers is an evolving field aiming to obtain accurate information to discriminate between high- and low-risk IPMNs leading to a sort of personalized medicine. Cystic fluid biomarkers obtained by EUS-FNA would be integrated into the management guidelines (based only on specific clinical, imaging, and laboratory parameters), helping in the clinical decision-making to timely send to surgery high-risk lesions, avoid high-risk surgical procedures in low-risk lesions that could be also followed-up with this combined approach including cyst fluid analyses.

3.7 Clinical and Surgical Management According to Published Guidelines

IPMNs are frequently found lesions carrying the potential of harboring or developing malignancy that has to be accurately evaluated by high-resolution imaging techniques and EUS to select patients for surgery and apply an adequate surveillance protocol [55].

To fulfil these two goals, several guidelines have been published (Tables 3.2 and 3.3) [21, 25, 38, 56], with differences between them regarding optimal indications for surgery, surveillance protocols, and the decision to stop follow-up [55].

Therefore, appropriate indication for surgery and surveillance will be based on high-risk stigmata/worrisome features balanced with the patient's age/comorbidities.

Table 3.2 Indications for surgery, diagnostic techniques, and management

Guideline	Year	Possible Indications for surgery	Diagnostic technique	Management
IAP I [56]	2006	Symptoms Cyst size ≥3 cm Mural nodule MPD ≥5 mm Positive cytology	CT scan MRI/MRCP EUS + FNA	Surgery
AGA [38]	2015	High risk features – Cyst size ≥3 cm – Presence of solid component – Dilated MPD – HGD or cancer on cytology	(CT scan) MRI/MRCP EUS + FNA	Surgery
IAP III[a] [25]	2017	High risk stigmata – Jaundice – Enhancing mural nodule ≥5 mm – MPD ≥10 mm – HGD or cancer on cytology	(CT scan) MRI/MRCP	Surgery
		Worrisome features – Cyst size ≥3 cm – Acute pancreatitis (due to IPMN) – Enhancing mural nodule <5 mm – Thickened and enhancing cyst wall – MPD dilation 5–9 mm – Abrupt change of MPD calibre with distal pancreatic atrophy – Presence of lymphadenopathy – Elevated serum CA 19–9 – Cyst growth rate >5 mm/2 years	(CT scan) MRI/MRCP EUS + FNA: required after imaging	Surgery versus close surveillance

(continued)

Table 3.2 (continued)

Guideline	Year	Possible Indications for surgery	Diagnostic technique	Management
European [21]	2018	Absolute indications – Jaundice – Enhancing mural nodule ≥5 mm – MPD ≥10 mm – HGD or cancer on cytology – Solid mass	(CT scan) (EUS + FNA) MRI/MRCP	Surgery
		Relative indications – Cyst size ≥4 cm – Enhancing mural nodule <5 mm – MPD dilation 5–9.9 mm – Serum CA 19.9 ≥37 U/ml – Cyst growth rate >5 mm/years – Acute pancreatitis (due to IPMN) – New onset of diabetes	(CT scan) (EUS + FNA) MRI/MRCP	Surgery

Adapted from the International European and American Gastroenterological Association (AGA) guidelines [55]

CT computed tomography, *EUS* endoscopic ultrasound, *FNA* fine needle aspiration, *HGD* high-grade dysplasia, *IAP* International Association of Pancreatology, *IPMN* intraductal papillary mucinous neoplasm, *MPD* main pancreatic duct, *MRCP* magnetic resonance with cholangiopancreatography, *MRI* magnetic resonance imaging

[a]A second revision of the International guidelines was made in 2012; since the guidelines did not change significantly—particularly when considering indications for surgery/surveillance—the last and updated version of the International guidelines has been included in this review

Table 3.3 Different surveillance strategies

Guideline	Year	Indications for surveillance	Methods of follow-up	Timing
IAP I [56]	2006	BD-IPMNs ≤30 mm without – Symptoms – Mural nodules – Positive cytology	MRI/MRCP or CT scan	Cyst size ≤20 mm • Every 6–12 months[a] Cyst size 20–30 mm • Every 3–6 months Lifetime surveillance • The interval follow-up can be outstreched if there are no changes after after a period of 2 years
AGA [38]	2015	BD-IPMNs ≤30 mm without – Solid component – Dilated MPD – HGD or cancer on cytology	MRI	Years 1, 2, 5 from initial diagnosis
IAP III[b] [25]	2017	No high-risk stigmata or worrisome features Cyst size <10 mm	(CT scan) MRI/MRCP	• At 6 months from diagnosis • Every 2 years (if no change)
		No high-risk stigmata or worrisome features	(CT scan) MRI/MRCP	• At 6–12 months from diagnosis • Yearly × 2 years • Every 2 years (if no change)
		No high-risk stigmata or worrisome features Cyst size 20–30 mm	MRI/MRCP EUS	• EUS in 3–6 months • Yearly follow-up alternating EUS and MRI
		No high-risk stigmata Presence of worrisome features including cyst size <30 mm	MRI/MRCP EUS	• Every 3–6 months alternating EUS and MRI
		Lifetime surveillance—consider surveillance discontinuation only in patients who become unfit for surgery		

Table 3.3 (continued)

Guideline	Year	Indications for surveillance	Methods of follow-up	Timing
European [21]	2018	No absolute or relative indications for surgery	MRI/MRCP or EUS Serum CA 19.9	• Every 6 months for the first year • Yearly thereafter
		No absolute indications for surgery One relative indication in patients with significant comorbidities	MRI/MRCP or EUS Serum CA 19.9	• Every 6 months

Adapted from International, European, and American Gastroenterological Association (AGA) guidelines [55]

BD branch duct, *CT* computed tomography, *EUS* endoscopic ultrasound, *FNA* fine needle aspiration, *HGD* high-grade dysplasia, *IAP* International Association of Pancreatology, *IPMN* intraductal papillary mucinous neoplasm, *MPD* main pancreatic duct, *MRCP* magnetic resonance with cholangiopancreatography, *MRI* magnetic resonance imaging

[a]The interval of follow-up can be lengthened after two years of no change

[b]A second revision of the International guidelines was made in 2012; since the guidelines did not change significantly— particularly when considering indications for surgery/surveillance—the last and updated version of the International guidelines has been included in this review

Different studies [57, 58] have demonstrated that, although high-risk stigmata or worrisome features are not observed in the diagnosis, after a median follow-up of 5 years, an important number of patients can develop malignancy or high-risk stigmata.

Finally, The addition of taking into account molecular markers into the management of these lesions would lead to a better individualized making-decision algorithm, especially in identifying high-risk lesions in otherwise patients presenting with low-risk lesions on conventional imaging parameters, being needed controlled studies and refining techniques.

References

1. Adsay V, Mino-Kenudson M, Furukawa T, et al. Pathologic evaluation and reporting of intraductal papillary mucinous neoplasms of the pancreas and other tumoral intraepithelial neoplasms of pancreatobiliary tract: recommendations of verona consensus meeting. Ann Surg. 2016;263(1):162–77.
2. Itai Y, Ohhashi K, Nagai H, et al. "Ductectatic" mucinous cystadenoma and cystadenocarcinoma of the pancreas. Radiology. 1986;161(3):697–700.
3. Klibansky DA, Reid-Lombardo KM, Gordon SR, et al. The clinical relevance of the increasing incidence of intraductal papillary mucinous neoplasm. Clin Gastroenterol Hepatol. 2012;10(5): 555–8.
4. Laffan TA, Horton KM, Klein AP, et al. Prevalence of unsuspected pancreatic cysts on MDCT. AJR Am J Roentgenol. 2008;191(3):802–7.
5. Spinelli KS, Fromwiller TE, Daniel RA, et al. Cystic pancreatic neoplasms: observe or operate. Ann Surg. 2004;239(5):651–7. discussion 7–9
6. Zhang XM, Mitchell DG, Dohke M, et al. Pancreatic cysts: depiction on single-shot fast spin-echo MR images. Radiology. 2002;223(2):547–53.
7. Girometti R, Intini SG, Cereser L, et al. Incidental pancreatic cysts: a frequent finding in liver-transplanted patients as assessed by 3D T2-weighted turbo spin echo magnetic resonance cholangiopancreatography. JOP. 2009;10(5):507–14.
8. Del Chiaro M, Segersvärd R, Pozzi Mucelli R, et al. Comparison of preoperative conference-based diagnosis with histology of cystic tumors of the pancreas. Ann Surg Oncol. 2014;21(5):1539–44.
9. Hao S, Takahashi C, Snyder RA, et al. Stratifying intraductal papillary mucinous neoplasms by cyst fluid analysis: present and future. Int J Mol Sci. 2020;21(3):1147.
10. Kosmahl M, Pauser U, Peters K, et al. Cystic neoplasms of the pancreas and tumor-like lesions with cystic features: a review of 418 cases and a classification proposal. Virchows Arch. 2004;445(2):168–78.
11. Allen PJ, D'Angelica M, Gonen M, et al. A selective approach to the resection of cystic lesions of the pancreas: results from 539 consecutive patients. Ann Surg. 2006;244(4):572–82.
12. Lee CJ, Scheiman J, Anderson MA, et al. Risk of malignancy in resected cystic tumors of the pancreas < or =3 cm in size: is it safe to observe asymptomatic patients? A multi-institutional report. J Gastrointest Surg. 2008;12(2):234–42.
13. Fukushima N, Mukai K. Pancreatic neoplasms with abundant mucus production: emphasis on intraductal papillary-mucinous tumors and mucinous cystic tumors. Adv Anat Pathol. 1999;6(2):65–77.
14. Capurso G, Boccia S, Salvia R, et al. Risk factors for intraductal papillary mucinous neoplasm (IPMN) of the pancreas: a multicentre case-control study. Am J Gastroenterol. 2013;108(6):1003–9.

15. Sato N, Rosty C, Jansen M, et al. STK11/LKB1 Peutz-Jeghers gene inactivation in intraductal papillary-mucinous neoplasms of the pancreas. Am J Pathol. 2001;159(6):2017–22.

16. Maire F, Hammel P, Terris B, et al. Intraductal papillary and mucinous pancreatic tumour: a new extracolonic tumour in familial adenomatous polyposis. Gut. 2002;51(3):446–9.

17. Poley JW, Kluijt I, Gouma DJ, et al. The yield of first-time endoscopic ultrasonography in screening individuals at a high risk of developing pancreatic cancer. Am J Gastroenterol. 2009;104(9):2175–81.

18. Buscail E, Cauvin T, Fernandez B, et al. Intraductal papillary mucinous neoplasms of the pancreas and European guidelines: importance of the surgery type in the decision-making process. BMC Surg. 2019;19(1):115.

19. Han Y, Lee H, Kang JS, et al. Progression of pancreatic branch duct intraductal papillary mucinous neoplasm associates with cyst size. Gastroenterology. 2018;154(3):576–84.

20. Lafemina J, Katabi N, Klimstra D, et al. Malignant progression in IPMN: a cohort analysis of patients initially selected for resection or observation. Ann Surg Oncol. 2013;20(2):440–7.

21. European Study Group on Cystic Tumours of the Pancreas. European evidence-based guidelines on pancreatic cystic neoplasms. Gut. 2018;67(5):789–804.

22. Tanaka M, Fernández-del Castillo C, Adsay V, et al. International consensus guidelines 2012 for the management of IPMN and MCN of the pancreas. Pancreatology. 2012;12(3):183–97.

23. Sereni E, Luchini C, Salvia R, et al. Molecular and clinical patterns of local progression in the pancreatic remnant following resection of pancreatic intraductal papillary mucinous neoplasm (IPMN). Chin Clin Oncol. 2019;8(2):21.

24. Koshita S, Fujita N, Noda Y, et al. Invasive carcinoma derived from "flat type" branch duct intraductal papillary mucinous neoplasms of the pancreas: impact of classification according to the height of mural nodule on endoscopic ultrasonography. J Hepatobiliary Pancreat Sci. 2015;22(4):301–9.

25. Tanaka M, Fernández-Del Castillo C, Kamisawa T, et al. Revisions of international consensus Fukuoka guidelines for the management of IPMN of the pancreas. Pancreatology. 2017;17(5):738–53.

26. Morales-Oyarvide V, Fong ZV, Fernández-Del Castillo C, et al. Intraductal papillary mucinous neoplasms of the pancreas: strategic considerations. Visc Med. 2017;33(6):466–76.

27. Fritz S, Fernandez-del Castillo C, Mino-Kenudson M, et al. Global genomic analysis of intraductal papillary mucinous neoplasms of the pancreas reveals significant molecular differences compared to ductal adenocarcinoma. Ann Surg. 2009;249:440–7.

28. Wu J, Jiao Y, Dal Molin M, et al. Whole-exome sequencing of neoplastic cysts of the pancreas reveals recurrent mutations in components of ubiquitin-dependent pathways. Proc Natl Acad Sci U S A. 2011;108(52):21188–93.

29. Amato E, Molin M, Mafficini A, et al. Targeted next-generation sequencing of cancer genes dissects the molecular profiles of intraductal papillary neoplasms of the pancreas. J Pathol. 2014;233(3):217–27.

30. Nasca V, Chiaravalli M, Piro G, et al. Intraductal pancreatic mucinous neoplasms: a tumor-biology based approach for risk stratification. Int J Mol Sci. 2020;21(17):6386.

31. Patra KC, Bardeesy N, Mizukami Y. Diversity of precursor lesions for pancreatic cancer: the genetics and biology of intraductal papillary mucinous neoplasm. Clin Transl Gastroenterol. 2017;8(4):e86.

32. Yamaguchi K, Kanemitsu S, Hatori T, et al. Pancreatic ductal adenocarcinoma derived from IPMN and pancreatic ductal adenocarcinoma concomitant with IPMN. Pancreas. 2011;40(4):571–80.

33. Grützmann R, Niedergethmann M, Pilarsky C, et al. Intraductal papillary mucinous tumors of the pancreas: biology, diagnosis, and treatment. Oncologist. 2010;15(12):1294–309.

34. Morales-Oyarvide V, Mino-Kenudson M, Ferrone CR, et al. Diabetes mellitus in intraductal papillary mucinous neoplasm of the pancreas is associated with high-grade dysplasia and invasive carcinoma. Pancreatology. 2017;17(6):920–6.

35. Fritz S, Hackert T, Hinz U, et al. Role of serum carbohydrate antigen 19-9 and carcinoembryonic antigen in distinguishing between benign and invasive intraductal papillary mucinous neoplasm of the pancreas. Br J Surg. 2011;98(1):104–10.

36. Wang W, Zhang L, Chen L, et al. Serum carcinoembryonic antigen & carbohydrate antigen 19-9 for prediction of malignancy and invasiveness in intraductal papillary mucinous neoplasms of the pancreas: a meta-analysis. Biomed Rep. 2015;3:43–50.

37. Crippa S, Bassi C, Salvia R, et al. Low progression of intraductal papillary mucinous neoplasms with worrisome features and high-risk stigmata undergoing non-operative management: a mid-term follow-up analysis. Gut. 2017;66(3):495–506.

38. Vege SS, Ziring B, Jain R, et al. American gastroenterological association institute guideline on the diagnosis and management of asymptomatic neoplastic pancreatic cysts. Gastroenterology. 2015;148(4):819–22.

39. Fernández-del Castillo C, Adsay NV. Intraductal papillary mucinous neoplasms of the pancreas. Gastroenterology. 2010;139(3):708–13. 13.e1–2

40. Kitano M, Sakamoto H, Komaki T, et al. New techniques and future perspective of EUS for the differential diagnosis of pancreatic malignancies: contrast harmonic imaging. Dig Endosc. 2011;23(Suppl 1):46–50.

41. Napoleon B, Palazzo M, Lemaistre A-I, et al. Needle-based confocal laser endomicroscopy of pancreatic

cystic lesions: a prospective multicenter validation study in patients with definite diagnosis. Endoscopy. 2019;51(09):825–35.

42. Barthet M, Giovannini M, Lesavre N, et al. Endoscopic ultrasound-guided radiofrequency ablation for pancreatic neuroendocrine tumors and pancreatic cystic neoplasms: a prospective multicenter study. Endoscopy. 2019;51(9):836–42.

43. Zhang ML, Arpin RN, Brugge WR, et al. Moray micro forceps biopsy improves the diagnosis of specific pancreatic cysts. Cancer Cytopathol. 2018;126(6):414–20.

44. Correa-Gallego C, Warshaw AL, Fernandez-del Castillo C. Fluid CEA in IPMNs: a useful test or the flip of a coin? Am J Gastroenterol. 2009;104:796–7.

45. Cao S, Hu Y, Gao X, et al. Serum carbohydrate antigen 19-9 in differential diagnosis of benign and malignant pancreatic cystic neoplasms: a meta-analysis. PLoS One. 2016;11(11):e0166406.

46. Scourtas A, Dudley JC, Brugge WR, et al. Preoperative characteristics and cytological features of 136 histologically confirmed pancreatic mucinous cystic neoplasms. Cancer Cytopathol. 2017;125(3):169–77.

47. Jones M, Zheng Z, Wang J, et al. Impact of next-generation sequencing on the clinical diagnosis of pancreatic cysts. Gastrointest Endosc. 2016;83(1):140–8.

48. Wu J, Matthaei H, Maitra A, et al. Recurrent GNAS mutations define an unexpected pathway for pancreatic cyst development. Sci Transl Med. 2011;3(92):92ra66.

49. Kim GE, Bae HI, Park HU, et al. Aberrant expression of MUC5AC and MUC6 gastric mucins and sialyl Tn antigen in intraepithelial neoplasms of the pancreas. Gastroenterology. 2002;123(4):1052–60.

50. Maker AV, Katabi N, Qin LX, et al. Cyst fluid interleukin-1beta (IL1beta) levels predict the risk of carcinoma in intraductal papillary muci-

nous neoplasms of the pancreas. Clin Cancer Res. 2011;17(6):1502–8.

51. Schmidt CM, Yip-Schneider MT, Ralstin MC, et al. PGE(2) in pancreatic cyst fluid helps differentiate IPMN from MCN and predict IPMN dysplasia. J Gastrointest Surg. 2008;12(2):243–9.

52. Yip-Schneider MT, Carr RA, Wu H, et al. Prostaglandin E(2): a pancreatic fluid biomarker of intraductal papillary mucinous neoplasm dysplasia. J Am Coll Surg. 2017;225(4):481–7.

53. Wang J, Paris PL, Chen J, et al. Next generation sequencing of pancreatic cyst fluid microRNAs from low grade-benign and high grade-invasive lesions. Cancer Lett. 2015;356(2, Part B):404–9.

54. Das KK, Geng X, Brown JW, et al. Cross validation of the monoclonal antibody das-1 in identification of high-risk mucinous pancreatic cystic lesions. Gastroenterology. 2019;157(3):720–30.e2.

55. Crippa S, Arcidiacono PG, De Cobelli F, et al. Review of the diagnosis and management of intraductal papillary mucinous neoplasms. United European Gastroenterol J. 2020;8(3):249–55.

56. Tanaka M, Chari S, Adsay V, et al. International consensus guidelines for management of intraductal papillary mucinous neoplasms and mucinous cystic neoplasms of the pancreas. Pancreatology. 2006;6(1-2):17–32.

57. Crippa S, Pezzilli R, Bissolati M, et al. Active surveillance beyond 5 years is required for presumed branch-duct intraductal papillary mucinous neoplasms undergoing non-operative management. Am J Gastroenterol. 2017;112(7):1153–61.

58. Pergolini I, Sahora K, Ferrone CR, et al. Long-term risk of pancreatic malignancy in patients with branch duct intraductal papillary mucinous neoplasm in a referral center. Gastroenterology. 2017;153(5):1284–94.e1.

Pancreatic Neuroendocrine Tumors: Diagnosis, Management, and Intraoperative Techniques

4

Baltasar Pérez-Saborido, Martín Bailón-Cuadrado,
Francisco Javier Tejero-Pintor,
Ekta Choolani-Bhojwani, Pablo Marcos-Santos,
and David Pacheco-Sánchez

4.1 Background

Pancreatic neuroendocrine tumors (pNETs) represent up to 2% of all pancreatic neoplasms. After pancreatic ductal adenocarcinoma, they are the second most common primary pancreatic malignant tumors. Pancreatic neuroendocrine tumors (pNETs) are overall rare; they have an incidence of ≤ 1 case per 100,000 individuals per year and account for 1–2% of all pancreatic tumors. pNETs represent less than 3% of primary pancreatic neoplasms. Incidence rates have been increasing over the last two decades, but it is mainly related to increased detection of asymptomatic disease on cross-sectional imaging and endoscopy done for other reasons [1–3]. pNETs are classified as *functional* when associated with hormone secretion and a clinical syndrome or *non-functioning*. Over 50% of pNETs are non-functional in contemporary studies [4–7]. The aim of this chapter is to illustrate the main concepts of pNETs concerning diagnosis, medical management, and surgical approach.

4.2 Diagnosis of pNETs: Imagining and Histological Diagnosis

Depending on the clinical presentation the diagnostic sequence varies, so a combination of laboratory tests and imaging studies are needed for its diagnosis [8].

4.2.1 Imaging Studies

4.2.1.1 Ultrasound (US)

pNETs are visualized in abdominal ultrasound (US) as well as circumscribed and hypoechoic tumors with smooth margins and can demonstrate a hypervascular enhancement with intravenous contrast [9, 10]. US can be useful to

B. Pérez-Saborido (✉) · M. Bailón-Cuadrado
F. J. Tejero-Pintor · E. Choolani-Bhojwani
P. Marcos-Santos · D. Pacheco-Sánchez
Hepatobiliopancreatic Surgical Unit, General and
Digestive Surgical Department, "Rio Hortega"
University Hospital, Valladolid, Spain
e-mail: ps.baltasar@gmail.com;
mbailonc@saludcastillayleon.es;
ftejeropintor@saludcastillayleon.es;
echoolanibhojwanic@saludcastillayleon.es;
pmarcoss@saludcastillayleon.es;
dpachecos@saludcastillayleon.es

perform a percutaneous needle biopsy of doubtful liver metastases. Ultrasound is an accepted first-line study in symptomatic patients but cannot replace other elaborate imaging modalities like CT or MRI, as it cannot differentiate between different types of pancreatic solid tumors [11].

4.2.1.2 Computed Tomography

Most pNETs appear as solid hypervascular neoplasms that often enhance on arterial or occasionally portal venous phase imaging [12, 13]. Dynamic CT has a sensitivity of 64–81% for pNETs diagnosis [14]. Small tumors as 4 mm can be visualized with CT; its sensitivity is decreased for those smaller than 2 cm [14]. The sensitivity approaches almost 100% in symptomatic but non-functioning tumors, VIPomas, and glucagonomas that present as large tumors (>3 cm) at the time of diagnosis [15].

4.2.1.3 Magnetic Resonance Imaging

On Magnetic Resonance Imaging (MRI), they appear with low signal on T1-weighted sequence, intermediate to high signal on T2-weighted sequence, hyper-enhancing on post-contrast, and diffusion restricting [16]. It presents an overall sensitivity of 74–94% and specificity of 78–100% for tumor detection [17]. As with CT scans, early arterial phase imaging following the injection of gadolinium contrast is critical for the detection of small hypervascular liver metastases [18].

4.2.1.4 Endoscopic Ultrasonography

Endoscopic ultrasonography (EUS) provides excellent sensitivity and specificity and it can detect lesions as small as 2–3 mm in diameter [19]. On EUS, pNETs usually appear as defined orbed, hypoechoic lesions with a homogeneous pattern and clear regular margins [20]. ENETS Consensus guidelines considered EUS as the imaging study of choice to be performed after other negative non-invasive imaging studies [21].

One of the benefits of this technique is the possibility to perform EUS-guided fine needle aspiration (FNA) biopsy of the pancreatic lesions for subsequent histological confirmation. EUS-FNA presents a sensitivity between 80 and 90%, specificity of 96%, and a sampling adequacy rate of 83–93%, therefore, this method is considered the primary sampling technique for pancreatic tumors [22]. It is important to assess the difficulty visualizing the pancreatic tail, thus a highly skilled endoscopist is often required.

4.2.1.5 Somatostatin Receptor-Based Imaging and Positron Emission Tomography

Most well-differentiated pNETs express high levels of somatostatin receptors which make functional imaging tests based on the expression of somatostatin receptors using radiolabelled somatostatin analogues a good option. The first imaging technique to visualize somatostatin receptor expressing tumors used 111-In pentetreotide to produce a scintigraphic image (OctreoScan). Following the advent of Positron Emission Tomography/Computed Tomography (PET/CT) systems, the development of several PET tracers for somatostatin receptor imagining such as 68-GaDOTATE and 68-Ga DOTATOC and metabolic markers (18F-FDG) have improved the detection of staging of these tumors [23, 24].

68-Ga DOTATATE or 68-Ga DOTATOC PET/CT is preferred for most pNETs, especially for staging, detection of lymph node, and bone metastases and identification of the primary tumor. Indeed, it provides a predictive clinical response to therapy with somatostatin analogues and peptide receptor radionuclide therapy and it can help in identifying an otherwise occult primary site [25].

Other procedures, such as digestive endoscopy, invasive approaches, or intraoperative ultrasonography may be required in rare cases. Procedures like arterial stimulation with venous sampling (ASVS) or arterial stimulation with transhepatic portal venous sampling (THPVS) have turned relatively obsolete given the improved sensitivity of preoperative imaging, especially 68-Ga DOTATATE PET and EUS and might be used as adjuncts of imagining in patients where pNETs cannot be identified or localized preoperatively.

Most pNETs are non-functioning, about 30–50% of them, but they frequently synthesize a variety of peptide markers, including chromogranin A (CgA), Neuron-Specific Enolase (NSE), ghrelin, neurotensin, subunits of human chorionic gonadotropin and pancreatic polypeptide (PP); that may be used in the follow-up of patients with pancreatic neuroendocrine tumors [26]. CgA has been correlated with tumor mass and metastasis of well-differentiated PNETs, as well as a prognostic marker, however, CgA is sensitive but not specific [27]. Due to suboptimal sensitivity and specificity of these markers a confirmed diagnosis requires histologic analysis.

Functional pNETs typically present with specific clinical syndromes related to peptide hypersecretion (i.e., insulin, proinsulin, glucagon, gastrin, and vasoactive intestinal polypeptide) than can be measured. These hormone levels can be correlated with changes in tumor size and might behave as specific tumor markers [28].

4.2.2 Histological Diagnosis

Focusing on their histopathological characteristics, pNETs are a heterogeneous group of tumors. It was thought that these neoplasms arose from neuroendocrine cells that migrated from the neural crest and initially these tumors were referred to as islet cell tumors because of its similarity to the islet of Langerhans. However, it is now known that enteropancreatic neuroendocrine cells originated from multipotent stem cells [29].

pNETs possess electron-dense granules with multiple peptides/amines, neuron-specific enolase, synaptophysin, and chromogranin. Histologically, they characteristically display small cells with uniform nuclei and low rates of mitotic figures [30].

Pancreatic endocrine tumors can present a variety of growth patterns like gyriform patterns; solid or medullary patterns and glandular patterns. They may also present with sarcomatous or anaplastic growth patterns, and many tumors show multiple growth patterns. Cytologically, they usually are composed of monomorphic cells with clear to eosinophilic cytoplasm and variable mitotic activity. No correlation has been described between growth pattern and biological behavior or between growth pattern and functional type [31].

pNETs have malignant potential and it is necessary to predict their biological behavior with its pathologic characterization of tumor grade and cell differentiation. To assess tumor grading and risk for malignancy several factors are studied such as tumor size, mitotic rate, presence of metastatic disease, local invasion, perineural spread, angioinvasion, and Ki-67 proliferation index. However, malignancy can only be confirmed by the presence of local spread, vascular invasion, lymphadenopathy, or metastasic disease [32].

4.3 Classification

Attending to the production of metabolically active hormones we can divide pancreatic neuroendocrine tumors into two types: non-functioning and hyperfunctioning tumors [33]. These tumors are related to diverse clinical syndromes that will be explained ahead in this chapter.

pNETs can be stratified into two groups attending to its histological grade well-differentiated tumors or pancreatic neuroendocrine tumors (pNETs) and poorly differentiated pancreatic tumors which are called pancreatic neuroendocrine carcinomas (pNECs) [34].

In the 2010 World Health Organization (WHO) classification system, pNETs were divided into three grades based on two factors: mitotic count and ki-67 labeling index. The system also divided pNETs into well-differentiated tumors, made up of grades 1 and 2, and poorly differentiated tumors, where grade 3 was included. However, the development of several studies has proved wrong the assumption that poorly differentiated histology and high tumor grade were equivalent. The most recent 2019

WHO classification of NENs of the digestive system now recognizes a category of high-grade but well-differentiated GEP NENs. According to the 2019 World Health Organization consensus criteria, the classification of pancreatic neoplasms is based on the following tumor characteristics: histology, differentiation, and grade [based on mitotic rate and proliferative index (Ki-67%)] (Table 4.1) [34–36].

Although pNETs were isolated from pancreatic adenocarcinoma in the seventh edition of the AJCC staging system published in 2010, the same staging classification criteria in pancreatic adenocarcinoma were applied to pNETs. Due to its different biological behaviors and prognosis, the revised eighth edition introduced another classification criterion asserted by the European Neuroendocrine Tumour Society (ENETS). However, some controversies remain in this staging system and a modified ENETS (mENETS) staging classification was proposed by maintaining the ENETS Tm N and M definitions but adopting the seventh AJCC edition's staging definitions (Table 4.2) [37].

Table 4.1 Adapted from the World Health Organization's (WHO) classification system of Pancreatic Neuroendocrine Neoplasm (PaNENs) [35]

Terminology	Differentiation	Grade	Mitotic rate (mitoses/2 mm^2	KI-67 proliferation index (%)
Pancreatic neuroendocrine tumor	Well differentiated	Low (G1)	<2	<3
		Intermediated (G2)	2–20	3–20
		High (G3)	>20	>20
Pancreatic neuroendocrine carcinoma small-cell type	Poorly differentiated	High	>20	>20
Pancreatic neuroendocrine carcinoma large-cell type	Poorly differentiated	High	>20	>20
Pancreatic mixed neuroendocrine non-neuroendocrine neoplasm	Well or poorly differentiated	Variable	Variable	Variable

Table 4.2 Definitions of American Joint Committee on Cancer, European Neuroendocrine Tumor Society, and modified European Neuroendocrine Tumor Society staging for pancreatic neuroendocrine tumors

Stage	AJCC 7th staging classification			AJCC 8th and ENETS staging classification			mENETS		
	T	N	M	T	N	M	T	N	M
IA	T1	N0	M0	T1	N0	M0	T1	N0	M0
IB	T2	N0	M0	T2	N0	M0	T2	N0	M0
IIA	T3	N0	M0	T3	N0	M0	T3	N0	M0
IIB	T1–T3	N1	M0	T4	N0	M0	T1–T3	N1	M0
III	T4	Any N	M0	Any T	N1	M0	T4	Any N	M0
IV	Any T	Any N	M1	Any T	Any N	M1	Any T	Any N	M1

Adapted from Ma et al. [37]

AJCC American Joint Committee on cancer, *ENETS* European Neuroendocrine Tumor Society, *mENETS* Modified European neuroendocrine Tumor society

4.4   Neuroendocrine Syndromes

As mentioned previously in this chapter, according to the specific hormone secretion, we divide these tumors into functioning pNETs which include insulinomas, gastrinomas, VIPomas, glucagonomas, and others resulting in a myriad of hormonal hypersecretion syndromes. Nevertheless, non-functioning pNETs comprise the largest group of pNETs and do not produce syndromes of hormonal excess; rather, they cause morbidity and mortality by invading normal tissue and metastasizing [38, 39].

We herein assemble the main pNETs features.

4.4.1   Functioning Pancreatic Neuroendocrine Tumors

4.4.1.1 Insulinoma

Insulinomas are the most common functioning pancreatic endocrine tumors. They are rare (approximately four cases per million per year) but are the most common cause of hyperinsulinemic hypoglycemia in adults. It has a slight female predominance, and the median age at diagnosis is in the fifth decade of life. Insulinomas are typically solitary pancreatic lesions that are small (90% are less than 2 cm), well-circumscribed, and equally distributed throughout the pancreas. Rarely, insulinomas occur as multiple lesions (8% of the total insulinoma cases); these are usually associated with MEN1.

To begin the work-up of a hyperinsulinemic hypoglycemia patient, Whipple's triad must first be established. Patients should have symptoms of hypoglycemia with concomitant low blood glucose levels (<50 mg/dL). In addition, symptoms should resolve with glucose intake or correction of the low blood glucose levels. Once Whipple's triad is confirmed, insulin levels should be checked. Inappropriately normal or elevated insulin levels in the presence of hypoglycemia are typically diagnostic of insulinoma after other factors such as exogenous insulin or hypoglycemic drugs have been ruled out [40].

4.4.1.2 Gastrinoma

Gastrinoma is a NET of the pancreas or duodenum that secretes gastrin and gastrin precursors (progastrins) that mimic the action of gastrin secreted by the G cells of the gastric antrum. Gastrinoma syndrome, also known as Zollinger-Ellison syndrome (ZES), is a rare disease (1–3 cases per million per year). It has a slight male predominance and is generally diagnosed in the fifth decade of life. Peptic ulcer is the most common presentation of ZES. Interestingly, diarrhea occurs in up to 75% of patients and is occasionally the foremost complaint. Most gastrinomas are sporadic, but in up to 20–30% of the cases, it is associated with MEN1. Approximately 50–60% of gastrinomas are in the pancreas, and 40–50% are in the duodenum. Approximately 60–90% of gastrinomas are malignant, and up to 50% of patients will have distant liver metastases at the time of diagnosis. The 5-year survival rate for all gastrinoma patients ranges between 62 and 75%.

Gastrinoma is suspected in patients with resistant or multiple peptic ulcers. Biochemical diagnosis of gastrinoma is challenging because gastrin levels increase for many reasons, such as the use of proton pump inhibitors, *H. pylori* infection, renal failure, and gastric outlet obstruction. Fasting gastrin level detection should be the first laboratory screening test. Normal gastrin levels rule out gastrinoma, and fasting gastrin levels >500 pg/mL or greater than fivefold the upper limit of normal suggest gastrinoma. In addition, fasting gastrin levels >1000 pg/mL are highly suggestive of gastrinoma, especially if the patient has an acidic gastric pH (<2). Because many other conditions increase gastrin levels, a provocative test must be performed to confirm the diagnosis. The most common provocative tests use secretin or calcium gluconate infusion. Secretin does not stimulate gastrin release from G cells of the stomach but does stimulate gastrin release from gastrinomas. An increase in fasting gastrin level higher than 200 pg/mL after secretin infusion is considered diagnostic [40].

4.4.1.3 VIPoma

VIPoma is a vasoactive intestinal polypeptide (VIP)—secreting tumor that commonly arises from the gastrointestinal tract. VIPoma syndrome is also known as WDHA syndrome and includes watery diarrhea, hypokalemia, and achlorhydria. VIPomas are rare and occur at a rate of 1 per 10 million per year. The median age at diagnosis is in the fifth decade of life, and there is a slight female predominance. Approximately 90% of these tumors are located in the pancreas, mostly in the body or tail. VIPomas are usually solitary (70–80%) and have a diameter of 1–7 cm. Many tumors are larger than 2 cm at the time of diagnosis, and symptoms typically appear after the tumor reaches a certain size. Typically, these tumors are metastatic at the time of diagnosis.

The diagnosis of VIPomas requires recognition of the VIPoma syndrome and exclusion of more common causes of chronic diarrhea, such as chronic gastrointestinal infection, inflammatory bowel disease, microscopic colitis, malabsorption syndrome, and laxative abuse. Fasting VIP levels greater than 200 pg/mL are required to confirm the diagnosis. Most patients with VIPomas have much higher VIP levels, sometimes as high as 7000 pg/mL [40].

4.4.1.4 Glucagonoma

Glucagonoma is a rare type of functioning pNETs, with an estimated incidence of 1 per 20 million per year. Glucagonoma syndrome is characterized by a skin rash known as necrolytic migratory erythema, diabetes mellitus, weight loss, anemia, stomatitis, thromboembolism, gastrointestinal disturbances, and neuropsychiatric symptoms. Glucagonomas vary in size from 2 to 25 cm and predominantly occur in the tail of the pancreas. Most glucagonomas have already metastasized to the liver at the time of diagnosis.

The diagnosis of glucagonoma requires a high index of suspicion. Non-specific elevations in glucagon levels are common under physiologic stress or in carcinoid syndrome, but glucagon levels are usually less than 500 pg/mL (upper limit of normal <100 pg/mL). Glucagonoma is associated with a markedly elevated serum glucagon level (>500 pg/mL, mean ~1400 pg/mL), and glucagon levels above 1000 pg/mL are diagnostic of glucagonoma if the patient has glucagonoma syndrome [41].

4.4.2 Non-functioning Pancreatic Neuroendocrine Tumors

Non-functioning pNETs are clinically defined as pNETs that are not associated with a clear hormonal hypersecretion syndrome. Non-functioning pNETs produce and secrete hormones, but the quantity and the biological activity of these hormones do not produce a distinct syndrome. Non-functioning pNETs result in non-specific symptoms resulting from tumor mass effects. Sometimes, non-functioning pNETs are discovered incidentally during abdominal imaging for other purposes. Non-functioning pNETs are usually diagnosed in the fourth or fifth decades of life and have often already metastasized to the liver at the time of diagnosis [42].

4.5 Localized pNETs Management

Treatment decisions of pNETs are based on whether the tumor is or not functioning, candidacy for surgical therapy, and treatment of metastatic disease. Surgical resection remains the only curative approach and must therefore be regarded as the current standard of care even in many cases where advanced disease is found [43]. The ideal aim of surgical resection is removal of the primary tumor and any affected lymph nodes [8, 44–46].

4.5.1 How Should Small Non-functioning (NF) pNETs Be Treated?

There are no truly prospective or randomized investigations and all recommendations and consensus are based on retrospective series and systematic reviews.

There are some good experiences with non-operative treatment in patients with small lesions (<4 cm in Mayo Clinic or <3 cm in Sloan Memorial Kettering Center) that remain stable on imaging and suggest that non-operative management could be an option [36, 47, 48]. Other studies are in favor of resection, having shown recurrence or lymph node involvement even in small tumors [49–51].

Size correlates with the potential for malignancy [52] and incidental finding goes against the potential for malignancy [53, 54]. Different series in the literature demonstrate the low potential for progression, malignancy, and the presence of lymphatic metastases in small lesions [36, 52, 55–57]. However, there are also studies that show 6% of malignant tumors [52] or 8% disease recurrence [7] with tumors <2 cm.

A recent study combining data from 16 European centers reviewed results of 210 patients undergoing surgical resection for sporadic, non-metastatic, NF-pNETs <2 cm. 10.6% had positive nodes (but only 3% between patients with grade 1 lesions) and 5.9% developed recurrence with a 5-year survival rate of 96% with tumors <20 mm. Concluded that patients with ductal dilatation, grade 2 or 3 tumors should undergo resection, while in other patients with small pNETs <2 cm, surveillance is a reasonable strategy [58].

ENETS, the Canadian Expert National Group and the NCCN Clinical Practical Guidelines suggested that incidentally discovered NF-pNETs <2 cm could be selectively observed [4, 59, 60]. For the Canadian Expert National Group is important to have low Ki-67 and no evidence of invasion or metastatic disease could be considered for surveillance [59] and NCCN recommended that surgical risk, site of tumor, and patients morbidities be considered in deciding observation vs. resection [60]. Recently, The North American Neuroendocrine Tumor Society Consensus published that initial observation is an acceptable treatment strategy for asymptomatic patients with pNETs <1 cm in size. The decision in patients with pNETs between 1 and 2 cm in size must be individualized considering criteria like age, comorbidities, tumor growth, estimated risk of symptom development, imaging, grade, the extent of surgical resection required, patient's wishes and access to long-term follow-up [59, 61, 62]. In selected patients when life-long surveillance is troublesome for them, it could be an option the treatment with endoscopic ultrasound-guide ablation with ethanol-lipiodol or radiofrequency. There are some good experiences published with complete necrosis in more than 60% of the cases [63, 64].

4.5.2 How Should Functional Lesions Be Treated?

Surgical treatment is recommended for all functioning pNETs regardless of their size [62, 65] with two goals: management of the endocrine syndrome to control symptoms and tumor control to improve survival. Two scenarios are possible: the PNET may be identified (localized) or not.

In the presence of a localized functional PNET without distant metastases, resection is indicated [61]. When resection is undertaken, removing the regional lymphatic nodes (LNs) should be considered, although the prognostic and therapeutic roles of nodal disease have been studied most extensively for NF-pNETs. In gastrinomas, LNs resection increases the chances of biochemical cure and improves overall survival [66, 67].

If the pNET is not localized preoperatively, exploration with intraoperative US should be performed in a center where there is specialized surgical expertise for this procedure and pNETs [61]. Experienced surgeons are able to localize >95% of lesions intraoperatively with the use of intraoperative US and hormonal testing in patients [68]. Partial pancreatic resection is favored once the tumor has been localized, total pancreatectomy along with splenectomy and/or duodenectomy may be necessary depending on tumor size or spread [9, 69]. While surgical exploration had been traditionally proposed for patients with non-localized functional pNETs [70, 71] actually and blind resection is not indicated [46, 61].

In insulinomas, vipomas, and somatostinomas, parenchyma-sparing surgery can be performed whenever possible, however, gastrinomas are considered more aggressive tumors and sparing-parenchyma surgeries are more controversial [43, 72, 73].

4.5.3 What Is the Role of Parenchymal-Sparing Surgical Techniques (PSRs)?

The most appropriate surgical technique in each case is not well established, not even if it's necessary to perform standard surgical techniques (cephalic pancreaticoduodenectomy (PD) or distal pancreatectomy (DP) with or without splenectomy or on the other hand to count up for parenchymal-sparing surgical techniques [enucleation or central pancreatectomies (CP)]. PSRs have been advocated in select pNETs patients in an effort to minimize morbidity and maintain pancreatic endocrine and exocrine function.

Enucleation consists of tumor excision, preserving the underlying tissue. Indications for enucleation, compared to extended resection of pNETs have not been the subject of rigorous review. A systematic review of 838 patients having enucleation for "benign" lesions discussed that tumor size >3–4 cm and the proximity of tumors to the main pancreatic duct were the most commonly accepted limitations for enucleation [74]. The distance from the main pancreatic duct should be 2–3 mm to be safe [73, 75]. In a recent meta-analysis that included 1148 patients, enucleation demonstrated improved operative times, estimated blood loss, length of stay, and rates of postoperative endocrine and exocrine insufficiency. There were no differences in mortality, overall complications, or reoperation rate. Formal resection demonstrated a reduction in postoperative pancreatic fistula [76].

For most authors, enucleation would be indicated in tumors <2 cm in stage I-II according to the TNM classification system of the ENETS [73, 75, 77] but others advocate enucleation between 2 and 4 cm if there are no obvious lymph nodes [78]. The North American Neuroendocrine Tumor Society Consensus recommends that enucleations should be reserved for smaller tumors (insulinoma or NF-pNETs <2 cm) and localized more than 2–3 mm from the main pancreatic duct. For larger tumors with risk of LN involvement formal resection with lymphadenectomy should be considered [61].

Central pancreatectomy may be indicated in patients with small, low-grade pNETs deeply located in the neck or proximal body of the pancreas that cannot be enucleated due to proximity to the main pancreatic duct, and in which the left pancreatic remnant is long enough to maintain sufficient pancreatic function (generally about 5 cm) [61, 75]. The management of the two pancreatic remnants offers several possibilities: derivation of the proximal and distal remnant to a Roux-en-Y bowel loop, suture of the proximal remnant, and diversion of the distal to a Roux-en-Y loop or to the stomach [79]. Patients with larger lesions, diffuse pancreatitis, and high-grade malignant tumors are not suitable candidates for CP. Central pancreatectomy has obvious advantages over DP and PD by preserving postoperative pancreatic endocrine and exocrine function but with higher morbidity and risk of postoperative pancreatic fistula [61].

PSRs are associated with a lower rate of de novo diabetes, better exocrine function, lower intraoperative morbidity, shorter surgical time, lower blood loss, and shorter hospital stay, compared to DP and these differences are minor with PD. However, they are associated with a higher rate of pancreatic fistula, postoperative morbidity, and reoperations [7, 73, 80–82]. A recent systematic review and meta-analysis of 50 studies with 1305 patients undergoing CP compared the clinical outcomes of CP vs. DP or PD [83]. When CP was compared to DP, it favored CP with regard to less blood loss ($P = 0.001$), lower rates of endocrine (OR, 0.13; $P < 0.001$), and exocrine insufficiency (OR, 0.38; $P < 0.001$). There was higher morbidity with CP than DP (OR, 1.93) as well as a higher POPF rate (OR, 1.5). When compared with PD the same trends persisted, with CP having a lower risk of endocrine (OR, 0.14; $P < 0.001$) and exocrine insufficiency (OR, 0.14; $P < 0.001$), but a higher POPF rate (OR, 1.6; $P = 0.015$). Although the POPF rate of CP was 35%, most cases of POPF were in grades A and B.

From the oncological point of view, sparing parenchyma surgery does not obscure the prognosis, it implies a higher quality of life with prolonged survival. A limitation of PSRs is the limited LNs sampling, however, the routine performance and extent of lymphadenectomy in the management of pNETs are unclear. However, if there are malignant pNETs with lymphatic involvement, radical resections should be performed [73, 75, 84].

4.5.4 What Is the Role of Splenic Preservation During DP as the Management of pNETs?

Patients with low-risk sporadic pNETs are unlikely to have nodal metastases, patients predict to have long survival, and young patients with pNETs may potentially benefit from splenic preservation. Splenectomy may be necessary for many pNETs patients with distal tumors, and it is indicated in patients with large pNETs, chronic pancreatitis, tumors abutting, or invading the splenic vasculature, bleeding during attempting vessel preservation, tumor thrombus, peripancreatic inflammation following the effects of neoadjuvant chemotherapy and high risk of nodal metastases. In the case of splenic preservation, there is conflicting evidence on the benefits of splenic vessel preservation over the Warshaw technique [61].

4.5.5 What Is the Role of Lymphadenectomy in pNETs?

The extent of lymphadenectomy in the management of pNETs remains controversial since the relationship between nodal metastases and survival has been inconsistent [85, 86].

The ENETS guidelines of 2016 recommended not to perform lymphadenectomy in insulinoma and always to perform it in gastrinoma (prognostic value and improvement of symptoms). There is limited data available to discuss the need for lymphadenectomy in other types of functioning tumors, but due to the high malignant potential and in the presence of symptoms, lymphadenectomy is recommended [62, 87–89].

Referring non-functioning tumors, there is a clear association with tumor size, tumors located in the head of the pancreas, higher grade, Ki-67 levels, and poor differentiation with LN involvement and lymphadenectomy should be done in cases of G2 tumors (with high Ki67). In the other cases, although the presence of metastasis lymph nodes seems to indicate a worse prognosis, the role of lymphadenectomy is highly controversial, since the removal of the affected nodes does not clearly correspond to a global survival benefit [67, 69, 90–92]. Fernández-Cruz et al. propose enucleation for NF-pNETs ≤3 cm, but always associated with a sampling of locoregional LNs from different lymphatic stations depending on the location of the tumor and complete lymphadenectomy in case of appearance metastasis after histological analysis [93]. Recently, a predictive lymph node metastasis score has been published, applied in patients with pNETs <2 cm combining tumor location and Ki-67 than can be used to guide future strategies of treatment [94].

If formal surgical resection (PD or DP) is planned for pNETs, oncologic resection with removal of 11–15 LNs should be performed for accurate nodal staging. If PSRs are planned for smaller pNETs (<2 cm), removal of suspicious nodes seen on preoperative imaging is warranted, and LN sampling may be considered if imaging is negative [61].

4.5.6 What Is the Role of Minimally Invasive Surgery in the Treatment of pNETs?

Recently, Drymousis et al. published a systematic review and meta-analysis comparing resection of pNETs between open and laparoscopic and conclude that laparoscopy presents advantages in terms of reduction of global complications, blood loss, and hospital stay, although it does not present differences in terms of pancreatic fistula, operative time or mortality [95, 96].

Level 1 evidence suggests that intra- and postoperative parameters of the laparoscopic approach for DP are improved and long-term outcomes are comparable to an open approach for appropriately selected patients (T1–T2) when these operations are performed in centers with appropriate expertise. Patients requiring multi-visceral resection, larger tumors, significant lymphadenopathy, and significant venous tumor thrombus are currently more likely to be better managed by an open approach. Robotic PD has demonstrated equivalent and even improved perioperative outcomes in retrospective series when compared to open PD in the hands of highly experienced surgeons past their learning curve of 80 cases. Robotic PD is associated with decreased conversion rates when compared to laparoscopic PD [61].

Similarly, a randomized controlled trial of robotic-assisted vs. open CP suggested that the robotic approach was associated with a significantly shorter hospital stay, reduced intraoperative time, less intraoperative blood loss, lower clinical PF rate, and expedited postoperative recovery [97]. There are also good experiences published with robotic enucleation on pNETs [98].

4.5.7 How Should We Manage pNETs in MEN1 Syndrome and Other Familial Diseases?

In patients with MEN1 and gastrinomas or NF-pNETs <2 cm, surveillance could be a good option, but with a lesion >2 cm enucleation remains the generally recommended surgery. In all patients with insulinomas without non-resectable metastatic disease surgical exploration should be performed. Multicentricity of pNETs renders surgical decision-making complex and unlikely to eliminate all diseases in the long term. Therefore, removal of the dominant lesion and potentially other easily accessible lesions that might be present should be the goal, balanced by preservation of pancreatic function and reducing the risk of complications [61, 62].

In the case of familial pNETs the broad principles in the management include parenchyma-sparing operations, watchful surveillance when appropriate for low-risk tumors, enucleation or minimal pancreatic resection for intermediate-risk tumors when feasible and effective, and reserving major pancreatic resection for locally invasive, anatomically difficult, or high-risk lesions. VHL patients with pNETs <3 cm, with doubling times >500 days and mutations outside of exon 3 can be safely observed with serial imaging every 1–2 years. Patients with one risk factor (>3 cm; doubling times <500 days or mutations in exon 3) should be considered for surgery vs. surveillance every 6 months and those with two or more risk factors should be considered for surgical management [61].

4.6 Management of Metastatic pNETS

4.6.1 Primary Tumor Resection in Patients with Metastatic PNET

Several papers have established the benefit of primary tumor resection in patients with metastatic pNETs. Zheng et al. [99] reported 1547 patients with NET and liver metastases (501 were pNETs). Primary tumor resection was performed in 33.5% of pNETs and it was statistically correlated to improved 5-year OS. In all patients, 5-year OS was significantly higher in patients in whom primary tumor resection was carried out (57.0 vs. 15.4%, $P < 0.001$). Keutgen et al. [100] presented 882 patients with metastatic pNETs, of which 34% had their primary tumor removed. In this group, median OS was statistically higher (65 vs. 10 months, $P < 0.0001$). In multivariate analysis, primary tumor resection was significantly associated to longer survival ($P < 0.0001$). So, it seems that surgical removal of primary tumor has an evident benefit on survival for patients with metastatic pNETs.

4.6.2 Hepatic Cytoreduction

Around 64% of patients with pNETs have synchronous liver metastases. In these cases, hepatic debulking decreases hormone levels, improve symptoms, and delays the main cause of death (liver failure secondary to hepatic replacement) [101]. However, this is not globally accepted, as most series are retrospective and have selection bias.

Even when acceptable cytoreductions, recurrence rates are 84–95% in 5 years, probably due to the existence of microscopic metastases that cannot be detected in radiology tests [102]. Ongoing debates about the threshold of hepatic disease you should resect to achieve a survival benefit exist.

Some decades ago, Foster et al. established that survival benefit was achieved when more than 95% of liver disease was able to be resected [103, 104]. In 2003, Sarmiento et al. reported 170 patients with NETLM (31% from pNETs) with more than 90% cytoreduction. 5-year OS rate was 61%, much higher than 30–40% for historical series, despite 56% of interventions were considered incomplete [105]. This way, they recommend cytoreduction when you predict you may achieve this limit of 90% debulking, in order to improve survival in these patients.

Nevertheless, other authors defend that 70% cytoreduction is a reasonable threshold for hepatic debulking. Graff-Baker et al. observed no difference in PFS with more than 70% cytoreduction, in a group of patients with metastatic GINET, thus defending this limit for hepatic debulking [106]. Morgan et al. presented 42 patients with metastatic NET who underwent cytoreduction in three groups (70–90%, 90–99%, and 100%). They concluded that there were no differences in OS or PFS among groups, adding evidence to lowering cytoreduction threshold to more than 70% [107].

Maxwell et al. reported 108 patients with metastatic GEPNET in whom a cytoreduction procedure was carried out. For PFS, both 70 and 90% limits reached statistical significance, while only 70% threshold was significant for OS [108]. Scott et al. presented 188 cytoreduction procedures in patients with metastatic GEPNET. They established three groups (less than 70%, 70–90%, and more than 90%). Results in OS and PFS were significantly worse in the first group, without differences between the last two groups [109].

Taking all these data into account, we might improve survival in these patients when more than 70% cytoreduction may be obtained [61]. Although this recommendation has a poor evidence level.

4.6.3 Liver Transplantation

Liver transplantation provides adequate survival rates in highly selected patients with NET with liver metastases (Milan criteria for liver transplantation in patients with hepatic metastases from neuroendocrine tumors [110]). Moris et al. reported 1-, 3-, and 5-year overall survival was 89%, 69%, and 63%, respectively. However, pancreatic origin was associated to worse survival [111]. This, added to the graft unavailability and the lack of evidence, makes this indication unclear and randomized studies would be necessary to elucidate this question.

4.6.4 Combined Pancreatectomy and Liver Debulking

When considering simultaneous pancreatectomy and hepatic procedure, we must consider that both interventions may have high complication rates (depending on the extension of the resection). So, combining both might increase substantially morbidity [61].

Morgan et al. presented 42 patients with metastatic pancreatic or periampullary NET in whom pancreatectomy and hepatic resection were performed (around 50% simultaneously and 50% in a staged way). There were no differences regarding complications or length of stay [107]. This way, authors conclude that combining pancreatectomy and hepatic debulking might be safe in selected patients and in experienced centers.

If pancreatic resection consists of Whipple procedure, must we take into account that liver abscesses are more frequent after this intervention, due to the existence of biliary-enteric anastomosis [61]?

De Jong et al. reported 126 patients with metastatic NET who underwent Whipple and hepatic procedures (resection, ablation, embolization, or irradiation). Forty-five percent were performed simultaneously and 55% in staged way (Whipple was carried out first in 90%). Appearance of liver abscesses was significantly more frequent in staged procedures (14.5 vs. 7%, $P < 0.05$) [112]. Consequently, these authors recommend a simultaneous approach or, in case of staged procedures, perform hepatic therapy before Whipple procedure.

4.6.5 Removing Primary Tumor When Unresectable Metastatic Disease Is Present

While removing primary pNETs does increase the quality of life in patients with symptomatic tumors, there exists debate about the paper of resecting the primary tumor in asymptomatic patients, since pancreatic surgery has high complication rates.

Huttner et al. reported 442 patients with metastatic pNETs. They observed that 5-year OS was significantly higher in those patients in whom primary tumor was resected (52.5 vs. 20.6%) [113]. Similar results were observed by Ye et al. with 392 patients with metastatic pNETs. Median OS was significantly higher in primary tumor resection group (78 vs. 21 months, $P < 0.001$) [114]. In the same way, Tierney et al. presented 6548 patients with metastatic pNETs. Median OS was also higher if primary tumor was resected (63.6 vs. 14.2 months, $P < 0.001$) [115].

However, in the last two publications, only 19.9 and 7.6% of primary tumors were resected. So, selection bias might decrease evidence quality about the benefit of resecting the primary tumor in pNETs with unresectable metastatic disease [61].

Some recent studies have observed interesting results in survival rates in patients in whom primary tumor resection was performed before peptide receptor radionuclide therapy (PRRT) with ^{90}Y or ^{177}Lu [61].

Kaemmerer et al. reported 889 patients with metastatic NET (38% were pNETs). Fifty-five percent underwent primary tumor resection before PRRT and 45% only had PRRT. Median OS was significantly higher in resection group (140 vs. 58 months, $P < 0.001$). Median PFS was also better in this group (18 vs. 14 months, $P = 0.012$) [116].

4.6.6 Primary Tumor Resection or Hepatic Cytoreduction When There Is Extrahepatic Disease

As the main cause of death in patients with pNETs is hepatic replacement causing liver failure, extrahepatic disease might not be an absolute contraindication for hepatic cytoreduction [61].

Morgan et al. reported 42 patients with pNETs who underwent hepatic cytoreduction. Extrahepatic disease was not statistically associated to OS or PFS. Most deaths were secondary to liver failure due to hepatic replacement [107]. Lewis et al. observed that 45.4% of patients with metastatic GINET (from the California Cancer Registry) had extrahepatic disease. Median OS was significantly higher in those in whom primary tumor was resected (57 vs. 12 months, $P < 0.001$) [117]. However, there exist selection bias, such as only 11% of patients had their primary tumors removed, or only 43.6% were pNETs.

However, other authors, such as Mayo et al. and Xiang et al., have observed that extrahepatic disease was statistically correlated to worse survival in patients with metastatic NET [102, 118]. Although less than half of these patients were pNETs.

4.7 Systemic Therapy

Systemic treatment is required in many patients with advanced, recurrent, or metastatic pancreatic neuroendocrine tumors (pNETs) that are not candidates for surgical intervention (see Fig. 4.1). Also, there may be a benefit in R2 resections of symptomatic tumors. However, in patients with asymptomatic or non-functional disease is controversial [60].

4.7.1 Symptoms-Directed Therapy in pNETs

- Insulinoma: Food fractionation suppression of insulin secretion has a key role in hypoglycemia control, as well as diazoxide.

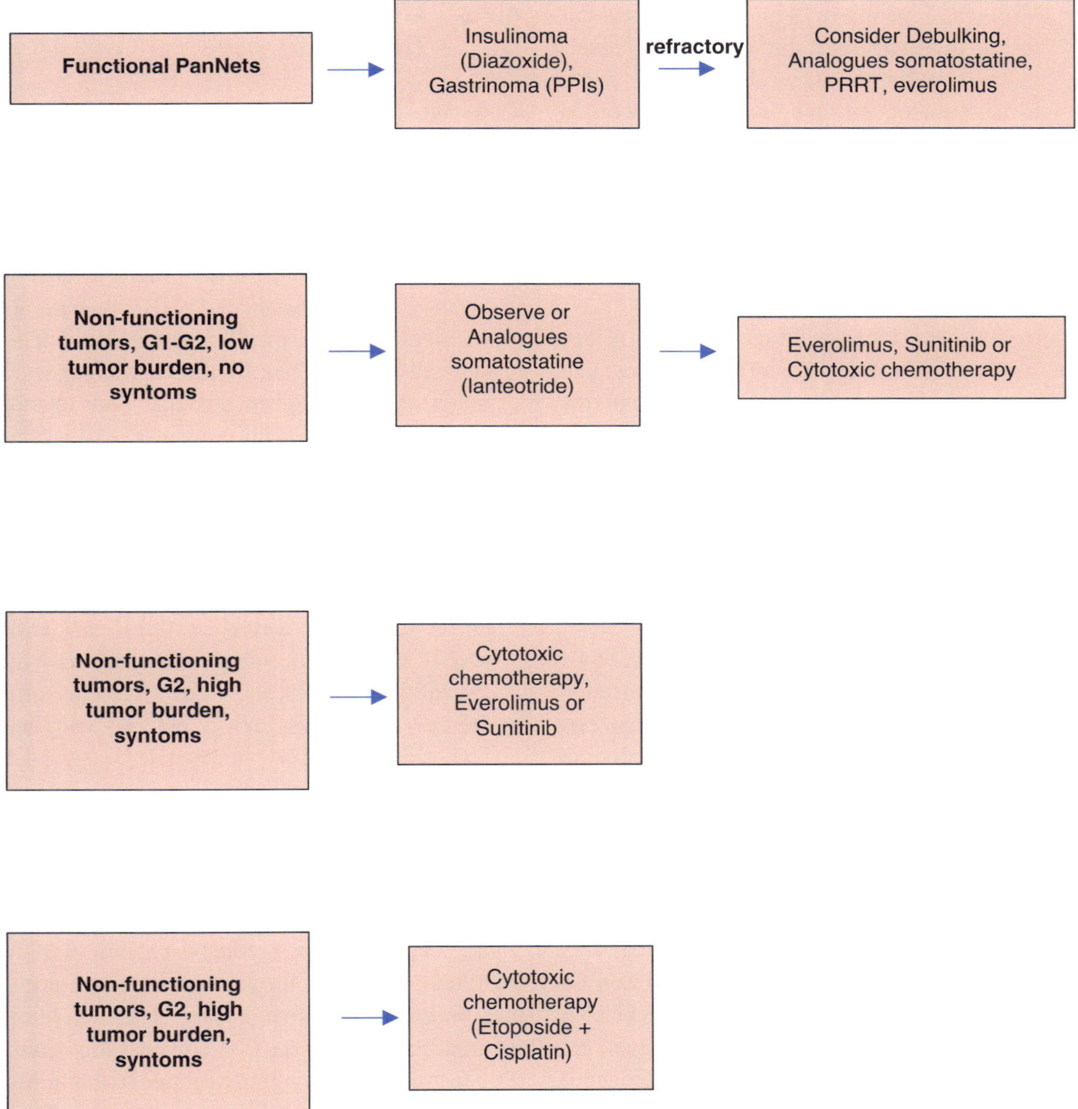

Fig. 4.1 Systemic treatment algorithm for advanced PanNETs [119]

Approximately 30–50% of patients respond to somatostatin analogues, although careful monitoring is required due to some patients can paradoxically aggravate hypoglycemia through suppression of glucagon greater than insulin. Several recent studies have shown that everolimus manages to reduce hypoglycemic episodes through anti-proliferative activity, a reduction in insulin secretion, and by promoting insulin resistance [120]. Treatment with sunitinib, chemoembolization, or peptide receptor radionuclide therapy (PRRT) has also shown efficacy in this setting.

- Gastrinoma: Proton pump inhibitors are effective in the symptomatic control of these patients. In exceptional cases, somatostatin analogues may also be useful.
- Glucagonoma: It is necessary to consider nutritional support, prophylactic anticoagulation especially prior to surgery.

- VIPoma: Hydration (with meticulous monitoring of electrolytes and acid–base balance before starting any surgical treatment), somatostatin analogues, and glucose control are all important factors in the symptomatic management of these patients.

4.7.2 Somatostatin Analogues

Octreotide and Lanreotide have similar effects in terms of efficacy in symptomatic control, which is achieved in 40–70% of patients, mainly in glucagonomas or vipomas (95–100%) with a lesser effect in patients with somatostatinomas or gastrinomas [121]. The anti-proliferative efficacy of somatostatin analogue treatment in pNETs was confirmed in two phase III clinical trials.

- CLARINET trial [121]: This was a phase III, multinational, randomized, placebo-controlled, double-blind study, involving 204 patients with well-differentiated neuroendocrine tumors (Ki67 antigen <10%), originating in the pancreas or gastrointestinal location, with documented disease progression. Treatment with Lanreotide was associated with a significant prolonged progression-free survival, compared with placebo (progression-free survival at 24 months: 65.1% with Lanreotide (95% CI, 54.0–75.1 months) and 33.0% with placebo (95% CI, 23.0–43.3 months). However, the study did not prove a significant difference in overall survival between the active treatment and placebo groups.
- PROMID trial [122]: 85 patients with metastatic, well-differentiated intestinal NETs (95% with Ki67 <2%) were included, who were randomized to receive monthly intramuscular octreotide or placebo. The mean time to progression (primary endpoint) was significantly higher in the group that received octreotide (14.3 vs. 6 months, RH 0.34, $P = 0.00007$). There were no differences between functioning (39%) and non-functioning (61%) NETs.

4.7.3 Molecularly Targeted Therapies

Two agents have been shown to improve progression-free survival in patients with advanced pNETs, Sunitinib and Everolimus.

- Sunitinib: It is a tyrosine kinase inhibitor, which was approved for the treatment of progressive well-differentiated pNETs in patients with unresectable, locally advanced, or metastatic disease. A phase III clinical trial reported increased disease-free survival and overall survival with sunitinib compared to placebo [123].
- Everolimus: It is a mammalian target of rapamycin (mTOR) inhibitor. It is usually used as a second-line treatment in patients with metastatic pNETs. RADIANT-3 is a phase III trial, involving 410 patients with pNET with disease progression treated with Everolimus or placebo. The Everolius arm seemed to be superior to placebo and had higher disease-free survival (11 vs. 4.6 months, $P < 0.05$) [124].

4.7.4 Cytotoxic Chemotherapy

There is no consensus on the best chemotherapy treatment, and drugs for patients with symptomatic, and/or progressive disease. The indication for treatment must take into consideration multiple factors, including those related to the tumor (degree of histological differentiation, proliferative index, location of the primary tumor, volume of metastatic disease or symptoms, growth rate tumor), with the patient and with the experience and/or availability of other therapeutic alternatives. In general, Cytotoxic chemotherapy is preferred over Somatostatin analogues or targeted therapy in patients with large tumor volume and/or symptoms derived from it, in those with rapidly progressive disease, or in all patients with grade 3 neuroendocrine carcinomas [119].

4.7.5 Peptide Receptor Radionuclide Therapy (PRRT)

This therapy involves delivery of targeted radiotherapy to malignant neuroendocrine tumor cells that express somatostatin receptors to cause tumor shrinkage.

The phase III NETTER-1 trial has shown a significant benefit in disease-free survival of treatment with 177-Lu-DOTATATE compared to high doses of Somatostatin analogues in patients with advanced intestinal NETs progressing to conventional doses of ASS [119], but to date there are no data from randomized studies comparing PRRT vs. placebo or other therapies in patients with pNETs. Therefore, the efficacy data comes from long series of patients treated in referral centers that include NETs of both pancreatic and non-pancreatic origin.

References

1. Fraenkel M, Kim MK, Faggiano A, Valk GD. Epidemiology of gastroenteropancreatic neuroendocrine tumours. Best Pract Res Clin Gastroenterol. 2012;26(6):691–703.
2. Lawrence B, Gustafsson BI, Chan A, Svejda B, Kidd M, Modlin IM. The epidemiology of gastroenteropancreatic neuroendocrine tumors. Endocrinol Metab Clin N Am. 2011;40(1):1–18.
3. Halfdanarson TR, Rubin J, Farnell MB, Grant CS, Petersen GM. Pancreatic endocrine neoplasms: epidemiology and prognosis of pancreatic endocrine tumors. Endocr Relat Cancer. 2008;15(2):409–27.
4. Falconi M, Bartsch DK, Eriksson B, Klöppel G, Lopes JM, O'Connor JM, et al. ENETS consensus guidelines for the management of patients with digestive neuroendocrine neoplasms of the digestive system: well-differentiated pancreatic non-functioning tumors. Neuroendocrinology. 2012;95(2):120–34.
5. Kimura W, Kuroda A, Morioka Y. Clinical pathology of endocrine tumors of the pancreas. Analysis of autopsy cases. Dig Dis Sci. 1991;36(7):933–42.
6. Klöppel G, Willemer S, Stamm B, Häcki WH, Heitz PU. Pancreatic lesions and hormonal profile of pancreatic tumors in multiple endocrineneoplasia type I. An immunocytochemical study of nine patients. Cancer. 1986;57(9):1824–32.
7. Salaria SN, Shi C. Pancreatic neuroendocrine tumors. Surg Pathol Clin. 2016;9(4):595–617.
8. Scott AT, Howe JR. Evaluation and management of neuroendocrine tumors of the pancreas. Surg Clin North Am. 2019;99(4):793–814.
9. Parbhu SK, Adler DG. Pancreatic neuroendocrine tumors: contemporary diagnosis and management. Hosp Pract (1995). 2016;44(3):109–19.
10. Lewis RB, Lattin GEJ, Paal E. Pancreatic endocrine tumors: radiologic-clinicopathologic correlation. Radiogr Rev Publ Radiol Soc North Am Inc. 2010;30(6):1445–64.
11. Younan G. Pancreas solid tumors. Surg Clin North Am. 2020;100(3):565–80.
12. Dromain C, Déandréis D, Scoazec J-Y, Goere D, Ducreux M, Baudin E, et al. Imaging of neuroendocrine tumors of the pancreas. Diagn Interv Imaging. 2016;97(12):1241–57.
13. Fidler JL, Fletcher JG, Reading CC, Andrews JC, Thompson GB, Grant CS, et al. Preoperative detection of pancreatic insulinomas on multiphasic helical CT. AJR Am J Roentgenol. 2003;181(3):775–80.
14. Kim JH, Eun HW, Kim YJ, Lee JM, Han JK, Choi B-I. Pancreatic neuroendocrine tumour (PNET): staging accuracy of MDCT and its diagnostic performance for the differentiation of PNET with uncommon CT findings from pancreatic adenocarcinoma. Eur Radiol. 2016;26(5):1338–47.
15. Wang SC, Parekh JR, Zuraek MB, Venook AP, Bergsland EK, Warren RS, et al. Identification of unknown primary tumors in patients with neuroendocrine liver metastases. Arch Surg. 2010;145(3):276–80.
16. Rozenblum L, Mokrane F-Z, Yeh R, Sinigaglia M, Besson F, Seban R-D, et al. The role of multimodal imaging in guiding resectability and cytoreduction in pancreatic neuroendocrine tumors: focus on PET and MRI. Abdom Radiol (NY). 2019;44(7):2474–93.
17. Singh A, Hines JJ, Friedman B. Multimodality imaging of the pancreatic neuroendocrine tumors. Semin Ultrasound CT MR. 2019;40(6):469–82.
18. Barat M, Soyer P, Al Sharhan F, Terris B, Oudjit A, Gaujoux S, et al. MRI may be able to identify the origin of neuroendocrine tumor liver metastases. Neuroendocrinology. 2020;111(11):1099–110.
19. Puli SR, Kalva N, Bechtold ML, Pamulaparthy SR, Cashman MD, Estes NC, et al. Diagnostic accuracy of endoscopic ultrasound in pancreatic neuroendocrine tumors: a systematic review and meta analysis. World J Gastroenterol. 2013;19(23):3678–84.
20. Cosgrove D, Piscaglia F, Bamber J, Bojunga J, Correas J-M, Gilja OH, et al. EFSUMB guidelines and recommendations on the clinical use of ultrasound elastography. Part 2: clinical applications. Ultraschall Med. 2013;34(3):238–53.
21. Falconi M, Eriksson B, Kaltsas G, Bartsch DK, Capdevila J, Caplin M, et al. ENETS consensus guidelines update for the management of patients with functional pancreatic neuroendocrine tumors and non-functional pancreatic docrine tumors and non-functional pancreatic

neuroendocrine tumors. Neuroendocrinology. 2016;103(2):153–71.

22. Zilli A, Arcidiacono PG, Conte D, Massironi S. Clinical impact of endoscopic ultrasonography on the management of neuroendocrine tumors: lights and shadows. Dig liver Dis. 2018;50(1):6–14.

23. Crown A, Rocha FG, Raghu P, Lin B, Funk G, Alseidi A, et al. Impact of initial imaging with gallium-68 dotatate PET/CT on diagnosis and management of patients with neuroendocrine tumors. J Surg Oncol. 2020;121(3):480–5.

24. Panagiotidis E, Bomanji J. Role of 18F-fluorodeoxyglucose PET in the study of neuroendocrine tumors. PET Clin. 2014;9(1):43–55.

25. Hope TA, Bergsland EK, Bozkurt MF, Graham M, Heaney AP, Herrmann K, et al. Appropriate use criteria for somatostatin receptor pet imaging in neuroendocrine tumors. J Nucl Med. 2018;59(1):66–74.

26. Anderson CW, Bennett JJ. Clinical presentation and diagnosis of pancreatic neuroendocrine tumors. Surg Oncol Clin N Am. 2016;25(2):363–74.

27. Han X, Zhang C, Tang M, Xu X, Liu L, Ji Y, et al. The value of serum chromogranin A as a predictor of tumor burden, therapeutic response, and nomogram-based survival in well-moderate nonfunctional pancreatic neuroendocrine tumors with liver metastases. Eur J Gastroenterol Hepatol. 2015;27(5):527–35.

28. Perri G, Prakash LR, Katz MHG. Pancreatic neuroendocrine tumors. Curr Opin Gastroenterol. 2019;35(5):468–77.

29. Barker N, van Es JH, Kuipers J, Kujala P, van den Born M, Cozijnsen M, et al. Identification of stem cells in small intestine and colon by marker gene Lgr5. Nature. 2007;449(7165):1003–7.

30. Wolin EM, Jensen RT. Neuroendocrine tumors. In: Goldman L, editor. Goldman-Cecil medicine. Philadelphia: Elsevier, Twenty Six; 2020. p. 1520–8.

31. College of American Pathologists. Protocol for examination of specimens from patients with carcinoma of the endocrine pancreas.

32. Oberg K. Pancreatic endocrine tumors. Semin Oncol. 2010;37(6):594–618.

33. Kim JY, Hong S-M. Recent updates on neuroendocrine tumors from the gastrointestinal and pancreatobiliary tracts. Arch Pathol Lab Med. 2016;140(5):437–48.

34. Klöppel G, Perren A, Sipos BKD. Diagnostic histopathology of tumors. In: Fletcher C, editor. 5. Edimburg: Elsevier; 2020. p. 1395–411.

35. Li D, Rock A, Kessler J, Ballena R, Hyder S, Mo C, et al. Understanding the management and treatment of well-differentiated pancreatic neuroendocrine tumors: a clinician's guide to a complex illness. JCO Oncol Pract. 2020;16(11):720–8.

36. Lee LC, Grant CS, Salomao DR, Fletcher JG, Takahashi N, Fidler JL, et al. Small, nonfunctioning, asymptomatic pancreatic neuroendocrine tumors (PNETs): role for nonoperative management. Surgery. 2012;152(6):965–74.

37. Ma ZY, Gong YF, Zhuang HK, Zhou ZX, Huang SZ, Zou YP, et al. Pancreatic neuroendocrine tumors: a review of serum biomarkers, staging, and management. World J Gastroenterol. 2020;26(19):2305–22.

38. Uppin MS, Uppin SG, Sunil CSPV, Hui M, Paul TR, Bheerappa N. Clinicopathologic study of neuroendocrine tumors of gastroenteropancreatic tract: a single institutional experience. J Gastrointest Oncol. 2017;8(1):139–47.

39. Schimmack S, Svejda B, Lawrence B, Kidd M, Modlin IM. The diversity and commonalities of gastroenteropancreatic neuroendocrine tumors. Langenbeck's Arch Surg. 2011;396(3):273–98.

40. Grant CS. Insulinoma. Best Pract Res Clin Gastroenterol. 2005;19(5):783–98.

41. Chastain MA. The glucagonoma syndrome: a review of its features and discussion of new perspectives. Am J Med Sci. 2001;321(5):306–20.

42. Ro C, Chai W, Yu VE, Yu R. Pancreatic neuroendocrine tumors: biology, diagnosis, and treatment. Chin J Cancer 2013;32(6):312–324.

43. D'Haese JG, Tosolini C, Ceyhan GO, Kong B, Esposito I, Michalski CW, et al. Update on surgical treatment of pancreatic neuroendocrine neoplasms. World J Gastroenterol. 2014;20(38):13893–8.

44. Metz DC, Jensen RT. Gastrointestinal neuroendocrine tumors: pancreatic endocrine tumors. Gastroenterology. 2008;135(5):1469–92.

45. Ishida H, Lam AKY. Pancreatic neuroendocrine neoplasms: the latest surgical and medical treatment strategies based on the current World Health Organization classification. Crit Rev Oncol Hematol. 2020;145(September 2019):102835.

46. Ito T, Igarashi H, Jensen RT. Pancreatic neuroendocrine tumors: clinical features, diagnosis and medical treatment: advances. Best Pract Res Clin Gastroenterol. 2012;26(6):737–53.

47. Sadot E, Reidy-Lagunes DL, Tang LH, Do RKG, Gonen M, D'Angelica MI, et al. Observation versus resection for small asymptomatic pancreatic neuroendocrine tumors: a matched case–control study. Ann Surg Oncol. 2016;23(4):1361–70.

48. Partelli S, Cirocchi R, Crippa S, Cardinali L, Fendrich V, Bartsch DK, et al. Systematic review of active surveillance versus surgical management of asymptomatic small non-functioning pancreatic neuroendocrine neoplasms. Br J Surg. 2017;104(1):34–41.

49. Sharpe SM, In H, Winchester DJ, Talamonti MS, Baker MS. Surgical resection provides an overall survival benefit for patients with small pancreatic neuroendocrine tumors. J Gastrointest Surg. 2015;19(1):117–23. discussion 123

50. Finkelstein P, Sharma R, Picado O, Gadde R, Stuart H, Ripat C, et al. Pancreatic neuroendocrine tumors (panNETs): analysis of overall survival of non-surgical management versus surgical resection. J Gastrointest Surg. 2017;21(5):855–66.

51. Haynes AB, Deshpande V, Ingkakul T, Vagefi PA, Szymonifka J, Thayer SP, et al. Implications of incidentally discovered, nonfunctioning pancreatic

endocrine tumors: short-term and long-term patient outcomes. Arch Surg. 2011;146(5):534–8.

52. Bettini R, Partelli S, Boninsegna L, Capelli P, Crippa S, Pederzoli P, et al. Tumor size correlates with malignancy in nonfunctioning pancreatic endocrine tumor. Surgery. 2011;150(1):75–82.

53. Cheema A, Weber J, Strosberg JR. Incidental detection of pancreatic neuroendocrine tumors: an analysis of incidence and outcomes. Ann Surg Oncol. 2012;19(9):2932–6.

54. Strosberg JR, Cheema A, Weber J, Han G, Coppola D, Kvols LK. Prognostic validity of a Novel American Joint Committee on Cancer staging classification for pancreatic neuroendocrine tumors. J Clin Oncol. 2011;29(22):3044–9.

55. Gaujoux S, Partelli S, Maire F, D'Onofrio M, Larroque B, Tamburrino D, et al. Observational study of natural history of small sporadic nonfunctioning pancreatic neuroendocrine tumors. J Clin Endocrinol Metab. 2013;98(12):4784–9.

56. Toste PA, Kadera BE, Tatishchev SF, Dawson DW, Clerkin BM, Muthusamy R, et al. Nonfunctional pancreatic neuroendocrine tumors <2 cm on preoperative imaging are associated with a low incidence of nodal metastasis and an excellent overall survival. J Gastrointest Surg. 2013;17(12):2105–13.

57. Busquets J, Ramírez-Maldonado E, Serrano T, Peláez N, Secanella L, Ruiz-Osuna S, et al. Surgical treatment of non-functioning pancreatic neuroendocrine tumours based on three clinical scenarios. Cir Esp. 2016;94(10):578–87.

58. Sallinen VJ, Le Large TYS, Tieftrunk E, Galeev S, Kovalenko Z, Haugvik S-P, et al. Prognosis of sporadic resected small (≤2 cm) nonfunctional pancreatic neuroendocrine tumors—a multi-institutional study. HPB. 2018;20(3):251–9.

59. Singh S, Dey C, Kennecke H, Kocha W, Maroun J, Metrakos P, et al. Consensus recommendations for the diagnosis and management of pancreatic neuroendocrine tumors: guidelines from a Canadian National Expert Group. Ann Surg Oncol. 2015;22(8):2685–99.

60. Shah MH, Goldner WS, Halfdanarson TR, Bergsland E, Berlin JD, Halperin D, et al. NCCN guidelines insights: neuroendocrine and adrenal tumors, version 2.2018. J Natl Compr Cancer Netw. 2018;16(6):693–702.

61. Howe JR, Merchant NB, Conrad C, Keutgen XM, Hallet J, Drebin JA, et al. The North American Neuroendocrine Tumor Society consensus paper on the surgical management of pancreatic neuroendocrine tumors. Pancreas. 2020;49:1–33.

62. Rindi G, Falconi M, Eriksson B, Kaltsas G, Bartsch D, Capdevila J, et al. Consensus guidelines update for the management of functional p-NETs (F-p-NETs) and non-functional p-NETs (NF-p-NETs). Neuroendocrinology. 2016;103(2):153–71.

63. Choi JH, Park DH, Kim MH, Hwang HS, Hong SM, Song TJ, et al. Outcomes after endoscopic ultrasound-guided ethanol-lipiodol ablation of small pancreatic neuroendocrine tumors. Dig Endosc. 2018;30(5):652–8.

64. Barthet M, Giovannini M, Lesavre N, Boustiere C, Napoleon B, Koch S, et al. Endoscopic ultrasound-guided radiofrequency ablation for pancreatic neuroendocrine tumors and pancreatic cystic neoplasms: a prospective multicenter study. Endoscopy. 2019;51(9):836–42.

65. Kimura W, Tezuka K, Hirai I. Surgical management of pancreatic neuroendocrine tumors. Surg Today. 2011;41(10):1332–43.

66. Partelli S, Gaujoux S, Boninsegna L, Cherif R, Crippa S, Couvelard A, et al. Pattern and clinical predictors of lymph node involvement in nonfunctioning pancreatic neuroendocrine tumors (NF-PanNETs). JAMA Surg. 2013;148(10):932–9.

67. Tsutsumi K, Ohtsuka T, Mori Y, Fujino M, Yasui T, Aishima S, et al. Analysis of lymph node metastasis in pancreatic neuroendocrine tumors (PNETs) based on the tumor size and hormonal production. J Gastroenterol. 2012;47(6):678–85.

68. Hiramoto JS, Feldstein VA, LaBerge JM, Norton JA. Intraoperative ultrasound and preoperative localization detects all occult insulinomas; discussion 1025-6. Arch Surg. 2001;136(9):1020–5.

69. Akerström G, Hellman P, Hessman O, Osmak L. Surgical treatment of endocrine pancreatic tumours. Neuroendocrinology. 2004;80(Suppl 1):62–6.

70. Norton JA, Fraker DL, Alexander HR, Venzon DJ, Doppman JL, Serrano J, et al. Surgery to cure the Zollinger-Ellison syndrome. N Engl J Med. 1999;341(9):635–44.

71. Norton JA, Fraker DL, Alexander HR, Jensen RT. Value of surgery in patients with negative imaging and sporadic Zollinger-Ellison syndrome. Ann Surg. 2012;256(3):509–17.

72. Lopez CL, Falconi M, Waldmann J, Boninsegna L, Fendrich V, Goretzki PK, et al. Partial pancreaticoduodenectomy can provide cure for duodenal gastrinoma associated with multiple endocrine neoplasia type 1. Ann Surg. 2013;257(2):308–14.

73. Watzka FM, Laumen C, Fottner C, Weber MM, Schad A, Lang H, et al. Resection strategies for neuroendocrine pancreatic neoplasms. Langenbeck's Arch Surg. 2013;398(3):431–40.

74. Beger HG, Siech M, Poch B, Mayer B, Schoenberg MH. Limited surgery for benign tumours of the pancreas: a systematic review. World J Surg. 2015;39(6):1557–66.

75. Cherif R, Gaujoux S, Couvelard A, Dokmak S, Vuillerme M-P, Ruszniewski P, et al. Parenchyma-sparing resections for pancreatic neuroendocrine tumors. J Gastrointest Surg. 2012;16(11):2045–55.

76. Hüttner FJ, Koessler-Ebs J, Hackert T, Ulrich A, Büchler MW, Diener MK. Meta-analysis of surgical outcome after enucleation versus standard resection for pancreatic neoplasms. Br J Surg. 2015;102(9):1026–36.

77. Falconi M, Zerbi A, Crippa S, Balzano G, Boninsegna L, Capitanio V, et al. Parenchyma-preserving resections for small nonfunctioning pancreatic endocrine tumors. Ann Surg Oncol. 2010;17(6):1621–7.

78. Casadei R, Ricci C, Rega D, D'Ambra M, Pezzilli R, Tomassetti P, et al. Pancreatic endocrine tumors less than 4 cm in diameter: resect or enucleate? A single-center experience. Pancreas. 2010;39(6):825–8.

79. Sabater Orti L, Ausania F Martín Pérez E. Neoplasia de Páncreas. In: Programa ET y procedimientos quirúrgicos. Pancreático, 4. edn; 2015. BM.

80. Song KB, Kim SC, Park K-M, Hwang DW, Lee JH, Lee DJ, et al. Laparoscopic central pancreatectomy for benign or low-grade malignant lesions in the pancreatic neck and proximal body. Surg Endosc. 2015;29(4):937–46.

81. Song KB, Kim SC, Hwang DW, Lee JH, Lee DJ, Lee JW, et al. Enucleation for benign or low-grade malignant lesions of the pancreas: single-center experience with 65 consecutive patients. Surgery. 2015;158(5):1203–10.

82. Hackert T, Hinz U, Fritz S, Strobel O, Schneider L, Hartwig W, et al. Enucleation in pancreatic surgery: indications, technique, and outcome compared to standard pancreatic resections. Langenbeck's Arch Surg. 2011;396(8):1197–203.

83. Xiao W, Zhu J, Peng L, Hong L, Sun G, Li Y. The role of central pancreatectomy in pancreatic surgery: a systematic review and meta-analysis. HPB. 2018;20(10):896–904.

84. Zerbi A, Capitanio V, Boninsegna L, Delle Fave G, Pasquali C, Rindi G, et al. Treatment of malignant pancreatic neuroendocrine neoplasms: middle-term (2-year) outcomes of a prospective observational multicentre study. HPB. 2013;15(12):935–43.

85. Wong J, Fulp WJ, Strosberg JR, Kvols LK, Centeno BA, Hodul PJ. Predictors of lymph node metastases and impact on survival in resected pancreatic neuroendocrine tumors: a single-center experience. Am J Surg. 2014;208(5):775–80.

86. Lee L, Ito T, Jensen RT. Prognostic and predictive factors on overall survival and surgical outcomes in pancreatic neuroendocrine tumors: recent advances and controversies. Expert Rev Anticancer Ther. 2019;19(12):1029–50.

87. Bartsch DK, Waldmann J, Fendrich V, Boninsegna L, Lopez CL, Partelli S, et al. Impact of lymphadenectomy on survival after surgery for sporadic gastrinoma. Br J Surg. 2012;99(9):1234–40.

88. Krampitz GW, Norton JA, Poultsides GA, Visser BC, Sun L, Jensen RT. Lymph nodes and survival in pancreatic neuroendocrine tumors. Arch Surg. 2012;147(9):820–7. Available from: https://pubmed.ncbi.nlm.nih.gov/22987171

89. Ito T, Igarashi H, Jensen RT. Therapy of metastatic pancreatic neuroendocrine tumors (pNETs): recent insights and advances. J Gastroenterol. 2012;47(9):941–60.

90. Gratian L, Pura J, Dinan M, Roman S, Reed S, Sosa JA. Impact of extent of surgery on survival in patients with small nonfunctional pancreatic neuroendocrine tumors in the United States. Ann Surg Oncol. 2014;21(11):3515–21.

91. Hashim YM, Trinkaus KM, Linehan DC, Strasberg SS, Fields RC, Cao D, et al. Regional lymphadenectomy is indicated in the surgical treatment of pancreatic neuroendocrine tumors (PNETs). Ann Surg. 2014;259(2):197–203.

92. Curran T, Pockaj BA, Gray RJ, Halfdanarson TR, Wasif N. Importance of lymph node involvement in pancreatic neuroendocrine tumors: impact on survival and implications for surgical resection. J Gastrointest Surg. 2015;19(1):152–60. discussion 160

93. Fernández-Cruz L, Molina V, Vallejos R, Jiménez Chavarria E, Lõpez-Boado MA, Ferrer J. Outcome after laparoscopic enucleation for non-functional neuroendocrine pancreatic tumours. HPB. 2012;14(3):171–6.

94. Lopez-Aguiar AG, Ethun CG, Zaidi MY, Rocha FG, Poultsides GA, Dillhoff M, et al. The conundrum of < 2-cm pancreatic neuroendocrine tumors: a preoperative risk score to predict lymph node metastases and guide surgical management. Surgery. 2019;166(1):15–21.

95. Drymousis P, Raptis DA, Spalding D, Fernandez-Cruz L, Menon D, Breitenstein S, et al. Laparoscopic versus open pancreas resection for pancreatic neuroendocrine tumours: a systematic review and meta-analysis. HPB. 2014;16(5):397–406.

96. Fernández-Cruz L, Blanco L, Cosa R, Rendón H. Is laparoscopic resection adequate in patients with neuroendocrine pancreatic tumors? World J Surg. 2008;32(5):904–17.

97. Chen S, Zhan Q, Jin J-B, Wu Z-C, Shi Y, Cheng D-F, et al. Robot-assisted laparoscopic versus open middle pancreatectomy: short-term results of a randomized controlled trial. Surg Endosc. 2017;31(2):962–71.

98. Di Benedetto F, Magistri P, Ballarin R, Tarantino G, Bartolini I, Bencini L, et al. Ultrasound-guided robotic enucleation of pancreatic neuroendocrine tumors. Surg Innov. 2019;26(1):37–45.

99. Zheng M, Li Y, Li T, Zhang L, Zhou L. Resection of the primary tumor improves survival in patients with gastro-entero-pancreatic neuroendocrine neoplasms with liver metastases: a SEER-based analysis. Cancer Med. 2019;8(11):5128–36.

100. Keutgen XM, Nilubol N, Glanville J, Sadowski SM, Liewehr DJ, Venzon DJ, et al. Resection of primary tumor site is associated with prolonged survival in metastatic nonfunctioning pancreatic neuroendocrine tumors. Surgery. 2016;159(1):311–8.

101. Kulke MH, Anthony LB, Bushnell DL, de Herder WW, Goldsmith SJ, Klimstra DS, et al. NANETS treatment guidelines: well-differentiated neuroendocrine tumors of the stomach and pancreas. Pancreas. 2010;39(6):735–52.

102. Mayo SC, de Jong MC, Pulitano C, Clary BM, Reddy SK, Gamblin TC, et al. Surgical management of hepatic neuroendocrine tumor metastasis: results from an international multi-institutional analysis. Ann Surg Oncol. 2010;17(12):3129–36.

103. Foster JH, Berman MM. Solid liver tumors. Major Probl Clin Surg. 1977;22:1–342.

104. Foster JH, Lundy J. Liver metastases. Curr Probl Surg. 1981;18(3):157–202.

105. Sarmiento JM, Heywood G, Rubin J, Ilstrup DM, Nagorney DM, Que FG. Surgical treatment of neuroendocrine metastases to the liver: a plea for resection to increase survival. J Am Coll Surg. 2003;197(1):29–37.

106. Graff-Baker AN, Sauer DA, Pommier SJ, Pommier RF. Expanded criteria for carcinoid liver debulking: maintaining survival and increasing the number of eligible patients. Surgery. 2014;156(6):1367–9.

107. Morgan RE, Pommier SJ, Pommier RF. Expanded criteria for debulking of liver metastasis also apply to pancreatic neuroendocrine tumors. Surgery. 2018;163(1):218–25.

108. Maxwell JE, Sherman SK, O'Dorisio TM, Bellizzi AM, Howe JR. Liver-directed surgery of neuroendocrine metastases: what is the optimal strategy? Surgery. 2016 Jan;159(1):320–33.

109. Scott AT, Breheny PJ, Keck KJ, Bellizzi AM, Dillon JS, O'Dorisio TM, et al. Effective cytoreduction can be achieved in patients with numerous neuroendocrine tumor liver metastases (NETLMs). Surgery. 2019;165(1):166–75.

110. Mazzaferro V, Pulvirenti A, Coppa J. Neuroendocrine tumors metastatic to the liver: how to select patients for liver transplantation? J Hepatol. 2007;47(4):460–6.

111. Moris D, Tsilimigras DI, Ntanasis-Stathopoulos I, Beal EW, Felekouras E, Vernadakis S, et al. Liver transplantation in patients with liver metastases from neuroendocrine tumors: a systematic review. Surgery. 2017;162(3):525–36.

112. De Jong MC, Farnell MB, Sclabas G, Cunningham SC, Cameron JL, Geschwind J-F, et al. Liver-directed therapy for hepatic metastases in patients undergoing pancreaticoduodenectomy: a dual-center analysis. Ann Surg. 2010;252(1):142–8.

113. Hüttner FJ, Schneider L, Tarantino I, Warschkow R, Schmied BM, Hackert T, et al. Palliative resection of the primary tumor in 442 metastasized neuroendocrine tumors of the pancreas: a population-based, propensity score-matched survival analysis. Langenbeck's Arch Surg. 2015;400(6):715–23.

114. Ye H, Xu HL, Shen Q, Zheng Q, Chen P. Palliative resection of primary tumor in metastatic nonfunctioning pancreatic neuroendocrine tumors. J Surg Res. 2019;243:578–87.

115. Tierney JF, Chivukula SV, Wang X, Pappas SG, Schadde E, Hertl M, et al. Resection of primary tumor may prolong survival in metastatic gastroenteropancreatic neuroendocrine tumors. Surgery. 2019;165(3):644–51.

116. Kaemmerer D, Twrznik M, Kulkarni HR, Hörsch D, Sehner S, Baum RP, et al. Prior resection of the primary tumor prolongs survival after peptide receptor radionuclide therapy of advanced neuroendocrine neoplasms. Ann Surg. 2019;274(1):e45–53.

117. Lewis A, Raoof M, Ituarte PHG, Williams J, Melstrom L, Li D, et al. Resection of the primary gastrointestinal neuroendocrine tumor improves survival with or without liver treatment. Ann Surg. 2019;270(6):1131–7.

118. Xiang J-X, Zhang X-F, Beal EW, Weiss M, Aldrighetti L, Poultsides GA, et al. Hepatic resection for non-functional neuroendocrine liver metastasis: does the presence of unresected primary tumor or extrahepatic metastatic disease matter? Ann Surg Oncol. 2018;25(13):3928–35.

119. Pavel M, O'Toole D, Costa F, Capdevila J, Gross D, Kianmanesh R, et al. ENETS consensus guidelines update for the management of distant metastatic disease of intestinal, pancreatic, bronchial neuroendocrine neoplasms (NEN) and NEN of unknown primary site. Neuroendocrinology. 2016;103(2):172–85.

120. Bernard V, Lombard-Bohas C, Taquet M-C, Caroli-Bosc F-X, Ruszniewski P, Niccoli P, et al. Efficacy of everolimus in patients with metastatic insulinoma and refractory hypoglycemia. Eur J Endocrinol. 2013;168(5):665–74.

121. Caplin ME, Pavel M, Ćwikła JB, Phan AT, Raderer M, Sedláčková E, et al. Lanreotide in metastatic enteropancreatic neuroendocrine tumors. N Engl J Med. 2014;371(3):224–33.

122. Rinke A, Müller H-H, Schade-Brittinger C, Klose K-J, Barth P, Wied M, et al. Placebo-controlled, double-blind, prospective, randomized study on the effect of octreotide LAR in the control of tumor growth in patients with metastatic neuroendocrine midgut tumors: a report from the PROMID Study Group. J Clin Oncol Off J Am Soc Clin Oncol. 2009;27(28):4656–63.

123. Raymond E, Dahan L, Raoul J-L, Bang Y-J, Borbath I, Lombard-Bohas C, et al. Sunitinib malate for the treatment of pancreatic neuroendocrine tumors. N Engl J Med. 2011;364(6):501–13.

124. Yao JC, Shah MH, Ito T, Bohas CL, Wolin EM, Van Cutsem E, et al. Everolimus for advanced pancreatic neuroendocrine tumors. N Engl J Med. 2011;364(6):514–23.

Pancreatic Adenocarcinoma: Current Status in Diagnostic Methods, Surgical Techniques, Complications, and Short/Long-Term Survival

Angel Nogales Muñoz,
Inmaculada Sanchez-Matamoros Martin,
Juan Manuel Castillo Tuñon, and Juan Bellido-Luque

5.1 Epidemiology and Risk Factors

Pancreatic adenocarcinoma (PADC) and its variants account for 90% of all pancreatic cancers (PC) [1]. Approximately 60–70% of them arise in the head and the rest are found in the body (15%) and tail (15%).

The latest data recorded for 2020, with 495,773 new cases of pancreatic cancer worldwide and 8697 in Spain, representing 2.6% of all cancers [2], being slightly more common in men (5.5 per 100,000) than in women (4.0 per 100,000).

The incidence rate for both sexes increases with age [2, 3]; it is rarely diagnosed before the age of 55 years and can be defined as a disease of elderly populations because the highest incidence is found in people over 70 years of age [4].

To date, pancreatic cancer remains one of the most lethal neoplasms, with a bleak prognosis and a 94% mortality/incidence rate.

Due to its poor prognosis, pancreatic cancer is the seventh leading cause of cancer death in both men and women in industrialized countries [2]. Rates are 3–4 times higher in countries with a high level of development, with higher incidence rates in Europe, North America, and Australia/New Zealand [2].

Given that, in the European Union, rates are quite stable in relation to decreasing rates of breast cancer, it has been estimated that, in the future, pancreatic cancer will overtake breast cancer as the third leading cause of cancer death [2].

The etiology of pancreatic cancer has been studied extensively and today we know that more than 80% is due to sporadic mutations, approximately 75–90% of pancreatic cancer cases involve a point activation mutation in the KRAS oncogene [5] and only a small proportion are due to hereditary germline mutations.

BRCA2 mutations may be the most common inherited genetic alteration in familial pancreatic cancer. Substantial progress in understanding pancreatic cancer genomics holds promise for future management of the disease. We know that there are a number of risk factors detected and well confirmed so far for this type of cancer [6] such as chronic pancreatitis history, Hereditary Pancreatitis, or Familial cancer syndromes.

A. Nogales Muñoz (✉) · I. Sanchez-Matamoros Martin
J. M. C. Tuñon · J. Bellido-Luque
Hepatobiliopancreatic Unit Surgical Department,
Virgen Macarena University Hospital, Seville, Spain
e-mail: anogal@telefonica.net;
Macu.sm@hotmail.com; jmcastum@hotmail.com;
j_bellido_l@hotmail.com

© The Author(s), under exclusive license to Springer Nature Switzerland AG 2023
J. Bellido Luque, A. Nogales Muñoz (eds.), *Recent Innovations in Surgical Procedures of Pancreatic Neoplasms*, https://doi.org/10.1007/978-3-031-21351-9_5

In addition, there are other related factors, such as Diabetes Mellitus, *H. Pylori* infection, history of gastrectomy or cholecystectomy, non-O blood group, consumption of red and processed meat, foods and beverages containing fructose, foods containing saturated fatty acids, or alcohol consumption (more than three drinks/day) [6].

Smoking is the best-established exogenous cause of this disease and we know that smoking cessation leads to a reduction in excess risk [6].

Alcohol consumption has been studied as a risk factor associated with PC. A recent meta-analysis showed that moderate or low levels of consumption were not associated with an increased risk of PC, however, it found that high consumption does increase the risk of suffering from it by 15%, especially with the consumption of spirits [7].

Chronic pancreatitis has also been found to be an entity that increases the risk of suffering from PC, reaching 5% of them suffering it throughout their lives [8].

Obesity has become an important risk factor, with obese people (body mass index [BMI] of 30 or more) being approximately 20% more likely to develop pancreatic cancer [6]. In addition, in 2016, a meta-analysis observed an increase in mortality related to pancreatic cancer among obese people, compared to patients of normal weight, so that for each increase of 1 kg/m^2 in BMI, a 10% increase in mortality was associated [9].

The family history of pancreatic cancer in a first-degree relative represents an increase in risk 9 times greater than the general population; people with 3 or more first-degree relatives affected by pancreatic cancer, the risk increases 32-fold [10, 11].

All known risk factors can be divided into modifiable (tobacco, alcohol, obesity, and dietary factors) and non-modifiable (male sex, advanced age, family history of pancreatic cancer, genetic factors, and chronic pancreatitis) [6]. For most of these risk factors, the association with pancreatic cancer is generally modest (with a relative risk ranging from 1.2 to 1.8), which makes it difficult to identify a high-risk population group that could benefit from a screening program [12, 13].

The intestinal microbiota has also been associated with the development of pancreatic cancer and although the presence of certain intestinal flora profiles is associated with a high risk of pancreatic cancer, there is not enough evidence to establish it as a factor on which action can be taken [14].

More than 90% of the cancers that are located in the pancreas are ductal adenocarcinomas being often named as pancreatic cancers, however, there are other malignancies that affect this gland such as malignant neuroendocrine tumors, as well as acinar carcinomas of the pancreas.

The histological subtypes of pancreatic adenocarcinoma (PADC) and their main pathological characteristics according to the WHO classification are shown in Table 5.1 [15].

Table 5.1 Subtypes of pancreatic adenocarcinomas

Summary of the different subtypes of pancreatic ductal adenocarcinoma	
Adenosquamous carcinoma	Significant components of ductal/glandular and squamous differentiation (at least 30%). Considered to have a worse prognosis than pancreatic adenocarcinoma
Colloid/mucinous carcinoma	Production of copious amounts of extracellular stromal mucin. Most arise in association with intraductal papillary mucinous neoplasms; thought to have a more favorable prognosis than pancreatic adenocarcinoma
Undifferentiated/anaplastic carcinoma	Minimal or no differentiation; highly atypical cells which may appear spindle shaped or sarcomatoid, often admixed with osteoclast-like giant cells. One of the most aggressive forms of pancreatic cancer with extremely poor survival rates
Signet ring cell carcinoma	Discohesive, singly invasive cells with intracytoplasmic mucin that may displace the nucleus. Similar tumors throughout the gastrointestinal tract. A very rare form of pancreatic cancer with a prognosis similar to that of pancreatic adenocarcinoma
Medullary carcinoma	Syncytial arrangement of pleomorphic epithelial cells with associated intratumoral lymphoid infiltrate. Prognosis is slightly better than pancreatic adenocarcinoma
Hepatoid carcinoma	Morphological similarity to hepatocellular carcinoma. May produce bile. A very rare tumor with a poor prognosis similar to that of pancreatic adenocarcinoma

5.2   Clinical Symptoms and Early Diagnosis

Approximately 60–70% of pancreatic adenocarcinomas occur in the head of the pancreas, and the rest is found in the body (15%) and tail (15%) although at diagnosis most of them are in other locations outside the gland and this location will condition the symptomatology.

The diagnosis of pancreatic cancer is a real challenge in the initial stages, the absence of specific symptoms means that patients often are not studied. Symptoms often occur lately when the tumor may have reached a level of development and spread that prevents treatment with a chance of success.

The most common presenting symptoms are pain, jaundice, and weight loss. They are often accompanied by steatorrhea as a sign of the commonly associated pancreatic insufficiency.

The initial symptomatology will be greatly influenced by the location of the tumor. For tumors in cephalic location, painless jaundice is the most common form of presentation associated with consumptive symptoms, abdominal discomfort at the epigastric or periumbilical level and mood alterations often labeled as depressive symptoms [16].

The PADCs of corporocaudal localization usually reach greater size since by not causing jaundice. They remain asymptomatic for longer being the abdominal pain of pancreatic characteristics with irradiation in belt to the back the most common form of presentation. It is usually accompanied by constitutional syndrome with weight loss and sadness.

These symptoms usually mean progression of the tumor to the surrounding tissues, especially to the retroperitoneum and vascular structures that are intimately related or to distant organs, overshadowing the prognosis of the disease.

Accompanying this symptomatology, it is common to appreciate functional alterations of the pancreatic gland such as those derived from both endocrine and exocrine pancreatic insufficiency. A novo Diabetes Mellitus is not only a common symptom but sometimes precedes the onset of neoplasia and can become a warning sign that can lead to an earlier diagnosis of the disease [17].

Since the only therapeutic option with curative intent is tumor resection, resectability, and early diagnosis become a fundamental tool to improve survival. A multitude of efforts is currently aimed at finding a way to perform screening tests.

An ideal screening test for early pancreatic cancer would be a highly accurate blood marker that could be measured non-invasively. Much research has been done to find PC biomarkers and several have been proposed (CEA, CA19-9, CA125, microRNA, etc.), although the clinical applicability of these tests remains unclear [18, 19]. Unfortunately, none to date have proven to be specific enough for early diagnosis of this disease.

The only serological marker approved by the US FDA for the routine management of PC is CA 19-9 in blood, but its low positive predictive value detracts from its value for early diagnosis in screening of asymptomatic population. Several studies corroborate this statement, finding useful the elevation of CA 19-9 as a predictor of PC in patients who also present Diabetes Mellitus and elevation of bilirubin [20].

Pancreatic carcinoma has a low incidence that is around 1% of the population, so it would not be profitable to perform population screening tests due to its low performance and low cost efficiency value. Therefore, a great effort has been made to identify high-risk populations to selectively monitor them.

So far, a series of hereditary syndromes have been identified with a higher PC incidence than the general population [21, 22]. These are hereditary breast and ovarian cancer associated with BCRA2, Peutz-Jegher Syndrome (STK11 gene), Hereditary Pancreatitis, Familiar Melanoma associated with CDKN2A, and Hereditary Non-polypoid Colorectal Cancer associated with the MMR gene.

Another target population would be those patients with lesions with malignancy capacity such as Mucinous Cystic Neoplasms (MCN) and Papillary Intraductal Mucinous Neoplasms (PIMN).

The risk of MCNs containing invasive carcinoma is low, at 7–12% [23]. The risk of PIMN developing a carcinoma depends on the presence or risk characteristics such as dilation of the main duct greater than 10 mm, wall thickening of more than 5 mm, location in the pancreatic head with the appearance of jaundice or elevation of CA 19-9 in blood, etc. These clinical and radiological criteria are used to recommend or not surgery and approximately 30% of resected PIMNs present invasive disease [24].

Regarding the imaging techniques to establish follow-up in the population at risk, there is no clear consensus since some provide greater advantages than others and vice versa. MRI with Cholangiopancreatography (C-RNM) is an excellent technique for the surveillance of patients at high risk of PC, with high sensitivity and the absence of ionizing radiation. This has been established as the most useful imaging test in terms of diagnosis of PIMN, since its sensitivity is greater than that of the CT scan, exceeding 88% [25]. It also overcomes the limitations of the CT scan and could show the communication between injury and duct, an essential fact in the PIMN, as well as the dilation of the main duct, which is of vital importance to stratify the risk of injury considering that dilations greater than 10 mm suppose a high degree of malignancy [26].

There is an agreement between the findings of the C-RNM and those of the Endoscopic Ultrasonography (E-US) although the latter has a greater sensitivity to identify smaller lesions (<2 cm), to identify worrying characteristics, and to obtain samples for biochemical and cytological studies, all of which are useful to better characterize suspicious lesions [27].

The International Consensus Group for Screening of Pancreatic Cancer recommends the use of the combination of MRI and Eco-Endoscopy for the surveillance of risk groups as well as that such screening and subsequent management should be carried out in high-volume centers with multidisciplinary teams, with established protocols [27].

Recommendations in existing clinical practice guidelines on the early diagnosis of pancreatic cancer are inconsistent and based on limited evidence. Most of them support the blood measurement of CA 19-9 as a complementary test, but established that, although it is not useful for diagnosing early pancreatic cancer, it is recommended in the follow-up of operated patients. Currently, there are no other tumor-specific markers recommended for early diagnosis of pancreatic cancer [28].

Awareness campaigns should be carried out to establish a diagnosis of suspicion in the face of vague and non-specific symptoms, since most of the patients diagnosed with PC had presented vague symptoms even intermittently in the previous months with frequent consultations in this period. The signs and symptoms except painless jaundice are commonly poorly specified by the patient so a high degree of suspicion is necessary to establish a correct diagnosis [29].

5.3 Diagnostic Protocol

We should consider essential steps to treat patients with PC in the most successful way to establish a diagnosis as early as possible and clearly define resectability.

A high level of suspicion that includes, symptomatology of the patient, family history, and risk factors, will lead us to a diagnosis as early as possible and more accurately.

It is important to obtain abdominal imaging tests, establishing an order based on their diagnostic profitability.

It is quite common to start studies of a picture of abdominal pain with the performance of an abdominal ultrasound. The ultrasound of the abdomen is an affordable test that usually yields a high sensitivity for the detection of dilation of bile ducts, as well as the observation of pancreatic mass (>95%) in lesions of more than 3 cm. The sensitivity of ultrasound increases with the use of specific contrasts [30].

Multidetector CT scan with contrast and pancreatic protocol is the most appropriate technique for suspected PC and to evaluate vascular invasion and resectability. This CT scan should include pancreatic parenchymal and venous phase. The sensitivity to detect PC is 85–97%, although it falls to 65–70% for lesions of less than 2 cm [31].

However, its effectiveness is less in detecting small liver metastases or peritoneal implants. Several studies have shown that MRI increases the sensitivity to detect liver metastases, also helping to characterize indeterminate lesions [32].

The ECO-US endoscopic ultrasonography is more precise, but at the same time more invasive to detect pancreatic lesions, especially of small size <2 cm with a sensitivity and specificity of 95% in most publications. It also provides the advantage of being able to obtain samples for histological study through a fine needle puncture [33]. The drawbacks of this technique are its invasiveness and the possible adverse effects of the puncture, including pancreatitis, hemorrhage, or infection.

A meta-analysis of 15 studies involving 1860 patients found that overall, euS-FNA sensitivity for pancreatic cancer was 92%, and specificity was 96% [34].

There is currently a broad consensus on the non-need for histological confirmation in cases of lesions with very characteristic radiological findings and resectability criteria.

It is desirable to obtain histological confirmation, although your absence does not rule out surgery. Thus, in cases where a lesion with typical characteristics of PC is diagnosed and with extension studies with resectability criteria, preoperative histological confirmation is not necessary to decide on surgical resection. Only in cases where systemic therapies with neoadjuvant intent are to be used or in unresectable cases, will it be essential [35].

Similarly, in patients in whom autoimmune pancreatitis is suspected (history of autoimmunity) or before signs of chronic pancreatitis (excessive alcohol consumption, destructure of the entire pancreatic gland, etc.) we should try to histologically confirm pancreatic cancer to avoid unnecessary surgeries.

PET-FDG (Positron emission tomography) with 18-fluorodeoxyglucose can be used in association with CT for the study of PC. It has been shown to be useful in the detection of distant metastases and can detect 97% of these if they are larger than 1 cm, but fails to see smaller lesions. Its drawback is the false positives found in inflammatory lesions. There is currently no evidence to recommend the use of PET for routine use in the diagnosis or staging of PC [36].

Years ago the study of obstructive jaundices was continued with the performance of an ERCP (endoscopic retrograde cholangiopancreatography). At present, it has been relegated by the RNM with Cholangiography (C-RNM) for the morphological study of the bile ducts. C-RNM has a high sensitivity without the drawbacks of ERCP (need for anesthesia, complications, etc.).

ERCP continues to maintain its main role when it is necessary to place a prosthesis for decompression of the bile duct assuming that the placement of prostheses can artifact the assessment by CT, as well as eventually produce alterations of the head of the pancreas that hinder and increase the morbidity of subsequent surgery. It will be other chapters of this book that abound in the use and limitation of this exploration.

5.4 Resectability Assessment

Only 10–15% of patients are diagnosed with resectable disease. R0 resection associated with preoperative systemic therapy regimens is currently the best and only cure opportunity for resectable and Borderline patients with a 5-year survival of 25% [37].

A good staging of the PC is essential to establish adequate therapeutic management. The National Comprehensive Cancer Network (NCCN) recommends a multidisciplinary team of pancreatic cancer management specialists. Decisions determining resectability status should be made in committees, which include radiology experts, cancer surgeons, gastroenterologists, and medical oncologists.

Katz et al. [38] studied the survival effect of multidisciplinary care for resectable pancreatic cancer. They reported a 5-year survival rate of 27% in their patients, higher than they had previously in patients not evaluated by the multidisciplinary team, and attributed the best results to the use of objective criteria to define resectability, along with a standardized, multidisciplinary approach to patient care; however, since then, few reports have examined the impact of multidisciplinary care on survival [38].

The detection of remote invasion especially to the liver and peritoneum as well as to other organs at a distance constitutes a cause of unresectableness established unanimously included in all the guidelines including the NCCN in its latest version 2.2021 [39].

Vascular infiltration is the main cause of non-resectability in non-metastatic PC and is mainly due to the involvement of the superior mesenteric vessels both superior mesenteric vein (SMV) and superior mesenteric artery (SMA), celiac trunk (CT), inferior cava vein, or the aorta. The degree of circumferential involvement, as well as the intensity of that contact that may or may not deform the vascular wall are taken into account in these definitions.

Using this vascular involvement as well as the existence or not of distant metastases, the NCCN establishes three categories: resectable, borderline, and unresectable [40].

The NCCN 2020.2 establishes the *definition of resectable PC* as those that in the absence of distant metastases and involvement of the SMV or PV (portal vein) do not exist or is less than 180°, without arterial involvement in case there is no irregularity of said wall [40].

Locally advanced unresectable PC are considered those tumors that encompass the superior mesenteric veins or the portal vein without the possibility of resection and reconstruction or any involvement of the superior mesenteric artery or the Celiac trunk of more than 180° of its circumference, as well as involvement of the aorta or vena cava.

The definition of *Border-Line PC* included in the latest version of the *NCCN Guidelines* [40] is as follows:

For venous involvement: Tumor contacts the SMV or PV > 180° with irregularity of the venous wall or thrombosis of the vein with proximal and distal vein length that allows a complete and safe resection and reconstruction.

With regard to arterial involvement for tumors that are located in the head of the pancreas or uncinated process: Tumor that contacts the common hepatic artery without extension to the Celiac Trunk or the hepatic bifurcation that allows a safe and complete resection and reconstruction or tumor that contacts the SMA < 180°. For tumors of the body and pancreatic tail, those that contact the CT scan less than or equal to 180° or if the contact is greater than 180° with the CT but without involvement of either the Aorta or the Gastroduodenal Artery and that allows the *Appleby procedure* is considered.

5.5 Staging and Prognosis

For the staging of pancreatic cancer, the 8th Edition of the TNM Classification of the AJCC is currently used [41].

Because pancreatic adenocarcinoma is usually diagnosed in stage III or IV, it has a very poor prognosis, even for those cases that can be treated with surgery, the 5-year survival rate is 16% [42].

During the 2014–2018 period, data from the US National Cancer Institute for pancreatic cancer, in both sexes and all races, showed that 10% of people were diagnosed at an early stage I, having a 5-year survival rate of 32%. If the cancer was stage III, the 5-year survival rate was 12% and those diagnosed as stage IV (52%) had a 5-year survival rate of 3% [42].

The American Joint Cancer Committee's (AJCC) TNM staging system was updated in the eighth edition of 2018, where extrapancreatic extension (presented in the 7th edition) was excluded to focus directly on tumor size [41]. The eighth edition of the TNM staging system demonstrated a more equitable distribution between the stages and better prognostic accuracy in patients with resected pancreatic ductal adenocarcinoma compared to the seventh edition [43]. There is evidence to show that tumor size is an independent risk factor for the prognosis of patients with pancreatic cancer, regardless of extrapancreatic extent, with a lower survival in patients with tumors larger than 2 cm compared to those smaller than 2 cm [44].

There are few studies that evaluate the value of the marker Ca19.9 at the time of diagnosis, as a prognostic factor for survival, in patients who have their pancreatic tumor dried.

Asaoka et al. published a study conducted in patients undergoing surgery for pancreatic head cancer and conclude that the marker Ca 19.9 $\geq$ 230 U/ml can be considered an independent prognostic factor of low survival ($P = 0.025$) [45].

Following the indications of the *International Study Group for Pancreatic Surgery (ISGPS)* the evaluation of resectability should be based on a multidetector CT scan with a three-phase technique and cuts of 1–2 mm, a specific protocol for the pancreas in the arterial and venous phase that manages to define the normal pancreas, the tumor and assess the hepatic parenchyma and that manages to clearly identify the relationships of the tumor with the arterial and venous vascular structures [46].

The findings of this CT scan should be standardized and ordered in a template that could similarly collect the findings so that the results of various groups can be adequately contrasted. These are included in the NCCN Clinical Guidelines [39].

5.6 Surgical Management

Currently, surgery is the only curative option for Pancreatic Cancer, although only 10–20% of diagnosed patients can undergo surgery [47].

Cephalic duodenopancreatectomy (CPD) is the standard technique for the resection of tumors that are located in the head of the pancreas and uncinated process. The classical technique initially described by *Whipple in 1953* has undergone multiple variations, especially with regard to the different anastomoses for the reconstruction. One of the most relevant has been the Pancreatic Duodenectomy with pilorus preservation that is introduced to try to avoid bile reflux and Dumping syndrome without compromising the oncological radicality.

The choice and type of reconstruction depend largely on personal election, and there is cur-

rently no technique superior to the rest and that must be recommended globally. Although many articles have been published comparing different techniques and different types of anastomosis, none of them has been established in a forceful way to be universally recommended.

Distal Pancreatectomy with Splenectomy is the technique of choice for PCs located in the body or tail of the pancreas. Splenic preservation in CP is not recommended as it would compromise lymphadenectomy and oncological radicality.

Anterograde modular radical pancreatosplenectomy (*RAMPS*) has appeared in recent decades in an attempt to improve R0 resection rates and oncological results by initially addressing splenic vessels as well as parenchymal transection at the level of the pancreatic neck. According to several studies, this approach presents a lower blood loss, increasing the number of resected nodes, R0 resections and therefore with better oncological results [48].

In a meta-analysis that includes 285 patients (135 RAMPS vs. 150 PD), there are advantages in favor of RAMPS these do not reach statistical significance [49]. However, at present this approach is imposed in most groups mainly due to the rise of Laparoscopic Distal Pancreatectomies.

Resective surgery of pancreatic cancer, whose purpose is curative, should try to achieve resection with R0 margins (without micro or macroscopic tumor cells), since it has shown a significant improvement in survival with respect to R1 (presence of microscopic tumor cells), this being more evident in tumors located in the pancreatic head compared to those located in the body or tail [50].

This rate of R0 resections has increased with vascular resections. Venous resections allow to increase the percentage of R0 resections without increasing morbidity or mortality in the short term with respect to those who do not have venous resection when performed in reference centers [51].

These conclusions do not reach arterial resections whose performance increases the rates of complications so their indication should be evaluated within trials and centers with extensive experience.

There are wide differences in the literature in the reported rates of R1 resections therefore incomplete from 15 to 75%. These enormous differences are based on the great variability of the definitions as well as on the lack of standardization of the pathological studies of the resection pieces. The dyeing of the piece in the operating room by the surgeon should assist the pathologist in the study and interpretation as it clearly defines the pancreatic, venous, and arterial margins [52] (Fig. 5.1).

The approach to the mesenteric artery in the first place tries on the one hand to reduce the rate of R1 resections as well as to facilitate venous resections in cases where this is necessary. Tumor infiltration of AMS remains a contraindication to pancreatic resection. The approach of this structure in an initial way allows to identify this infiltration early and helps the surgeon to make an early decision before having made irreversible gestures such as pancreatic transection. There are several types of approaches depending on the place through which this artery is addressed and that will depend on both the location of the pancreatic lesion and the preferences of the surgeon [53]. A recently published meta-analysis concludes that this approach, especially by a later route, increases the rate of R0, decreases blood loss, and improves survival at 3 years [54]. Compared to a classic standard CPD approach, there appears to be a better postoperative evolu-

tion with a lower rate of transfusions, pancreatic fistulas, and delayed gastric emptying. In part, this may also be influenced by increased training and technical expertise of groups that systematically address AMS first [55].

The extent of lymphadenectomy in pancreatic cancer has also been subject to debate. Nodal involvement in patients with CP is an important predictor of survival. Extended lymphadenectomy appears as an attempt to reduce nodal recurrences by including a greater number of nodal stations. Numerous publications conclude that this extensive dissection associates with a higher rate of complications without providing a significant increase in patient survival. There has been intense debate about his recommendation against the so-called standard lymphadenectomy. At present and after the Consensus of the *International Group of Studies on Pancreatic Surgery* (ISGPS), it is established that standard lymphadenectomy is the one that should be recommended [56]. This consensus defines the extent of this standard lymphadenectomy by establishing the nodal stations that must be resected depending on the tumor location. For cephalic Duodenum-Pancreatectomy, the ganglion stations 5 (supra pyloric), 6 (infra pyloric), 8 (common hepatic arteria), 12b–c (bile duct and cystic), 13 a–b (along the head of the pancreas), 14 a–b (right part of AMS), and 17 a–b (anterior face of the pancreas). For cancers of the body and tail of the pancreas, they must be removed from seasons 10, 11, and 18 [56].

The retroperitoneal tissue must be completely removed with 360° circumferential dissection of the axis of the superior mesenteric vein-portal vein and of the right half of the 180° circumference of the superior mesenteric artery. removal of lymphofast tissue from the inter aorto-cavo space with cranial margin of the right renal vein [57]. This technique requires the intraoperative study of the margins of both the vascular contacts and the pancreatic and biliary edges of the section (Fig. 5.2).

At least 15 nodes should be resected for proper staging of the disease [58].

It is controversial whether intraoperatively cosigned tumor involvement of the nodes for aor-

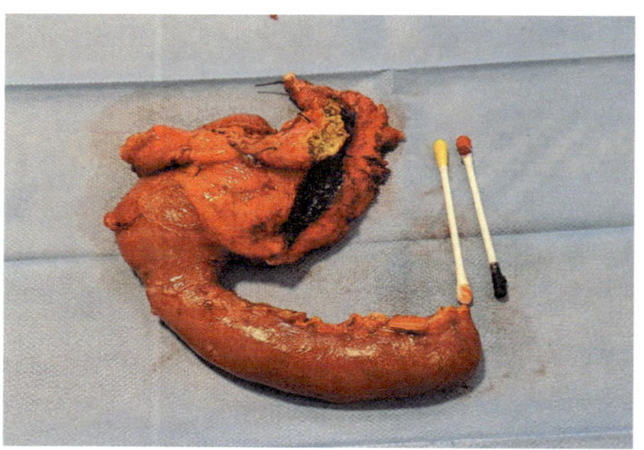

Fig. 5.1 Yellow border pancreatic section, Blue venous margin, Red arterial margin

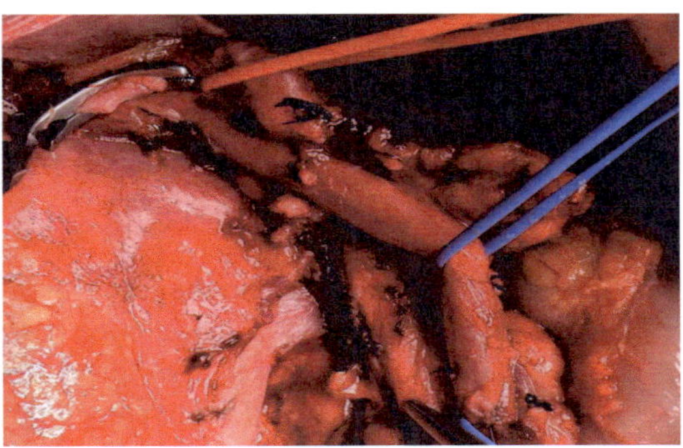

Fig. 5.2 Surgical field after resection. Blue ribbon: portal-mesenteric axis. Red ribbon: Proper hepatic artery. Common hepatic biliary stump is clamped

tic contraindicates surgical resection. Some teams do not perform CPD in case of positive involvement in the study by freezing and are based on the significant drop in the survival of patients in these cases. However, there is no international consensus to recommend CPD in case of positive paraaortic nodes [59, 60].

5.7 Complications and Postoperative Results

The morbidity rate after pancreatic surgery is high, in the range of 15–65%, although mortality has decreased to less than 5% due to recent advances in surgical techniques and perioperative management.

The concentration and referral of these patients to high-volume centers have improved the results, hand in hand with the increase in experience in surgeons. Innovations in technology and operative technique have sought to further reduce adverse outcomes and improve survival [61].

Postoperative pancreatic fistula (POPF) is defined as outflow by draining any volume of fluid with an amylase level >3 times the upper limit of the normal value of serum amylase. It is one of the most serious postoperative complications after pancreatic surgery associated with a higher incidence of life-threatening complications, such as abscess or intra-abdominal bleeding and sepsis [62].

In a systematic review of 40 studies, clinically relevant pancreatic fistula occurred in 13% of patients after pancreatic resections.

A Dutch study showed that mortality in patients with severe pancreatic fistula remains high (18%) [63].

The International Pancreatic Surgery Study (ISGPS) showed that postoperative pancreatic fistula ranges from 15 to 45% in patients undergoing pancreatic surgery. Several strategies have been proposed for the reduction of POPF:

- Pancreato-gastric anastomosis instead of the classic pancreatic-jejunal anastomosis.
- Trans-anastomotic tutors.
- Use of somatostatin analogues.

The results of the multiple published studies are inconclusive. A systematic review including 5323 patients undergoing CPD performed by 62 surgeons in 17 different centers found 29% of clinically relevant POPF. This review established as a pancreas high risk to present POPF those soft consistency pancreas with fine caliber pancreatic duct. In those types of pancreas, the placement of externalized trans-anastomotic tutors decreases the rate of POPF [64].

5.8 Medical Management

Although surgical resection is the only curative option in PADC, a multitude of treatments have been tried to improve the survival of these patients.

The multicenter phase III TRIAL CONKO-1 demonstrated that patients treated with adjuvant Gemcitabine for 6 cycles after pancreatic cancer surgery had longer disease-free survivals than those treated with surgery alone; from this study, the treatment would be surgical resection with the addition of chemotherapy in the adjuvant environment since this strategy improves survival rates [65]. This study demonstrated significantly better median disease-free survival (13.4 vs. 6.7 months) and 5-year overall survival of 20.7 vs. 10.4% and a 10-year survival of 12.2 vs. 7.7%.

However, despite these promising results, median overall survival only improved from 20 to 23 months ($P = 0.01$) [65].

Subsequently there are other trials that compare different adjuvant treatment protocols, but today adjuvant with Gemcitabine is the standard treatment, included by protocol in resected patients with pancreatic cancer.

FOLFIRINOX (irinotecan, oxaliplatin, and 5-FU infusion) has been shown to be more effective in response rate, improvement of progression-free survival, and overall survival against gemcitabine monotherapy, but is more toxic [66]. In patients with good general conditions, it is a treatment to be considered. Neoadjuvant protocols in resectable cancer are currently underway in an attempt to improve the poor survival outcomes that PC continues to present.

5.9 Recurrence in Ca Pancreas

Despite surgery and subsequent adjuvant chemotherapy with curative intent, tumor recurrence is the norm in this type of cancer; relapses in up to 80% of patients, mainly within 2 years after the operation [67]. For follow-up, a combination of serum CA 19-9 marker tests and routine imaging studies, such as CT or PET-CT, continues to be the most widely used surveillance strategy to assess early recurrence of the disease.

The management of recurrence at present is based on systemic therapies being so far accepted that both local and distant recurrence of CP should not opt for surgical treatment. However, there is currently a tendency to propose surgical resection in patients with isolated recurrence and in selected cases since it increases survival with respect to patients who in the same situation undergo only systemic therapies [68].

5.10 Conclusions

There is currently a relative increase in PC in recent years without observing substantial improvements in survival. If this tendency con-

tinues, by 2040 it will become the second leading cause of cancer death.

Identifying risk groups and follow-up strategies for early diagnosis in incipient stages of the disease are so far the most effective tools to reverse this trend.

Multidisciplinary management in high-volume hospitals is mandatory to improve outcomes. The expertise of teams with an interest in pancreatic cancer that include gastroenterologists, radiologists, surgeons, and oncologists will mean that at least maximum survival can be offered to patients with PC.

References

1. Feldmann G, Beaty R, Hruban RH, Maitra A. Molecular genetics of pancreatic intraepithelial neoplasia. J Hepato-Biliary-Pancreat Surg. 2007;14(3):224–32.
2. Bray F, Ferlay J, Soerjomataram I, Siegel RL, Torre LA, Jemal A. Global cancer statistics 2018: GLOBOCAN estimates of incidence and mortality worldwide for 36 cancers in 185 countries. CA Cancer J Clin. 2018;68(6):394–424.
3. Noone AM, Howlader N, Krapcho M, Miller D, Brest A, Yu M, Ruhl J, Tatalovich Z, Mariotto A, Lewis DR, Chen HS, Feuer EJ, Cronin KA, editors. SEER cancer statistics review, 1975–2015. Bethesda: National Cancer Institute.
4. Malvezzi M, Carioli G, Bertuccio P, Rosso T, Boffetta P, Levi F, et al. European cancer mortality predictions for the year 2016 with focus on leukaemias. Ann Oncol. 2016;27(4):725–31.
5. Vincent A, Herman J, Schulick R, Hruban RH, Goggins M. Pancreatic cancer. Lancet. 2011;378:607–20.
6. Adami H-O, Hunter DJ, Lagiou P, Mucci L, editors. Textbook of cancer epidemiology, vol. 1. Oxford: Oxford University Press; 2018.
7. Wang YT, Gou YW, Jin WW, Xiao M, Fang HY. Association between alcohol intake and the risk of pancreatic cancer: a dose-response meta-analysis of cohort studies. BMC Cancer. 2016;16(1):212.
8. Raimondi S, Lowenfels AB, Morselli-Labate AM, Maisonneuve P, Pezzilli R. Pancreatic cancer in chronic pancreatitis; aetiology, incidence, and early detection. Best Pract Res Clin Gastroenterol. 2010;24(3):349–58.
9. Majumder K, Gupta A, Arora N, Singh PP, Singh S. Premorbid obesity and mortality in patients with pancreatic cancer: a systematic review and meta-analysis. Clin Gastroenterol Hepatol. 2016;14:355–368.e2.

10. Klein AP, Brune KA, Petersen GM, Goggins M, Tersmette AC, Offerhaus GJA, et al. Prospective risk of pancreatic cancer in familial pancreatic cancer kindreds. Cancer Res. 2004;64(7):2634–8.

11. Brune KA, Lau B, Palmisano E, Canto M, Goggins MG, Hruban RH, et al. Importance of age of onset in pancreatic cancer kindreds. J Natl Cancer Inst. 2010;102(2):119–26.

12. Maisonneuve P, Lowenfels AB. Risk factors for pancreatic cancer: a summary review of meta-analytical studies. Int J Epidemiol. 2015;44(1):186–98.

13. Rosato V, Polesel J, Bosetti C, Serraino D, Negri E, La VC. Population attributable risk for pancreatic cancer in northern Italy. Pancreas. 2015;44(2):216–20.

14. McGuigan A, Kelly P, Turkington RC, Jones C, Coleman HG, McCain RS. Pancreatic cancer: a review of clinical diagnosis, epidemiology, treatment and outcomes. World J Gastroenterol. 2018;24:4846–61.

15. Bosman FT, Carneiro F, Hruban RH, Theise ND. WHO classification of tumours of the digestive system, 4 edn. 2010.

16. Porta M, Fabregat X, Malats N, Guarner L, Carrato A, De Miguel A, et al. Exocrine pancreatic cancer: symptoms at presentation and their relation to tumour site and stage. Clin Transl Oncol. 2005;7(5):189–97.

17. Pereira SP, Oldfield L, Ney A, Hart PA, Keane MG, Pandol SJ, et al. Early detection of pancreatic cancer. Lancet Gastroenterol Hepatol. 2020;5:698–710.

18. Gold DV, Goggins M, Modrak DE, Newsome G, Liu M, Shi C, et al. Detection of early-stage pancreatic adenocarcinoma. Cancer Epidemiol Biomark Prev. 2010;19(11):2786–94.

19. Chang JC, Kundranda M. Novel diagnostic and predictive biomarkers in pancreatic adenocarcinoma. Int J Mol Sci. 2017;18(3):667.

20. Choe JW, Kim HJ, Kim JS, Cha J, Joo MK, Lee BJ, et al. Usefulness of CA 19–9 for pancreatic cancer screening in patients with new-onset diabetes. Hepatobiliary Pancreat Dis Int. 2018;17(3):263–8.

21. Del Chiaro M, Segersvärd R, Löhr M, Verbeke C. Early detection and prevention of pancreatic cancer: is it really possible today? World J Gastroenterol. 2014;20:12118–31.

22. Chen F, Roberts NJ, Klein AP. Inherited pancreatic cancer. Chin Clin Oncol. 2017;6(6):58.

23. Ren B, Liu X, Suriawinata AA. Pancreatic ductal adenocarcinoma and its precursor lesions: histopathology, cytopathology, and molecular pathology. Am J Pathol. 2019;189(1):9–21.

24. Pittman ME, Rao R, Hruban RH. Classification, morphology, molecular pathogenesis, and outcome of premalignant lesions of the pancreas. Arch Pathol Lab Med. 2017;141(12):1606–14.

25. Singhi AD, Koay EJ, Chari ST, Maitra A. Early detection of pancreatic cancer: opportunities and challenges. Gastroenterology. 2019;156(7):2024–40.

26. Pagliari D, Saviano A, Serricchio ML, Dal Lago AA, Brizi MG, Lanza F, et al. Up to date in the assessment and management of intraductal papillary mucinous neoplasms of the pancreas. Eur Rev Med Pharmacol Sci. 2017;21(12):2858–74.

27. Canto MI, Harinck F, Hruban RH, Offerhaus GJ, Poley JW, Kamel I, et al. International cancer of the pancreas screening (CAPS) consortium summit on the management of patients with increased risk for familial pancreatic cancer. Gut. 2013;62(3):339–47.

28. Takaori K, Bassi C, Biankin A, Brunner TB, Cataldo I, Campbell F, et al. International Association of Pancreatology (IAP)/European Pancreatic Club (EPC) consensus review of guidelines for the treatment of pancreatic cancer. Pancreatology. 2016;16(1):14–27.

29. Stapley S, Peters TJ, Neal RD, Rose PW, Walter FM, Hamilton W. The risk of pancreatic cancer in symptomatic patients in primary care: a large case-control study using electronic records. Br J Cancer. 2012;106(12):1940–4.

30. Kersting S, Roth J, Bunk A. Transabdominal contrast-enhanced ultrasonography of pancreatic cancer. Pancreatology. 2011;11(Suppl 2):20–7.

31. Al-Hawary MM, Francis IR, Chari ST, Fishman EK, Hough DM, Lu DS, et al. Pancreatic ductal adenocarcinoma radiology reporting template: consensus statement of the society of abdominal radiology and the American Pancreatic Association. Radiology. 2014;270(1):248–60.

32. Bhalla M, Aldakkak M, Kulkarni NM, O'Connor SD, Griffin MO, Christians KK, et al. Characterizing indeterminate liver lesions in patients with localized pancreatic cancer at the time of diagnosis. Abdom Radiol. 2018;43(2):351–63.

33. Yamashita Y, Kitano M, Ashida R. Value of endoscopy for early diagnosis of pancreatic carcinoma. Dig Endosc. 2020;32(1):27–36.

34. Chen J, Yang R, Lu Y, Xia Y, Zhou H. Diagnostic accuracy of endoscopic ultrasound-guided fine-needle aspiration for solid pancreatic lesion: a systematic review. J Canc Res Clin Oncol. 2012;138(9):1433–41.

35. Vera R, Díez L, Martín Pérez E, Plaza JC, Sanjuanbenito A, Carrato A. Surgery for pancreatic ductal adenocarcinoma. Clin Transl Oncol. 2017;19(11):1303–11.

36. Matsumoto I, Shirakawa S, Shinzeki M, Asari S, Goto T, Ajiki T, et al. 18-fluorodeoxyglucose positron emission tomography does not aid in diagnosis of pancreatic ductal adenocarcinoma. Clin Gastroenterol Hepatol. 2013;11(6):712–8.

37. Hackert T, Ulrich A, Büchler MW. Borderline resectable pancreatic cancer. Cancer Lett. 2016;375(2):231–7.

38. Katz MHG, Wang H, Fleming JB, Sun CC, Hwang RF, Wolff RA, et al. Long-term survival after multidisciplinary management of resected pancreatic adenocarcinoma. Ann Surg Oncol. 2009;16(4):836–47.

39. Tempero MA, Malafa MP, Al-Hawary M, Behrman SW, Benson AB, Cardin DB, et al. Pancreatic adenocarcinoma, version 2.2021, NCCN clinical practice guidelines in oncology. J Natl Compr Cancer Netw. 2021;19(4):439–57.

40. Tempero MA. NCCN guidelines updates: pancreatic cancer. J Natl Compr Canc Netw. 2019;17(5.5):603–5.

41. Chun YS, Pawlik TM, Vauthey JN. 8th edition of the AJCC cancer staging manual: pancreas and hepatobiliary cancers. Ann Surg Oncol. 2018;25(4):845–7.

42. Drouillard A, Manfredi S, Lepage C, Bouvier AM. Épidémiologie du cancer du pancréas [Epidemiology of pancreatic cancer]. Bull Cancer. 2018;105(1):63–9.

43. Van Roessel S, Kasumova GG, Verheij J, Najarian RM, Maggino L, De Pastena M, et al. International validation of the eighth edition of the American Joint Committee on Cancer (AJCC) TNM staging system in patients with resected pancreatic cancer. JAMA Surg. 2018;153(12):e183617.

44. Takahashi C, Shridhar R, Huston J, Meredith K. Correlation of tumor size and survival in pancreatic cancer. J Gastrointest Oncol. 2018;9(5):910–21.

45. Asaoka T, Miyamoto A, Maeda S, Tsujie M, Hama N, Yamamoto K, et al. Prognostic impact of preoperative NLR and CA19-9 in pancreatic cancer. Pancreatology. 2016;16(3):434–40.

46. Bockhorn M, Uzunoglu FG, Adham M, Imrie C, Milicevic M, Sandberg AA, et al. Borderline resectable pancreatic cancer: a consensus statement by the International Study Group of Pancreatic Surgery (ISGPS). Surgery. 2014;155(6):977–88.

47. Hartwig W, Werner J, Jäger D, Debus J, Büchler MW. Improvement of surgical results for pancreatic cancer. Lancet Oncol. 2013;14(11):476–85.

48. Abe T, Ohuchida K, Miyasaka Y, Ohtsuka T, Oda Y, Nakamura M. Comparison of surgical outcomes between radical antegrade modular pancreatosplenectomy (RAMPS) and standard retrograde pancreatosplenectomy (SPRS) for left-sided pancreatic cancer. World J Surg. 2016;40(9):2267–75.

49. Zhou Q, Fengwei-Gao GJ, Xie Q, Liu Y, Wang Q, Lei Z. Assessement of postoperative long-term survival quality and complications associated with radical antegrade modular pancreatosplenectomy and distal pancreatectomy: a meta-analysis and systematic review. BMC Surg. 2019;19(1):12.

50. Demir IE, Jäger C, Schlitter AM, Konukiewitz B, Stecher L, Schorn S, Tieftrunk E, Scheufele F, Calavrezos L, Schirren R, Esposito I, Weichert W, Friess H, Ceyhan GO. R0 versus R1 resection matters after pancreaticoduodenectomy, and less after distal or total pancreatectomy for pancreatic cancer. Ann Surg. 2018;268(6):1058–68.

51. Barreto SG, Windsor JA. Justifying vein resection with pancreatoduodenectomy. Lancet Oncol. 2016;17(3):e118–24.

52. Verbeke CS. Resection margins and R1 rates in pancreatic cancer—are we there yet? Histopathology. 2008;52(7):787–96.

53. Sanjay P, Takaori K, Govil S, Shrikhande SV, Windsor JA. 'Artery-first' approaches to pancreatoduodenectomy. Br J Surg. 2012;99(8):1027–35.

54. Jiang X, Yu Z, Ma Z, Deng H, Ren W, Shi W, Jiao Z. Superior mesenteric artery first approach can improve the clinical outcomes of pancreaticoduodenectomy: a meta-analysis. Int J Surg. 2020;73:14–24.

55. Negoi I, Hostiuc S, Runcanu A, Negoi RI, Beuran M. Superior mesenteric artery first approach versus standard pancreaticoduodenectomy: a systematic review and meta-analysis. Hepatobiliary Pancreat Dis Int. 2017;16(2):127–38.

56. Tol JAMG, Gouma DJ, Bassi C, Dervenis C, Montorsi M, Adham M, et al. Definition of a standard lymphadenectomy in surgery for pancreatic ductal adenocarcinoma: a consensus statement by the International Study Group on Pancreatic Surgery (ISGPS). Surgery. 2014;156(3):591–600.

57. Delpero JR, Bachellier P, Regenet N, Le Treut YP, Paye F, Carrere N, Sauvanet A, Autret A, Turrini O, Monges-Ranchin G, Boher JM. Pancreaticoduodenectomy for pancreatic ductal adenocarcinoma: a French multicentre prospective evaluation of resection margins in 150 evaluable specimens. HPB (Oxford). 2014;16(1):20–33.

58. Slidell MB, Chang DC, Cameron JL, Wolfgang C, Herman JM, Schulick RD, et al. Impact of total lymph node count and lymph node ratio on staging and survival after pancreatectomy for pancreatic adenocarcinoma: a large, population-based analysis. Ann Surg Oncol. 2008;15(1):165–74.

59. Zizzo M, Castro Ruiz C, Annessi V, Zanelli M. Prognostic role of pancreatic head cancer metastatic paraaortic lymph nodes detected intraoperatively. HPB (Oxford). 2020;22(6):935–6.

60. Sperti C, Gruppo M, Valmasoni M, Pozza G, Passuello N, Beltrame V, et al. Para-aortic node involvement is not an independent predictor of survival after resection for pancreatic cancer. World J Gastroenterol. 2017;23(24):4399–406.

61. Lynch SM, Vrieling A, Lubin JH, Kraft P, Mendelsohn JB, Hartge P, et al. Cigarette smoking and pancreatic cancer: a pooled analysis from the pancreatic cancer cohort consortium. Am J Epidemiol. 2009;170(4):403–13.

62. Bassi C, Marchegiani G, Dervenis C, Sarr M, Abu Hilal M, Adham M, Allen P, Andersson R, Asbun HJ, Besselink MG, Conlon K, Del Chiaro M, Falconi M, Fernandez-Cruz L, Fernandez-Del Castillo C, Fingerhut A, Friess H, Gouma DJ, Hackert T, Izbicki J, Lillemoe KD, Neoptolemos JP, Olah A, Schulick R, Shrikhande SV, Takada T, Takaori K, Traverso W, Vollmer CR, Wolfgang CL, Yeo CJ, Salvia R, Buchler M. International Study Group on Pancreatic Surgery (ISGPS). The 2016 update of the International Study Group (ISGPS) definition and grading of postoperative pancreatic fistula: 11 years after. Surgery. 2017;161(3):584–91.

63. Smits FJ, van Santvoort HC, Besselink MG, Batenburg MCT, Slooff RAE, Boerma D, Busch OR, Coene PPLO, van Dam RM, van Dijk DPJ, van Eijck CHJ, Festen S, van der Harst E, de Hingh IHJT, de Jong KP, Tol JAMG, Borel Rinkes IHM, Molenaar IQ, Dutch Pancreatic Cancer Group. Management

of severe pancreatic fistula after pancreatoduodenectomy. JAMA Surg. 2017;152(6):540–8.

64. Ecker BL, McMillan MT, Asbun HJ, Ball CG, Bassi C, Beane JD, et al. Characterization and optimal management of high-risk pancreatic anastomoses during pancreatoduodenectomy. Ann Surg. 2018;267(4):608–16.

65. Oettle H, Neuhaus P, Hochhaus A, Hartmann JT, Gellert K, Ridwelski K, et al. Adjuvant chemotherapy with gemcitabine and long-term outcomes among patients with resected pancreatic cancer: the CONKO-001 randomized trial. JAMA. 2013;310(14):1473–81.

66. Conroy T, Desseigne F, Ychou M, Bouché O, Guimbaud R, Bécouarn Y, et al. FOLFIRINOX versus gemcitabine for metastatic pancreatic cancer. N Engl J Med. 2011;364(19):1817–25.

67. Groot VP, Rezaee N, Wu W, Cameron JL, Fishman EK, Hruban RH, et al. Patterns, timing, and predictors of recurrence following pancreatectomy for pancreatic ductal adenocarcinoma. Ann Surg. 2018;267(5):936–45.

68. Kim YI, Song KB, Lee YJ, Park KM, Hwang DW, Lee JH, Shin SH, Kwon JW, Ro JS, Kim SC. Management of isolated recurrence after surgery for pancreatic adenocarcinoma. Br J Surg. 2019;106(7):898–909.

Role of Endoscopic Ultrasound and Endoscopic Retrograde Cholangiopancreatography in the Diagnosis and Treatment of Pancreatic Tumors

6

María Muñoz García-Borruel,
María Fernanda Guerra Veloz,
Estefanía Moreno Rincón,
and Manuel Rodríguez-Téllez

6.1 Introduction

Pancreatic cancer (PC) remains one of the most lethal malignancies with little improvement in survival over the past decades despite advances in diagnosis and treatment. The incidence of pancreatic cancer is increasing, with 458,918 new cases diagnosed worldwide and 432,242 deaths in 2018, according to the GLOBOCAN 2018 estimation [1]. Most patients diagnosed with PC present at an advanced stage of the disease when surgical treatment is no longer possible. Only 15–20% of patients present with potentially resectable tumors [2], but pancreatic surgery associates a high morbidity and mortality; thus, early diagnosis and accurate staging are necessary. To evaluate the resectability of PC, it is important that lymphovascular invasion and liver metastasis are appropriately evaluated. When the cancer is unresectable, oncologic treatment such as chemotherapy or radiotherapy could improve the quality of life and enhance overall survival.

Radial EUS provides cross-sectional imaging, similar to computed tomography (CT) and lineal type shows views in the same plane as the shaft of the endoscope, similar to trans-abdominal US. With EUS, it is possible to position the transducer in direct proximity to the pancreas. The lesions within of pancreatic head and uncinate process are visualized from duodenum, whereas lesions in the body and tail are best assessed from the gastro-esophageal junction (GOJ) and the stomach. High-resolution images of the pancreas are obtained using a frequency of 5–20 MHz to offer the best ratio between image resolution and depth of the field, without the disrupting effects of interfering gas, fat, and bone. The procedure is performed under sedation and usually with the patient on a left lateral position.

EUS is now an accurate method for staging malignancies of the pancreatico-biliary system and other digestive malignancies. The most valuable role of EUS is the ability to identify

M. Muñoz García-Borruel (✉) · M. F. Guerra Veloz
M. Rodríguez-Téllez
Gastroenterology and Endoscopy Department, Virgen
Macarena University Hospital, Seville, Spain
e-mail: m.munozgb@gmail.com;
maferguerrita@hotmail.com;
mrodrigueztellez@gmail.com

E. Moreno Rincón
Gastroenterology and Endoscopy Department,
Virgen Macarena University Hospital, Seville, Spain

Gastroenterology and Endoscopy Department,
The Royal London Hospital, London, UK
e-mail: estefania.mr.86@gmail.com

Table 6.1 EUS features of the main pancreatic lesions

	Adenocarcinoma	Neuroendocrine tumors (TNEs)	Cystic neoplasms
EUS	Hypoechogenic and heterogeneous	Hypoechoic, homogeneous, clearly demarcated, round	Mural thickening, microcalcifications, nodules, communication with the main pancreatic duct, septa, or microcysts
Doppler	Mainly arterial-type signals	Hypervascular	Avascular
CE-EUS	Isoenhancement or hypoenhancement, arterial irregularity, and absent venous vasculature	Clear hypersignal	Contrast enhancement of the walls/septa/nodule
Elastography	Blue pattern	Heterogeneous/blue-green pattern	–
Comments	80% of all pancreatic cancers 60–70% pancreatic head EUS-FNA: cytology/histology	Insulinomas and gastrinomas most common EUS-FNA: Ki-67	10–15% of pancreatic cystic lesions Heterogeneous group (IPMN, mucinous, cystadenoma, etc.) EUS-FNA: cytology, amylase, glucose, CEA, DNA

which patients will be unlikely to have a curative surgical excision due to vascular invasion or regional nodal metastasis. Nowadays, EUS and its associated procedures, including contrast-enhanced EUS (CE-EUS), EUS elastography, and EUS-guided fine needle aspiration (EUS-FNA) play an essential role in the clinical evaluation of PC, including the detection of small cancers, the differential diagnosis of pancreatic solid or cystic lesions and the staging of PC (Table 6.1).

6.2 Role of EUS for Diagnosis of Pancreatic Cancer

Multidetector computed tomography (MDCT) is the standard of care method for an initial evaluation of patients with suspicion of PC. MDCT can detect the primary tumor, assess the presence of vascular involvement and identify nodal or distant metastasis. MRI has similar sensitivity and specificity in PC diagnosis, but is less available and more expensive than CT. Nevertheless, MRI provides an exceptional view of the biliary and pancreatic duct. Also, it is superior to CT in evaluating isoattenuated pancreatic lesions and the characterization of indeterminate or small liver lesions.

PC without vascular involvement can receive surgical treatment, and a CT scan can obviate the need for EUS in these cases. Some authors recommend EUS to provide a second staging assessment to prevent major surgery. However, the EUS indication should not delay surgical intervention.

Multiple studies have demonstrated that EUS is shown more sensitive, specific, and accurate in detecting pancreatic lesions than high-quality cross-sectional imaging (sensitivity 100% for EUS vs. 86% for MDCT) [3–5], particularly with small diameter pancreatic lesions (0.5–2 cm). In addition, this technique can provide tissue sampling by EUS-guided fine needle aspiration (EUS-FNA) or fine needle biopsy (EUS-FNB).

EUS imaging findings supporting a PC diagnosis in chronic pancreatitis settings are the following: mass size above 2 cm, irregular dilatation of the main pancreatic duct and side branch ducts, vascularity of the mass, absence of cysts within and presence of lymphadenopathy and vascular invasion [6, 7]. However, EUS has some limitations in the differential diagnosis between PC and mass-forming chronic pancreatitis or autoimmune pancreatitis. Some ancillary techniques such as contrast-enhanced EUS (CE-EUS) and elastography can improve the characterization of these pancreatic lesions.

CE-EUS was first reported in 1995 with an intra-arterial infusion of CO_2. It is a technique that combines high-resolution endoscopy ultrasound waves with intravenous contrast. Contrast

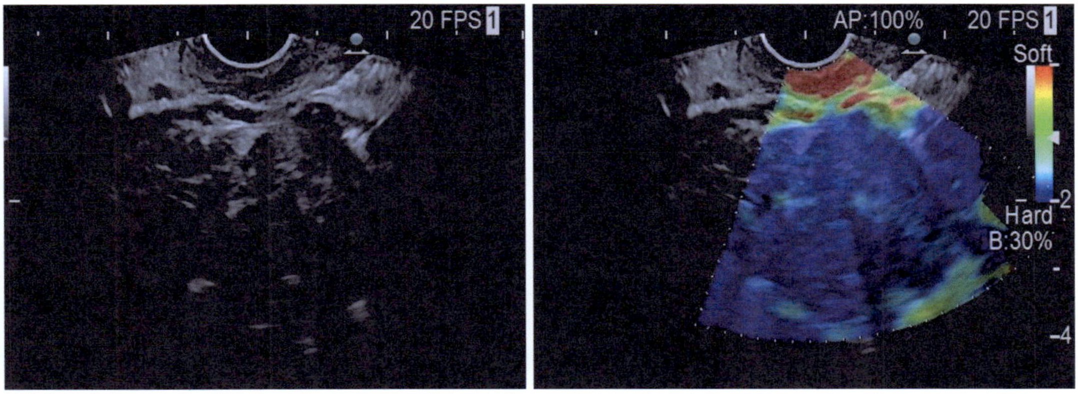

Fig. 6.1 Malignant pancreatic mass. With elastography it shows a blue pattern

agents consist of gas-filled microbubbles of approximately 2–5 ml in diameter, encapsulated by a phospholipid or lipid shell [8]. Many contrast agents are commercially available (Levovist®, Sonovue®, Sonazoid®) [9]. CE-EUS generates an acoustic signal when ultrasound waves interact with oscillating microbubbles in the intravenous contrast. Therefore, these acoustic signals provide information about echogenicity and help in the assessment of vascularity of pancreatic lesions. PC usually shows isoenhancement or hypoenhancement, arterial irregularity, and absent venous vasculature, while hyperenhanced lesions with preserved architecture of both arterial and venous microvasculature are a sign of chronic pancreatitis. CE-EUS provides a high accuracy in the differential diagnosis of PC and chronic pancreatitis (sensitivity 91%, specificity 93%, positive predictive value 100%, and negative predictive value 88%) [10, 11]. It helps in the differential diagnosis of cystic pancreatic lesions, such as mucinous cystic neoplasm (irregular enhancement of intralesional septum and nodule), serous cystadenoma (enhancement of intracystic septation), benign intraductal papillary mucinous neoplasms (IPMN) (polypoidal non-invasive papillary nodule) and malignancy IPMN (invasive and papillary mural nodule).

Elastography was first reported in 2006 [8]. It is a newer non-invasive technique that evaluates the stiffness or elasticity of a target lesion compared to the surrounding normal tissue. The equipment can be coupled with conventional EUS without the need for additional devices. EUS transducer sends a shearing wave through the pancreas and generates an elastogram by calculating the velocity faced by the shearing wave while passing through soft tissue [11]. Elastography may help in the differentiation between malignant and benign masses. The elastography data can be displayed qualitatively as a color overlay on the standard B-mode image. PCs are firm lesions appearing as blue (Fig. 6.1), inflammatory lesions appear as green or yellow and soft lesions as red. Three meta-analyses have reported a 95–97% pooled sensitivity and 67–76% specificity of EUS elastography in reliable solid PC diagnosis [12, 13].

In summary, the role of these ancillary techniques could be useful in clinical practice by allowing the differentiation between different pancreatic lesions. Furthermore, they enable targeted biopsies in complicated diagnostic situations.

6.2.1 EUS-Guided Tissue Diagnosis

The development of linear array endoscopes in the 1990s offered the possibility of performing fine needle aspiration biopsy during EUS (EUS-FNA), and this is the main advantage of EUS. It is an efficient technique with high diagnostic accuracy and good safety profile. The ability to obtain tissue confirmation plays a critical role in identifying those patients unsuitable for surgical treatment but who would benefit from palliative treatment. Another important application of EUS-FNA is the detection of malignant lymph nodes. The results of EUS-FNA of pancreatic masses are excellent because its accuracy is 85–92%, the sensitivity of 85–90%, and the specificity of 92–100% [11, 14].

A pathological diagnosis is needed when a cross-sectional imaging technique shows a pancreatic mass with a high suspicion of malignancy. Before the EUS, the acquisition of tissue was made by US or CT-guided percutaneous biopsy or ERCP-guided bile brush cytology or surgical exploration. Nowadays, EUS-FNA biopsy is the preferred method.

The needle is precisely introduced into the target lesion because it is advanced in the same plane as the US image (Fig. 6.2). Tissue acquisition from neck, body, and tail lesions can be obtained by positioning an echoendoscope in GOJ or proximal stomach. In contrast, tissue from the uncinate, head and neck lesions can be performed by positioning echoendoscope in the duodenal bulb or second portion of the duodenum.

The sample can be either a cytology specimen obtained through a hollow needle (fine needle aspiration, FNA) or a fine core of tissue acquired through a specially designed needle (fine needle biopsy, FNB). These needles are available in different diameters, from 19 to 25 G. Small caliber needles (25 G) have a similar cytology yield as larger caliber needles (19 G) with less blood contamination and greater flexibility. In the study of cystic pancreatic lesions, EUS-FNA can obtain cyst fluid analysis for cytology, mucin-containing goblet cells, tumor markers like carcinoembryonic antigen or CEA, amylase, glucose, and DNA genetic mutation analysis like K-ras [11], that may help to establish the diagnosis of cystic pancreatic lesions.

EUS-guided FNA targets the pancreatic lesion under direct vision. The recommendation is to obtain a tissue sample from different areas of the lesion, with the FNA needle close to the EUS probe. Although there is a risk of needle tract seeding with EUS-FNA, this is often not a concern because after the surgery the potential sites of seeding are removed and the patients with unresectable PC die mostly due to disease progression before any seeding is detected.

The rapid on-site evaluation (ROSE) of cytology specimens has reduced the need for multiple passes. If there is no on-site cytopathologist available, it is recommended to do at least 5–6 passes for pancreatic lesions and 2–3 passes for lymph nodes and metastasis to improve the diagnostic yield. The EUS-FNB provides core tissue with preserved architecture that could differentiate malignancy from other lesions such as autoimmune pancreatitis, chronic pancreatitis, pancreatic lymphoma, or tuberculosis. Besides, it could provide additional tissue for molecular profiling. The technical considerations and safety are the same as EUS-FNA but the diagnostic yield seems to be higher and it may eradicate the need for ROSE [11, 15].

There is consensus that it is reasonable to obtain a tissue diagnosis in patients with suspected PC who are poor surgical candidates. Histologic confirmation in such patients can help decide on chemotherapy or radiotherapy. More controversial is the role of EUS-FNA in patients whose pancreatic lesions seem to be resectable on other imaging studies.

6.2.1.1 Indications of EUS-FNA

1. To exclude tumors other than ductal adenocarcinomas, such as lymphoma, small cell metastasis, or neuroendocrine tumor because they will require a different management strategy.
2. To obtain cytological or histological confirmation of malignancy in patients with borderline operable and inoperable tumors, before neoadjuvant or palliative chemotherapy.

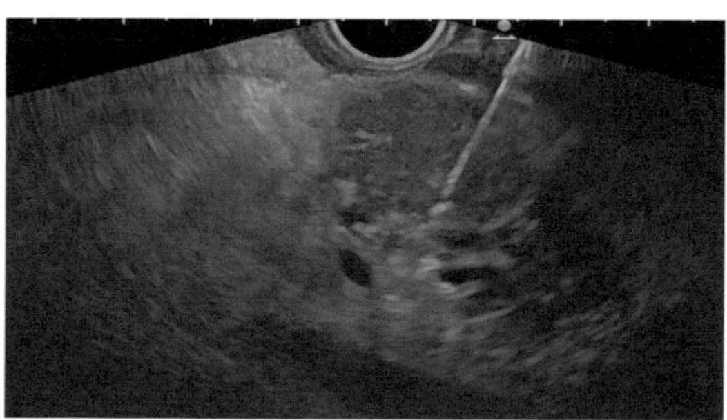

Fig. 6.2 EUS-FNA of solid lesion in pancreatic head

3. If the patient or the surgeon desire to obtain histological confirmation before performing a major surgery.
4. When the presence of malignancy is uncertain (e.g., fibrous nodule or an inflammatory pseudotumor in chronic calcific pancreatitis).

6.2.1.2 Safety and Complications

EUS-FNA is considered a safe procedure with a low rate of complications (overall 2.5%) [11]. It has been reported complications such as pancreatitis, which is the most common one (0–3.4%), bleeding, infection, and other rare but serious events such as intestinal perforation and biliary peritonitis. The current standard of care includes the administration of prophylactic antibiotics for patients undergoing FNA of cystic pancreatic lesions to decrease the risk of infection. As mentioned before, the risk of malignant peritoneal seeding is minimal compared with other techniques such as percutaneous biopsy (2.2 vs. 16.3%) [16]. The frequency and severity of these adverse events vary between centers and may be related to operator experience.

6.2.2 Pancreatic Cancer Screening

In pancreatic carcinogenesis, the normal pancreatic ductal epithelium evolves into infiltrative carcinoma in a sequential process. There are multiple risk factors for PC such as smoking (the most important, with active smokers having a twofold increased risk of developing PC), Ashkenazi Jewish descent, diabetes, and factors related to dietary habits (obesity, alcohol, red meat intake, low fruit, and vegetable intake). Furthermore, it is estimated that 5–10% of PCs arise due to genetic susceptibility and (or) familial aggregation, and patients with hereditary factors constitute high-risk individuals [5].

Pancreatic cancer screening in general population is not recommended given the low disease prevalence and lack of cost-effectiveness. However, some data suggest that an early diagnosis can lead to an increased survival in high-risk individuals. A recent American Gastroenterological Association Institute–commissioned clinical practice update, some experts describe the indications for screening for PC in high-risk individuals [17]:

- Consider PC screening in first-degree relatives of pancreatic cancer patients with ≥2 affected genetically related family members.
- Consider screening in patients with Peutz-Jeghers syndrome (PJS); hereditary pancreatitis; *CDKN2A*, *BRCA1*, *BRCA2*, *PALB2*, or *ATM* mutations; or ≥1 first-degree relative with PC with Lynch syndrome.
- Consider genetic testing and counseling for familial pancreatic cancer relatives.
- Pursue participation in an appropriate hepato-pancreato-biliary center or registry for high-risk patients.
- Average-risk individuals do not warrant screening for PC.
- In most high-risk individuals, it advisable to start screening at age 50 or 10 years before the affected relative's age of onset. In patients with CDKN2S and PRSS1 mutations it advisable to start screening at age 40 and in PJS at age 35.

AGA's experts recommend MRI and EUS together as the main screening modalities. Screening intervals of 12 months should be considered when there are no concerning pancreatic lesions, with shortened intervals and (or) the performance of EUS in 6–12 months directed to lesions determined to be low risk (by a multidisciplinary team). EUS evaluation should be performed within 3–6 months for indeterminate lesions and 3 months for high-risk lesions if surgical resection is not planned. It is recommended to stop screening when patients are no longer candidates for pancreatic surgery or have significant comorbidities.

6.3   Role of EUS for the Staging of Pancreatic Cancer

The cross-sectional imaging techniques (CT and MRI) are useful for accurate staging of the tumor and remain the first-line imaging of choice because of their non-invasive nature and widespread availability. Approximately 85% of PCs are inoperable at the time of diagnosis due to the existence of metastatic disease or major vessel invasion. If there is no metastatic disease, operability depends on the extent of local disease, particularly the presence or absence of vascular and lymph node involvement. According to the American Hepato-Pancreato-Biliary Association consensus report, and based on imaging results, the disease is categorized into three groups: operable, borderline operable, and locally advanced inoperable disease [18] (Fig. 6.3). Performance, nutritional status, and medical comorbidities are

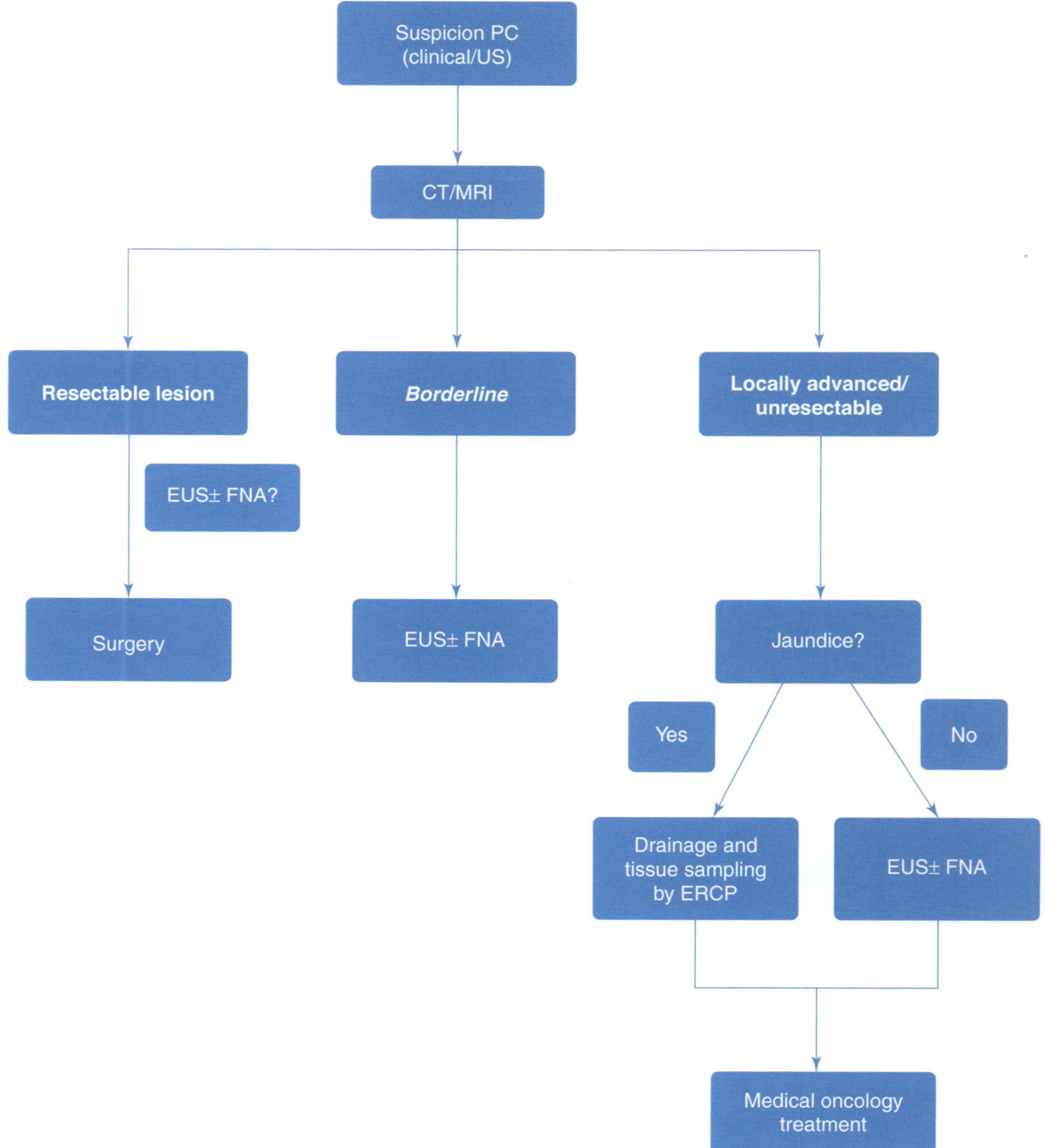

Fig. 6.3 Algorithm for the evaluation and management of patients with suspected pancreatic adenocarcinoma based on current guidelines

Table 6.2 The 8th edition of TNM staging system of pancreatic cancer

T1	Limited to the pancreas, tumor diameter ≤2 cm
T2	Limited to the pancreas, tumor diameter >2 cm and ≤4 cm
T3	Limited to the pancreas, tumor diameter >4 cm
T4	Tumor involves the coeliac axis, SMA, or common hepatic artery
N0	No regional lymph node metastasis
N1	Metastasis 1–3 regional lymph nodes
N2	Metastasis in ≥4 regional lymph nodes
M0	No distant metastasis
M1	Distant metastasis

SMA Superior mesenteric artery

Table 6.3 Echoendoscopic criteria for vascular invasion

The presence of collateral veins around a pancreatic mass erases the usual anatomical location of a portal vessel
Presence of tumor in the vascular lumen
Abnormal vascular profile due to compression of a vessel by the pancreatic mass. Also, by a loss of the hyperechoic interface between the vessel and the parenchyma

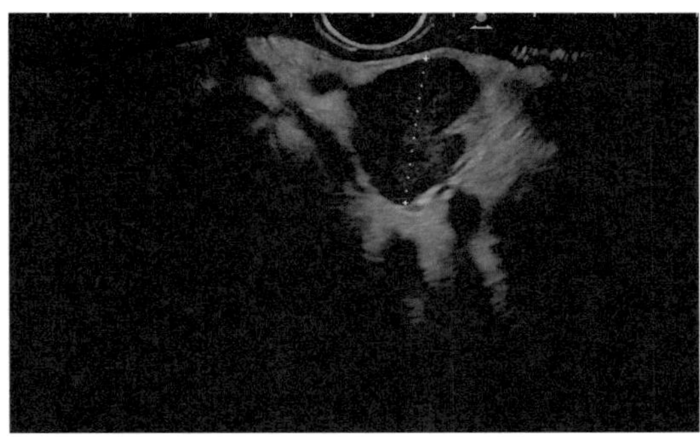

Fig. 6.4 Malignant lymphadenopathy located in celiac plexus

essential factors for all patients with PC considered for any significant treatment modality (surgery, chemotherapy, or radiation). Advanced age usually is not a contraindication for any of these treatments. Nowadays, PC staging is based on the tumor node metastasis (TNM) (Table 6.2).

EUS is now largely used in the staging of pancreatic adenocarcinoma. EUS can provide accurate loco-regional staging and complement the findings of cross-sectional imaging, especially in cases of borderline operable disease or in cases where CT and MRI cannot detect a mass due to the enhancement pattern of the lesion. EUS also provides additional objective data on perivascular cuffing, assessment of liver masses, and local lymph nodes for the staging of PCs, especially in those individuals who have undergone prior chemotherapy treatment. The great advantage of EUS is the EUS-FNA, which allows up to 95% diagnostic accuracy. Besides, this technique also permits the sampling of atypical lymph nodes (portocaval especially) to check for tumors with distant metastasis, a finding which would contraindicate radical resection. In addition, an emerging role for EUS is the detection of small, occult liver metastasis in patients with PC, which can be sampled.

T-Staging

EUS is superior to CT for T-staging with less risk of over staging because it is more sensitive and less specific than CT. The sensitivity for both techniques is 86% [19]. The sensitivity and specificity of EUS for detection of tumor vascular invasion range from 42% to 91% and 89% to 100%, respectively (Table 6.3) [8]. The sensitivity of the technique depends on the target vessel and is higher than CT for portal vein (around 80%) and lower for celiac artery and superior mesenteric vessels because it is technically difficult to provide entire images of these vessels [8, 20].

N-Staging

EUS is less accurate and sensitive for N-staging. The diagnostic accuracy varies from 64 to 82% and is superior in combination with EUS-FNA [21]. In a meta-analysis (16 studies) the pooled sensitivity was 69% and the specificity was 81% [22]. There are some criteria for identifying lymph node metastasis such as spherical shape, hypoechoic node, well-delineated boundaries, and 10 mm diameter or more (Fig. 6.4), although these features are usually not enough to exclude malignancy and EUS-FNA is often needed.

M-Staging

CT and MRI are superior to EUS. However, its high resolution and proximity to the left lobe and inferior right lobe of the liver can lead to the detection of small liver metastases. EUS may also identify and allow performing ascitic tap [23].

EUS has some limitations. Peritumoral inflammatory changes and attenuation of the ultrasound beam in large tumors may affect the accuracy of EUS staging, and, as a consequence, PC less than 3 cm are more accurately staged with EUS. Structures located more than 5 cm from the EUS probe are challenging to assess, and EUS has a limited role in assessing distant lymph nodes or metastatic disease. Furthermore, in cases where the anatomy is surgically altered or distorted by the presence of a biliary stent, it may not be possible to obtain optimal imaging. Similarly, in patients with chronic pancreatitis, the presence of pancreatic calcifications can significantly limit image quality.

In conclusion, EUS is an important tool in the evaluation of pancreatic lesions and should be considered complementary to other imaging modalities in establishing accurate staging of pancreatic cancer.

6.4 Role of EUS in Treatment

The therapeutic spectrum of EUS has turned endoscopy into an integral component of palliative treatment in patients with unresectable PC. There are currently emerging EUS-guided therapeutic techniques that play an essential role, providing biliary drainage, treating pain, and delivering implants and injections into pancreatic tumors.

6.4.1 Celiac Plexus Neurolysis/Block

Pain is one of the most prevalent symptoms in PC and its management is sometimes challenging. EUS-guided celiac plexus neurolysis is a technique used in patients with unresectable PC, with the objective of achieving pain control and reducing the need for opioids.

EUS identifies the location of the celiac plexus at the junction between the celiac trunk and aorta.

With a dedicated 20 G needle with multiple side holes, bupivacaine and dehydrated 98% alcohol or phenol are injected into the celiac plexus. There are central or bilateral techniques. In the central approach, the needle is directed centrally at the junction of the aorta and the celiac artery. In the bilateral approach, the echoendoscope is rotated clockwise to advance the needle adjacent to the celiac artery to the point of origin of SMA from the aorta [11].

EUS-guided celiac plexus neurolysis is a relatively safe alternative compared to CT or fluoroscopically guided plexus neurolysis. The main side effects are local pain, hypotension, and diarrhea.

6.4.2 EUS Fine Needle Injection and Radiofrequency Ablation

EUS fine needle injection (FNI) is a rapidly emerging technique used to deliver implants and injections into pancreatic lesions under direct EUS visualization. This technique is very safe and minimally invasive. EUS-guided implantation of fiducial markers into the pancreatic tumor or local lymph nodes enables stereotactic radiotherapy, and direct injection of antitumor agents may provide localized chemotherapy. Furthermore, the preoperative EUS-guided injection of dye (India ink, carbon particles, or indocyanine) to mark the lesion is increasingly used for the localization of operable pancreatic tumors.

Radiofrequency ablation is performed with an adapted probe designed to induce thermal necrosis of focal pancreatic lesions such as small PCs and NETs in patients who are not fit for surgery.

6.4.3 Biliary Drainage

ERCP-guided drainage is the most used technique for biliary drainage of PCs with a success rate of over 90% [24]. Sometimes this procedure is not possible because of duodenal distorted anatomy, postoperative changes, or abnormal ampulla, representing 3–10% of failure [25]. Alternatives to failed ERCP are percutaneous transhepatic biliary drainage or surgery, but they associate with a high risk of complications. EUS-guided drainage is a promising salvage technique with technical and clinical success rates comparable to ERCP. EUS-guided drainage presents a low risk of pancreatitis and longer stent patency, and the use of metal stents has reduced stent-related complications. This technique is considered safer than other alternative procedures [11]. Complications associated with EUS-biliary drainage are bleeding, perforation, bile leak, stent migration, and infection. However, the rate of complications can be reduced by performing this procedure in expert centers.

EUS-biliary drainage can be performed with either extrahepatic or intrahepatic techniques depending on the anatomy and technical feasibility. Both approaches are similar in technical and clinical success rates. EUS-guided choledocho-duodenostomy is an extrahepatic technique where the dilated CBD can be visualized from the antrum or duodenal bulb. After inserting a transduodenal needle into CBD, a needle track is created over guidewire and a transluminal or transpapillary stent is deployed (Fig. 6.5). The intrahepatic techniques are EUS-guided hepaticogastrostomy with antegrade stent placement, where the tip of the EUS scope is positioned along the gastric lesser curvature to visualize the dilated left hepatic duct. After inserting a 19 or 22 G transgastric needle into the lumen of the left hepatic duct under fluoroscopic and EUS guidance, the needle track is dilated over the guidewire with a 6.5-Fr cystotome to create a hepatogastric fistula and a fully covered or partially covered self-expandable metal stent (SEMS) can be deployed. A transpapillary stent could be deployed with antegrade advancement of the wire or with a EUS-guided rendezvous (EUS-RV) technique.

6.4.4 Role of EUS in Gastric Outlet Obstruction

Nonbilious vomiting, nausea, dehydration, and malnutrition are the initial symptoms of gastric outlet obstruction (GOO). In most patients, the progression of PC causes GOO due to extrinsic duodenal compression. Palliative treatment is aimed to improve the nutritional status and to resolve symptoms of GOO. EUS-gastrojejunostomy (GJ) is a minimally invasive endoscopic technique that can be an alternative to duodenal stenting and surgical GJ [11], and it should only be performed by advanced therapeutic endoscopists. There are two modalities, a balloon-assisted gastroenterostomy and direct EUS-gastroenterostomy [26].

EUS-GJ is a safe modality in the management of malignant GOO compared to surgical bypass, with higher technical and clinical success rates

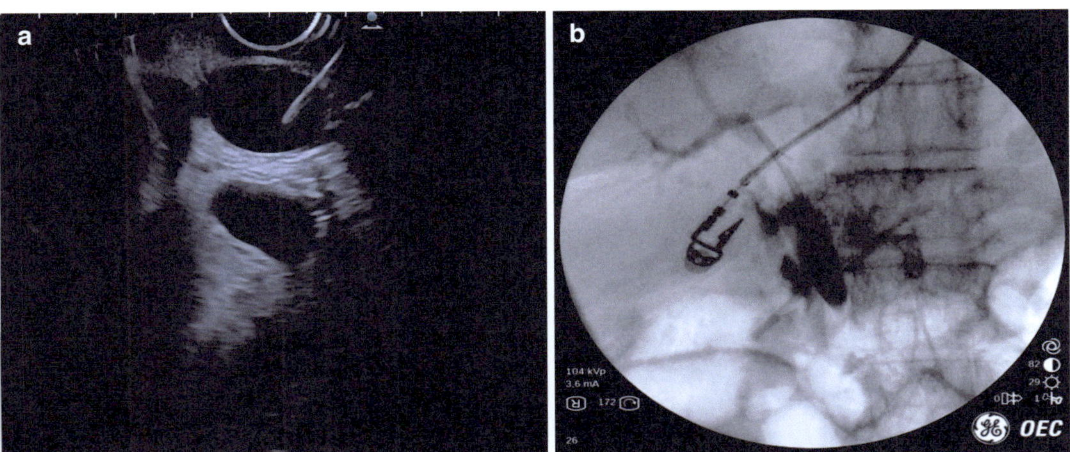

Fig. 6.5 EUS-guided choledochoduodenostomy (**a**) Needle into CBD, (**b**) Biliary stent deployed

and lower risk of adverse events [27]. Complications of EUS-GJ are perforation, bleeding, peritonitis, and luminal obstruction of the stent due to food impaction.

6.5 Role of ERCP in Pancreatic Cancer

The principal utility of ERCP in pancreatic tumors is centered in biliary drainage of unresectable tumors and preoperative drainage in resectable tumors [2]. Nowadays, with the advancement of diagnostic imaging modalities and EUS, the ERCP has a minor role in the initial diagnosis of PC [3]. ERCP-guided biliary tissue sampling in diagnosing PC is suggested if a therapeutic intervention during the same procedure is required [28].

Endoscopy is often combined with fluoroscopy and contrast medium, permitting a detailed visualization of the anatomy of the pancreaticobiliary ductal system.

6.5.1 Indications

1. In the initial diagnosis of pancreatic duct stenosis, or another abnormal pancreatic duct finding without mass lesions, that could not be characterized by other imaging techniques.
2. Preoperative endoscopic biliary drainage, in patients with resectable PC and active cholangitis, severe symptomatic jaundice, or in those whom resection for cure cannot be scheduled within 2 weeks of diagnosis.
3. Biliary drainage in patients with unresectable PC and jaundice.
4. Palliative option in patients with gastric outlet obstruction due to tumor progression.

6.6 Role of ERCP for Diagnosis of Pancreatic Cancer

MDCT, MRI, and EUS are recommended as a diagnostic tool in subjects with suspected PC [2]. However, ERCP can be considered pathognomonic when it shows a double stop on the main bile and pancreatic duct. Moreover, ERCP is recommended for the diagnosis of pancreatic duct stenosis, which is difficult to differentiate from inflammatory lesions by other imaging modalities or could be a manifestation of early PC [29].

Recently published Asian consensus guidelines recommended ERCP-guided biliary sampling for an unresectable mass when there is a concurrent need for biliary decompression, however, for resectable masses, or when ERCP tissue acquisition is unsuccessful, EUS-guided fine needle biopsy is preferred [28]. Fluoroscopy-guided biliary brush cytology, biliary biopsy, and cholangioscopy-guided biopsy are the most common ERCP techniques for tissue acquisition [30].

6.6.1 ERCP-Tissue Sampling

6.6.1.1 Brush Cytology
This technique remains the first line and most used method of acquiring tissue at the time of ERCP with minimal risk of adverse events such as pancreatitis and bile duct perforation. However, the technique is simple and easy to perform with an excellent specificity, however, its sensibility is not adequate, ranging from 30 to 57% according to some studies [31].

Theoretically, cytology from pancreatic duct brushing and pancreatic duct juice collection (after the administration of intravenous secretin) may increase the diagnostic rate of PC, nevertheless, it is considered technically difficult and has been found to be impossible in more than 25% of the time because of malignancy-related duct disruption [32]. In this scenario, post-ERCP pancreatitis rate was assumed to be higher in cases of benign stricture and relatively low in cases of malignancy, ranging from 0 to 21.5%.

Biliary brush cytology is obtained by advancing 6 or 8 Fr cytology brush over a guidewire beyond the stricture, especially biliary tree, using a specialized catheter. The brush is moved back and forth across the stricture to obtain an adequate sample, approximately 10 times. The brush is then withdrawn into the catheter before removal of the endoscope as a unit. It had showed that removing the brush and catheter together improves cancer detection and prevents contamination [31].

6.6.1.2 Endobiliary Forceps Biopsy

Fluoroscopic-guided biliary biopsy improves the diagnostic over simple biliary brush cytology by obtaining biliary tissue sampling deeper to the epithelial layer. Nonetheless, this remains a technically challenging and user-dependent procedure that is performed less frequently than brush cytology.

Forceps biopsy can be performed by passing 5–10 Fr biopsy forceps at the lower edge of stricture after a sphincterotomy or with an intact papilla. The optimum number of biopsy specimens to obtain has not been established, however, some authors suggest a minimum of three tissue samples [33].

Using this technique, a few adverse events, such as bleeding and perforation of common hepatic duct, secondary to a variety of factors—forceps size and stiffness, number of biopsy passes, and the technical capability of the endoscopist—could be expected examples [31].

6.6.1.3 Multimodal Tissue Sampling

Several studies have shown that the combination of multiple ERCP tissue sampling can improve the cancer detection rate. The combination of forceps biopsy and brush cytology has increased the sensibility and specificity with a pooled sensitivity of 63–86% and a specificity of 97–100%. Jailwala et al. [34] showed that patients who underwent sequential brushing, endoscopic FNA, and biopsy sampling (always in that order) had a cancer detection rate of 62%. This author suggests that at least two techniques should be used to obtain samples.

Another retrospective study of triple modality (brush cytology, forceps biopsy sampling, and fluorescence in situ hybridization (FISH)) showed an increase in the sensitivity to 82%, with 100% specificity. As expected, the individual sensitivities of the techniques were low [35].

FISH is a cytogenetic technique for detecting and locating a specific DNA sequence on a chromosome. It is known that most solid tumors are aneuploid or contain an abnormal number of chromosomes. These molecular abnormalities have been identified in approximately 80% of biliary and PC [36].

Several other molecular techniques (flow cytometry, digital image analysis, and molecular analysis) have demonstrated promise at one time or another but have not gained widespread use or have fallen out of favor entirely.

6.6.1.4 Cholangiopancreatoscopic-Guided Biopsy

This technique allows direct visualization of the lumen of the bile and pancreatic duct. Conventionally it involved a *"mother–baby"* scope setup, which required two endoscopists and had issues with scope fragility. However, with the introduction of ultra-slim gastroscope loaded with anchoring balloon (a slight modification in this technique) a single operator could perform this procedure without issues of scope fragility [31].

The Spyglass system involves the use of a disposable SpyScope with a tip-deflecting access catheter, working catheter, SpyBite biopsy forceps, and two irrigation channels enabling a single operator to perform the procedure.

ERCP-guided pancreatoscopy with biopsy may be helpful in the diagnosis of main pancreatic duct IPMN, particularly due to its classic, pathognomonic features of fish egg-like, villous, and prominent mucosal protrusions. Cholangioscopy has shown at 88–100% sensitive and 77–92% specific for the diagnosis of pancreatico-biliary malignancy [37]. This technique has twofold higher risk of therefore, it should be reserved for selected cases of inaccessible ductal lesions [38].

6.7   Role of ERCP in Treatment

6.7.1   ERCP in Preoperative Biliary Drainage in Resectable Pancreatic Cancer

Surgical resection is the only option for cure for patients newly diagnosed with PC. The decision as to whether patients with resectable pancreatic adenocarcinoma require preoperative biliary drainage for obstructive jaundice has long been debated. Some studies reported an increased risk of postoperative infectious complications, morbidity, and mortality after ERCP preoperative biliary drainage, however, in most of them the higher rate of complications came from the preoperative cholangitis and not from differences in postoperative complications related to jaundice [39].

ERCP-guided biliary drainage or decompression with transpapillary stenting is the backbone of management for patients with biliary obstruction and its related complications (Fig. 6.6). Current guidelines indicate preoperative biliary drainage (PBD) should be reserved for patients with cholangitis, severe symptomatic jaundice (e.g., intense pruritus), or delayed surgery, or for before neoadjuvant chemotherapy in jaundiced patients [2, 40].

For preoperative biliary drainage, the use of self-expandable metal stents (SEMS) should be preferred over plastic stents since they are associated with significantly lower complication rate and stent dysfunction, with a similar surgical complication rate [41]. Same results were shown for neoadjuvant therapy, the use of fully covered SEMS resulted in a longer stent patency duration and fewer days of delay in neoadjuvant therapy compared with plastic stents and uncovered SEMS [42, 43]. Moreover, fully covered SEMS present the advantage of being removable if surgical resection is finally not performed. SEMSs could prolong operative duration; however, these do not compromise R0 resection or increase the risk of local unresectability [44].

6.7.2 ERCP Biliary Drainage in Unresectable Pancreatic Cancer

Biliary obstruction secondary to tumor infiltration of the bile duct is a very common complication of PC (Fig. 6.7). Obstructive jaundice is often the first clinical sign of the disease, limiting the use of chemotherapy in unresectable cases. Therefore, biliary drainage becomes essential at this stage.

Endoscopic, percutaneous, and surgical biliary drainage are techniques that could be used in patients with unresectable tumors. ERCP biliary stenting vs. surgical biliodigestive anastomosis show similar technical success rate and long-term efficacy [45]. However, endoscopic biliary drainage is associated with less complications, shorter hospital stay, better quality of life, and lower cost than the

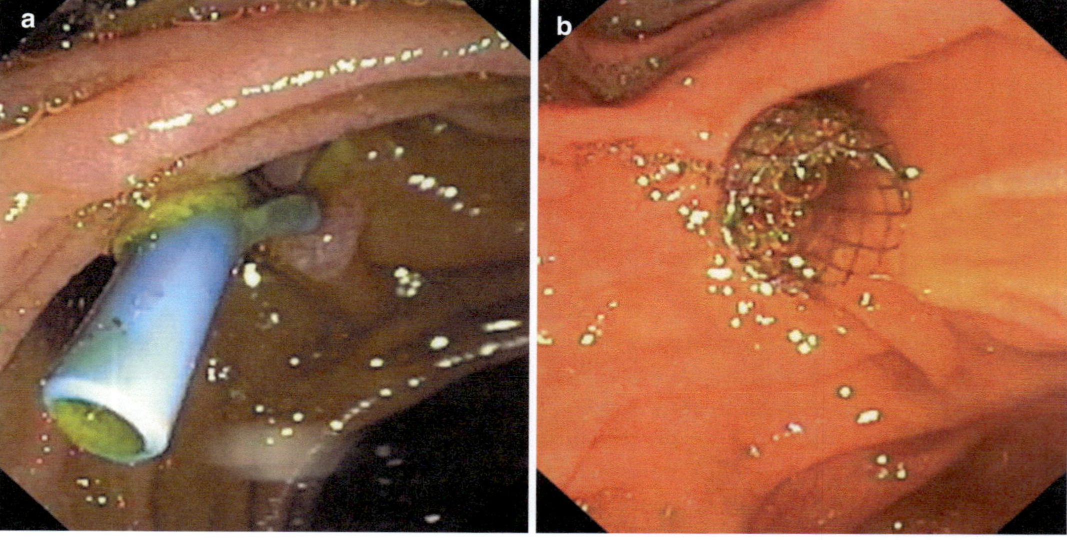

Fig. 6.6 Biliary drainage. (**a**) Plastic stent, (**b**) Uncovered metal stent

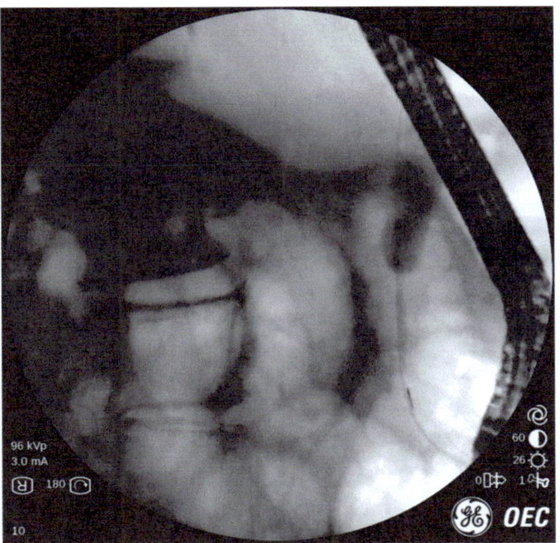

Fig. 6.7 Biliary stricture secondary to pancreatic cancer

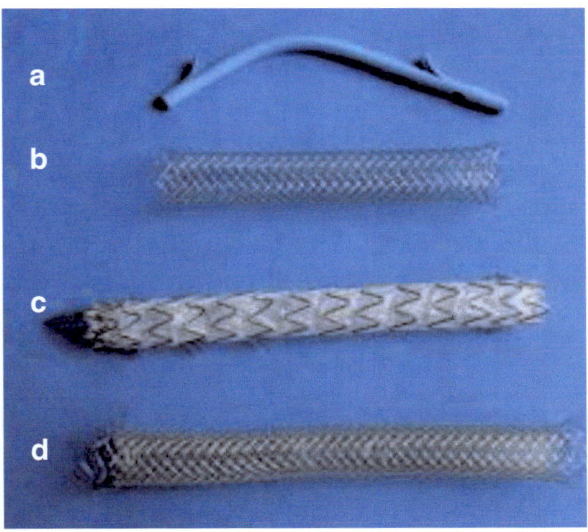

Fig. 6.8 Biliary stents. (**a**) Plastic stent, (**b**) Uncovered metal stent, (**c**) Fully covered metal stent, and (**d**) Partially covered metal stent

surgical palliative approach [46]. Moreover, biliary stenting through ERCP vs. percutaneous transhepatic biliary drainage shows lower adverse event rate, shorter hospitalization and lower total costs, longer patient survival, and less frequent peritoneal/liver recurrence [41, 47]. Biliary SEMS have a significantly longer patency rate than do plastic stents. Although it has been suggested that the use of SEMSs should be reserved for patients whose estimated survival is >3–6 months.

Current guidelines recommend that decompression of malignant extrahepatic biliary obstruction should be performed via ERCP using SEMS rather than by surgery or percutaneously. Also, they restrict the use of EUS-guided biliary drainage to cases where biliary drainage using standard ERCP techniques has failed, as mentioned before [40].

Type of Stent

Both SEMS and plastic stents are commercially available for endoscopic biliary drainage (Fig. 6.8). The selection of biliary stent subtype depends on multiple factors including dysfunction rate and need for reinterventions, complication rate, patient survival, and costs. SEMS are preferred over plastic stents because of longer luminal patency, lower rates of stent dysfunction, and overall cost.

– *Plastic stents*: Plastic biliary stents are usually made of polyethylene, polyurethane, or Teflon and these are available in different sized diameters including 7, 8.5, 10, and 11.5 Fr and lengths ranging from 5 to 15 cm. These stents are designed into various shapes—straight, curved, single, or double pigtails [30]. For decreasing the stent occlusion, a large diameter is chosen.

Plastic stents are preferred for benign lesions, whereas metal stents are favored in malignant lesions. Moreover, plastic stents offer the benefit of easy deployment, abrogate the need for biliary sphincterotomy, and are less expensive in the management of individuals with shorter life expectancies [48]. Therefore, these are not recommended in patients with longer life expectancy, as replacement is required every 10–12 weeks to sidestep stent occlusion.

– *Self-expanding metal stents*: Endoscopic biliary SEMS employ a large diameter stent (8–10 mm), which has been shown to significantly reduce the risk of stent occlusion. SEMS are manufactured as fully covered or partially covered devices. For addressing the stent dysfunction secondary to tumor ingrowth or occlusive biliary sludge showed with the first-generation SEMS (of uncovered metal), second-generation SEMS were manufactured as partially covered or fully covered devices with a polyurethane, polycaprolactone, or silicone membrane [30].

These stents had a significantly lower risk of tumor ingrowth and reduced difficulties associated with stent retrieval/removal, however, fully covered biliary SEMS present a high risk of stent migration and several specific anatomical restrictions, primarily due to their covered nature.

To summarize, uncovered SEMS are associated with higher rates of stent dysfunction due to tumor ingrowth whereas covered SEMS have a higher rate of stent migration and a lower risk of sludge-mediated occlusion. There were no differences in adverse events such as pancreatitis and cholecystitis between covered and uncovered SEMS [49].

Safety and Complications of ERCP-Guided Biliary Decompression

ERCP-guided biliary drainage is a relatively safe, minimally invasive intervention compared to percutaneous or surgical biliary decompression. The degree of obstructive jaundice, previous gastrointestinal surgeries, and multiple comorbidities have been identified as risk factors for high rates of complications during the procedure. Several complications including post-ERCP pancreatitis, cholangitis, cholecystitis, biliary ductal perforation, stent migration or obstruction, liver abscess, and hemorrhage could be expected. The complication rate is about 13% after both SEMS and plastic stents [46]. To avoid post-ERCP pancreatitis, current guidelines recommend routine administration of 100 mg of diclofenac or indomethacin intrarectally immediately before or immediately after ERCP in every patient with no contraindication.

Post-ERCP biliary infection is a serious complication that is fatal in 8–20% of cases and it is best prevented by complete biliary drainage. Routine antibiotic prophylaxis failed to show a decrease in sepsis/cholangitis after the procedure, therefore, antibiotic prophylaxis administration before biliary stenting is recommended in selected patients.

Identification of recurrent biliary obstruction due to stent occlusion is crucial. For those patients with a longer life expectancy a scheduled stent change is necessary. In case of biliary decompression using SEMS, a new procedure based on clinical criteria could be performed.

6.7.3 Role of ERCP in Gastric Outlet Obstruction

As mentioned above, an estimated 15% of patients with PC experience mechanical GOO during their disease, especially if malignant lesions involve the gastric antrum, proximal, or distal duodenum [49]. Treatment options for malignant GOO include surgical resection, surgical bypass, endoscopic stenting, and palliative decompressive gastrostomy with or without feeding tube placement. Surgery is the preferred strategy for those patients who are potential candidates for curative resection.

Endoscopic-guided enteral stent placement (SEMS placement by ERCP) is an effective palliative option in patients with a shorter life expectancy usually less than 6 months, reporting a technical success rate ranged from 91 to 100%, and clinical success from 63 to 95% [50].

Simultaneous obstructions of both gastroduodenal outlet and bile duct are often found in patients with advanced PC (Fig. 6.9). Current guidelines suggest endoscopic insertion of a biliary SEMS and an uncovered duodenal SEMS as primary treatment. The anatomical level of the malignant stricture helps to classify it into three types: type I involving proximal duodenum at the level of duodenal bulb or genu; type II second part of duodenum involving papilla; and type III or distal to papilla in the third part of duodenum. According to this classification in type I obstruction, ERCP biliary stenting should be performed prior to duodenal stent placement in cases without technical difficulties associated with endoscope passage through a duodenal stricture. In type II obstruction, ERCP-guided transpapillary stenting may be challenging due to difficulty in finding a papillary opening. In this situation, EUS-guided transmural or antegrade biliary stenting is recommended and duodenal stenting could be performed

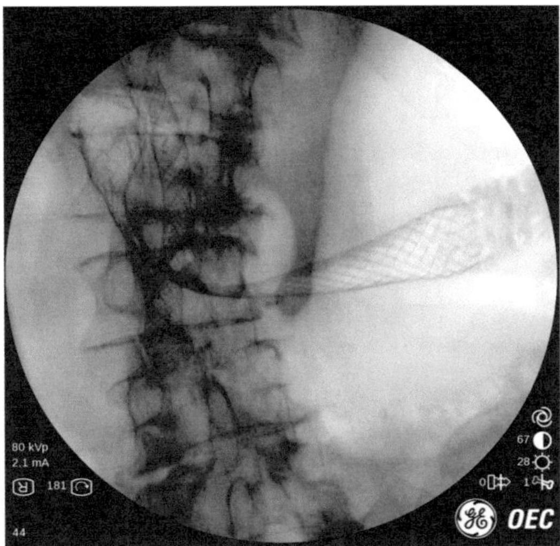

Fig. 6.9 Biliary and duodenal SEMS in a patient with pancreatic cancer and GOO

simultaneously. In type III obstruction, the sequence of either biliary or duodenal stent placement is not relevant [49]. ERCP-guided transpapillary stenting is associated with poor clinical outcomes in patients with combined biliary and GOO because of risk of cholangitis from duodenobiliar reflux of food particles and digestive juice.

Endoscopic enteral stenting should be performed in cases of a solitary malignant stricture without evidence of distal obstruction from the site of stent deployment.

Stent malfunction caused by tumor ingrowth, food impaction, or stent migration is the most reported complication and is typically managed by insertion of additional stents and/or clearance of the food impaction [50].

6.8   Conclusions

- Conventional EUS plays an important role in identifying pancreatic masses, particularly those of a small size.
- Appropriate staging of pancreatic cancer is essential to provide the correct management.
- EUS and CT are complementary methods in the staging and evaluation of resectability of pancreatic cancer.

- EUS offers a better assessment of T-staging and certain types of vascular invasion in patients with suspected pancreatic cancer.
- The possibility of obtaining samples from suspicious lesions or lymphadenopathies with EUS-FNA makes this technique essential in the management of pancreatic tumors.
- EUS-FNA allows the diagnosis of solid pancreatic lesions other than ductal adenocarcinoma, the staging of suspected or proven pancreatic cancer, and the cytological or histological study of unresectable pancreatic lesions.
- The diagnostic accuracy of conventional EUS and EUS-FNA increases with ancillary techniques such as CE-EUS and elastography.
- ERCP plays an essential role in the management of PC, principally in biliary drainage in those with resectable PC.
- In patients with unresectable PC, palliation with ERCP-guided biliary decompression by the placement of either plastic or self-expanding metal stents relieves symptoms to improve quality of life.
- ERCP-guided enteral stenting is the preferred modality over surgical gastrojejunostomy in the management of GOO in patients with poor performance and shorter life expectancy with excellent technical and clinical result.

References

1. World Health Organization. Cancer today. International Agency for Research on Cancer. Accessed November 2020. http://gco.iarc.fr/today/home
2. Ducreux M, Cuhna AS, Caramella C, Hollebecque A, Burtin P, Goéré D, et al. Cancer of the pancreas: ESMO Clinical Practice Guidelines for diagnosis, treatment and follow-up. Ann Oncol. 2015;26:v56–68.
3. Bhutani MS, Koduru P, Joshi V, Saxena P, Suzuki R, Irisawa A, et al. The role of endoscopic ultrasound in pancreatic cancer screening. Endosc Ultrasound. 2016;5:8–16. https://doi.org/10.4103/2303-9027.175876.
4. DeWitt J, Devereaux B, Chriswell M, McGreevy K, Howard T, Imperiale TF, et al. Comparison of endoscopic ultrasonography and multidetector computed tomography for detecting and staging pancreatic cancer. Ann Intern Med. 2004;141:753–63. https://doi.org/10.7326/0003-4819-141-10-200411160-00006.

5. Moutinho-Ribeiro P, Iglesias-Garcia J, Gaspar R, Macedo G. Dig Liver Dis. 2019;51(1):4–9. https://doi.org/10.1016/j.dld.2018.09.027.

6. Canto MI, Hruban RH, Fishman EK, et al. Frequent detection of pancreatic lesions in asymptomatic high-risk individuals. Gastroenterology. 2012;142:796–804. https://doi.org/10.1053/j.gastro.2012.01.005.

7. Das KK, Early D. Pancreatic cancer screening. Curr Treat Options Gastroenterol. 2017;15(4):562–75. https://doi.org/10.1007/s11938-017-0149-8.

8. Kitano M, Yoshida T, Itonaga M, Tamura T, Hatamaru K, Yamashita Y. Impact of endoscopic ultrasonography on diagnosis of pancreatic cancer. J Gastroenterol. 2019;54(1):19–32. https://doi.org/10.1007/s00535-018-1519-2.

9. Gonzalo-Marin J, Vila JJ, Pérez-Miranda M. Role of endoscopic ultrasound in the diagnosis of pancreatic cancer. World J Gastrointest Oncol. 2014;6(9):360–8. https://doi.org/10.4251/wjgo.v6.i9.360.

10. Kongkam P, Ang TL, Vu CKF, et al. Current status on the diagnosis and evaluation of pancreatic tumor in Asia with particular emphasis on the role of endoscopic ultrasound. J Gastroenterol Hepatol. 2013;28:924–30. https://doi.org/10.1111/jgh.12198.

11. Yousaf MN, Chaudhary FS, Ehsan A, et al. Endoscopicu ltrasound (EUS) and the management of pancreatic cancer. BMJ Open Gastroenterol. 2020;7:e000408. https://doi.org/10.1136/bmjgast-2020-000408.

12. Chaudhary V, Bano S. Imaging of the pancreas: recent advances. Indian J Endocrinol Metab. 2011;15:S25–32. https://doi.org/10.4103/2230-8210.83060.

13. Dewitt J, Devereaux BM, Lehman GA, et al. Comparison of endoscopic ultrasound and computed tomography for the preoperative evaluation of pancreatic cancer: a systematic review. Clin Gastroenterol Hepatol. 2006;4:717–25.

14. Mohan BP, Shakhatreh M, Garg R, et al. Comparison of Franseen and fork-tip needles for EUS-guided fine-needle biopsy of solid mass lesions: a systematic review and meta-analysis. Endosc Ultrasound. 2019;8:382–91. https://doi.org/10.4103/eus.eus_27_19.

15. Dietrich CF, Braden B, Hocke M, Ott M, Ignee A. Improved characterization of solitary solid pancreatic tumors using contrast enhanced trans-abdominal ultrasound. J Cancer Res Clin Oncol. 2008;134(6):635–43. https://doi.org/10.1007/s00432-007-0326-6.

16. van Heerde MJ, Biermann K, Zondervan PE, Kazemier G, van Eijck CHJ, Pek C, et al. Prevalence of auto-immune pancreatitis and other benign disorders in pancreatoduodenectomy for presumed malignancy of the pancreatic head. Dig Dis Sci. 2012;57:2458–65. https://doi.org/10.1007/s10620-012-2191-7.

17. Aslanian HR, Lee JH, Canto MI. AGA clinical practice update on pancreas cancer screening in high-risk individuals: expert review. Gastroenterology. 2020;159(1):358–62. https://doi.org/10.1053/j.gastro.2020.03.088.

18. Zar S, Kohoutová D, Bureš J. Pancreatic adenocarcinoma: epidemiology, Role of EUS in diagnosis, role of ERCP, endoscopic palliation. Acta Medica (Hradec Kralove). 2019;62(4):131–6. https://doi.org/10.14712/18059694.2020.1.

19. Arabul M, Karakus F, Alper E, Kandemir A, Celik M, Karakus V, Yucel K, Unsal B. Comparison of multidetector CT and endoscopic ultrasonography in malignant pancreatic mass lesions. Hepato-Gastroenterology. 2012;59(117):1599–603. https://doi.org/10.5754/hge11608.

20. Brugge WR, Lee MJ, Kelsey PB, Schapiro RH, Warshaw AL. The use of EUS to diagnose malignant portal venous system invasion by pancreatic cancer. Gastrointest Endosc. 1996;43(6):561–7. https://doi.org/10.1016/s0016-5107(96)70191-8.

21. Sakamoto H, Kitano M, Komaki T, Noda K, Chikugo T, Dote K, Takeyama Y, Das K, Yamao K, Kudo M. Prospective comparative study of the EUS guided 25-gauge FNA needle with the 19-gauge Trucut needle and 22-gauge FNA needle in patients with solid pancreatic masses. J Gastroenterol Hepatol. 2009;24(3):384–90. https://doi.org/10.1111/j.1440-1746.2008.05636.x.

22. Nawaz H, Fan CY, Kloke J, Khalid A, McGrath K, Landsittel D, Papachristou GI. Performance characteristics of endoscopic ultrasound in the staging of pancreatic cancer: a meta-analysis. JOP. 2013;14(5):484–97. https://doi.org/10.6092/1590-8577/1512.

23. Nguyen PT, Chang KJ. EUS in the detection of ascites and EUS-guided paracentesis. Gastrointest Endosc. 2001;54(3):336–9. https://doi.org/10.1067/mge.2001.117544.

24. Janssen J, Schlörer E, Greiner L. EUS elastography of the pancreas: feasibility and pattern description of the normal pancreas, chronic pancreatitis, and focal pancreatic lesions. Gastrointest Endosc. 2007;65(7):971–8. https://doi.org/10.1016/j.gie.2006.12.057.

25. Yarmohammadi H, Covey AM. Percutaneous biliary interventions and complications in malignant bile duct obstruction. Chin Clin Oncol. 2016;5(5):68. https://doi.org/10.21037/cco.2016.10.07.

26. Gohil VB, Klapman JB. Endoscopic Palliation of Pancreatic Cancer. Curr Treat Options Gastroenterol. 2017;15(3):333–48. https://doi.org/10.1007/s11938-017-0145-z.

27. Tringali A, Giannetti A, Adler DG. Endoscopic management of gastric outlet obstruction disease. Ann Gastroenterol. 2019;32(4):330–7. https://doi.org/10.20524/aog.2019.0390.

28. Nakai Y, Isayama H, Wang HP, et al. International consensus statements for endoscopic management of distal biliary stricture. J Gastroenterol Hepatol. 2020;35:967–79.

29. ASGE Standards of Practice Committee, Eloubeidi MA, Decker GA, Chandrasekhara V, et al. The role

of endoscopy in the evaluation and management of patients with solid pancreatic neoplasia. Gastrointest Endosc. 2016;83(1):17–28. https://doi.org/10.1016/j.gie.2015.09.009.

30. Yousaf MN, Ehsan H, Wahab A, et al. Endoscopic retrograde cholangiopancreatography guided interventions in the management of pancreatic cancer. World J Gastrointest Endosc. 2020;12(10):323–40. https://doi.org/10.4253/wjge.v12.i10.323.

31. Korc P, Sherman S. ERCP tissue sampling. Gastrointest Endosc. 2016;84(4):557–71. https://doi.org/10.1016/j.gie.2016.04.039.

32. McGuire DE, Venu RP, Brown R, et al. Brush cytology for pancreatic carcinoma: an analysis of factors influencing results. Gastrointest Endosc. 1996;44:300–4.

33. Tanaka H, Matsusaki S, Baba Y, Isono Y, Sase T, Okano H, Saito T, Mukai K, Murata T, Taoka H. Usefulness of endoscopic transpapillary tissue sampling for malignant biliary strictures and predictive factors of diagnostic accuracy. Clin Endosc. 2018;51(2):174–80. https://doi.org/10.5946/ce.2017.082.

34. Jailwala J, Fogel EL, Sherman S, Gottlieb K, Flueckiger J, Bucksot LG, Lehman GA. Triple-tissue sampling at ERCP in malignant biliary obstruction. Gastrointest Endosc. 2000;51(4 Pt 1):383–90. https://doi.org/10.1016/s0016-5107(00)70435-4.

35. Nanda A, Brown JM, Berger SH, Lewis MM, Barr Fritcher EG, Gores GJ, Keilin SA, Woods KE, Cai Q, Willingham FF. Triple modality testing by endoscopic retrograde cholangiopancreatography for the diagnosis of cholangiocarcinoma. Ther Adv Gastroenterol. 2015;8(2):56–65. https://doi.org/10.1177/1756283X14564674.

36. Barr Fritcher EG, Voss JS, Brankley SM, Campion MB, Jenkins SM, Keeney ME, Henry MR, Kerr SM, Chaiteerakij R, Pestova EV, Clayton AC, Zhang J, Roberts LR, Gores GJ, Halling KC, Kipp BR. An optimized set of fluorescence in situ hybridization probes for detection of pancreatobiliary tract cancer in cytology brush samples. Gastroenterology. 2015;149(7):1813–1824.e1. https://doi.org/10.1053/j.gastro.2015.08.046.

37. Chen YK, Pleskow DK. SpyGlass single-operator peroral cholangiopancreatoscopy system for the diagnosis and therapy of bile-duct disorders: a clinical feasibility study (with video). Gastrointest Endosc. 2007;65(6):832–41. https://doi.org/10.1016/j.gie.2007.01.025.

38. Sethi A, Chen YK, Austin GL, Brown WR, Brauer BC, Fukami NN, Khan AH, Shah RJ. ERCP with cholangiopancreatoscopy may be associated with higher rates of complications than ERCP alone: a single-center experience. Gastrointest Endosc. 2011;73(2):251–6. https://doi.org/10.1016/j.gie.2010.08.058.

39. Lee PJ, Podugu A, Wu D, Lee AC, Stevens T, Windsor JA. Preoperative biliary drainage in resectable pancreatic cancer: a systematic review and network meta-analysis. HPB (Oxford). 2018;20(6):477–86. https://doi.org/10.1016/j.hpb.2017.12.007.

40. Dumonceau JM, Tringali A, Papanikolaou IS, Blero D, Mangiavillano B, Schmidt A, Vanbiervliet G, Costamagna G, Devière J, García-Cano J, Gyökeres T, Hassan C, Prat F, Siersema PD, van Hooft JE. Endoscopic biliary stenting: indications, choice of stents, and results: European Society of Gastrointestinal Endoscopy (ESGE) Clinical Guideline—updated October 2017. Endoscopy. 2018;50(9):910–30. https://doi.org/10.1055/a-0659-9864.

41. Inamdar S, Slattery E, Bhalla R, Sejpal DV, Trindade AJ. Comparison of adverse events for endoscopic vs percutaneous biliary drainage in the treatment of malignant biliary tract obstruction in an inpatient national cohort. JAMA Oncol. 2016;2(1):112–7. https://doi.org/10.1001/jamaoncol.2015.3670.

42. Song TJ, Lee JH, Lee SS, Jang JW, Kim JW, Ok TJ, Oh DW, Park DH, Seo DW, Lee SK, Kim MH, Kim SC, Kim CN, Yun SC. Metal versus plastic stents for drainage of malignant biliary obstruction before primary surgical resection. Gastrointest Endosc. 2016;84(5):814–21. https://doi.org/10.1016/j.gie.2016.04.018.

43. Tol JA, van Hooft JE, Timmer R, Kubben FJ, van der Harst E, de Hingh IH, Vleggaar FP, Molenaar IQ, Keulemans YC, Boerma D, Bruno MJ, Schoon EJ, van der Gaag NA, Besselink MG, Fockens P, van Gulik TM, Rauws EA, Busch OR, Gouma DJ. Metal or plastic stents for preoperative biliary drainage in resectable pancreatic cancer. Gut. 2016;65(12):1981–7. https://doi.org/10.1136/gutjnl-2014-308762.

44. Cavell LK, Allen PJ, Vinoya C, Eaton AA, Gonen M, Gerdes H, Mendelsohn RB, D'Angelica MI, Kingham TP, Fong Y, Dematteo R, Jarnagin WR, Kurtz RC, Schattner MA. Biliary self-expandable metal stents do not adversely affect pancreaticoduodenectomy. Am J Gastroenterol. 2013;108(7):1168–73. https://doi.org/10.1038/ajg.2013.93.

45. Moss AC, Morris E, Leyden J, MacMathuna P. Malignant distal biliary obstruction: a systematic review and meta-analysis of endoscopic and surgical bypass results. Cancer Treat Rev. 2007;33(2):213–21. https://doi.org/10.1016/j.ctrv.2006.10.006.

46. Domínguez-Muñoz JE, Lariño-Noia J, Iglesias-Garcia J. Biliary drainage in pancreatic cancer: the endoscopic retrograde cholangiopancreatography perspective. Endosc Ultrasound. 2017;6(Suppl 3):S119–21. https://doi.org/10.4103/eus.eus_79_17.

47. Zorrón PL, de Moura EG, Bernardo WM, et al. Endoscopic stenting for inoperable malignant biliary obstruction: a systematic review and meta-analysis. World J Gastroenterol. 2015;21(47):13374–85. https://doi.org/10.3748/wjg.v21.i47.13374.

48. Moss AC, Morris E, Mac Mathuna P. Palliative biliary stents for obstructing pancreatic carcinoma. Cochrane Database Syst Rev. 2006;(1):CD004200. https://doi.org/10.1002/14651858.CD004200.pub2.

49. Nakai Y, Hamada T, Isayama H, Itoi T, Koike K. Endoscopic management of combined malignant biliary and gastric outlet obstruction. Dig Endosc. 2017;29(1):16–25. https://doi.org/10.1111/den.12729.
50. ASGE Standards of Practice Committee, Fukami N, Anderson MA, Khan K, Harrison ME, Appalaneni V, Ben-Menachem T, Decker GA, Fanelli RD, Fisher L, Ikenberry SO, Jain R, Jue TL, Krinsky ML, Maple JT, Sharaf RN, Dominitz JA. The role of endoscopy in gastroduodenal obstruction and gastroparesis. Gastrointest Endosc. 2011;74(1):13–21. https://doi.org/10.1016/j.gie.2010.12.003.

Interventional Biliary Radiology in Pancreatic Neoplasm

7

Antonio Linares Cuartero,
José Alberto Porfirio Camacho,
and Jesus Saenz de Zaitigui Fernández

Abbreviations

PTHC   Transhepatic Cholangiography
PTBD   Percutaneous Transhepatic Drainage
SEMS   Self-Expanding Metal Stent

7.1 Introduction

Surgical interventions were initially the only alternative for the treatment of benign or malignant diseases of the bile ducts; but these procedures had significant morbidity and mortality. These features changed with the introduction of interventional percutaneous techniques for the treatment of obstructive biliary tract pathology.

The procedures for the diagnosis and treatment of biliary pathology continue to evolve with the advances of minimally invasive techniques, provided by radiologists and endoscopists. Imaging technical advances have made it easier to select the best treatment options in a multidisciplinary setting. Therefore, interventional radiology plays a fundamental role in the treatment of bile ducts obstructive pathology through the application of advanced imaging techniques, which allow the diagnosis and planning of percutaneous procedures when endoscopic options are not feasible. The primary objective is to achieve the permeability of the biliary tract, either as a step prior to surgery or as a definitive or palliative treatment when the surgical risk is not acceptable.

7.2 Etiology

The most frequent causes of bile duct obstruction found in multiple series are malignant tumor lesions, between 75 and 84% of the published series [1, 2], over the benign ones [2]. Pancreatic head carcinoma represents the most frequent cause of malignant biliary obstruction and of these, approximately 80% are adenocarcinomas [3–5]. The second causes are hepatic and/or lymphatic metastatic involvement on the hepatic hilum and the third and fourth causes are cholangiocarcinoma [6, 7] and gallbladder carcinoma [8]. Other less common tumors are ampuloma, lymphomas, hepatocellular carcinoma, duodenal carcinoma, cystadenocarcinoma, and insular tumors of the pancreas.

A. Linares Cuartero (✉) · J. A. Porfirio Camacho
J. Saenz de Zaitigui Fernández
Interventional Radiology Unit, "Virgen Macarena"
University Hospital, Seville, Spain
e-mail: alinares330@gmail.com;
joseporfirio76@yahoo.es; zaitigui80@gmail.com

© The Author(s), under exclusive license to Springer Nature Switzerland AG 2023
J. Bellido Luque, A. Nogales Muñoz (eds.), *Recent Innovations in Surgical Procedures of Pancreatic Neoplasms*, https://doi.org/10.1007/978-3-031-21351-9_7

7.3 Diagnostic Imaging

The usual noninvasive imaging technique for bile duct stenosis/obstruction diagnosis is ultrasound with a sensitivity to detect bile duct obstruction between 90 and 95% and specificity to classify benign or malignant between 30 and 70% [9]. Multidetector CT (Computed Tomography) scan has a sensitivity >90% to detect obstruction and specificity of 60–90% to define benignity or malignancy [10, 11]. MR (Magnetic Resonance) or MR cholangiopancreatography [12, 13] shows sensitivity higher than 95% and specificity of 30–90%. When bile stenosis length is mandatory to identify, both CT and MR are superior to ultrasound with 75% and 95%, respectively [10, 12].

7.4 Management of Malignant Stenosis of the Bile Ducts

When we faced a bile duct malignant stenosis and the nature of the tumor is known, the first step is to establish the tumor stage in order to consider a curative surgical resection, a medical therapy, and/or minimally invasive palliative interventions. In case of opting for curative surgery, in most cases a bile duct decompression is performed preoperatively to clinically stabilize the patient or in cases with associated cholangitis. In studies conducted, preoperative PTBD (Percutaneous Transhepatic Biliary Drainage) is performed between 87 and 94% of cases [14, 15]. Controversy exists regarding preoperative biliary drainage in different studies. Some authors show no improvement in morbidity and surgical mortality [16, 17] and that this procedure can increase morbidity related to infection [18–20].

Other studies support preoperative PTBD, especially in cases of planned pancreatic head resection, with lower hospitalization and postoperative morbidity [21, 22]. PTBD is preferable to preoperative endoscopic drainage given the lower incidence of infectious complications [23].

Generally in most patients and depending on the experience, endoscopic biliary drainage (EBD) tends to be the first option, when anatomically possible.

7.5 Biliary Drainage Technique

The placement of biliary drainage is a basic procedure to solve an obstructive jaundice and a first step to perform other procedures. It helps to solve the biliary obstruction, either in a single act or in several sessions. It will depend on several factors; some are dependent on the clinical presentation of obstructive jaundice and the patient (degree of jaundice, cholangitis, altered liver function, adjuvant medical treatment, etc.) and others are dependent on the tumor nature, stage, and therapeutic options to be performed.

7.5.1 Patient Preparation

No oral intake at least 8 hours previous to the procedure with adequate hydration is indicated. Once informed consent is signed, the patient is taken to the radiology room. The anesthesiologist is part of the team that performs biliary interventional techniques. Coagulation and blood test studies are routinely taken from the patient previously and antibiotic prophylaxis is done during the procedure and 2 days later according to working standards of the *Spanish Society of Vascular and Interventional Radiology* [24].

7.5.2 Percutaneous Transhepatic Cholangiography

Percutaneous transhepatic cholangiography (PTHC) is a technique that allows to identify the biliary tract, as a step prior to other percutaneous procedures and is always performed in the same act with the biliary drainage is performed. The patient is under general anestesia and also treated with local anestesia in the skin and abdominal wall. A puncture with fine needle (22 G), under radioscopic and/or ultrasound control (Fig. 7.1) is performed. Peripheral biliary radical tract is punctured in order to obtain a map of the biliary tree to plan the best approach. It allows to identify the anatomy of the biliary tract, level and length of the obstruction/stenosis, and presence of other associated alterations such as fistulas, abscesses, or anatomical variants. Success rates are higher with dilated (99%) than no dilated bile duct (75%) [25].

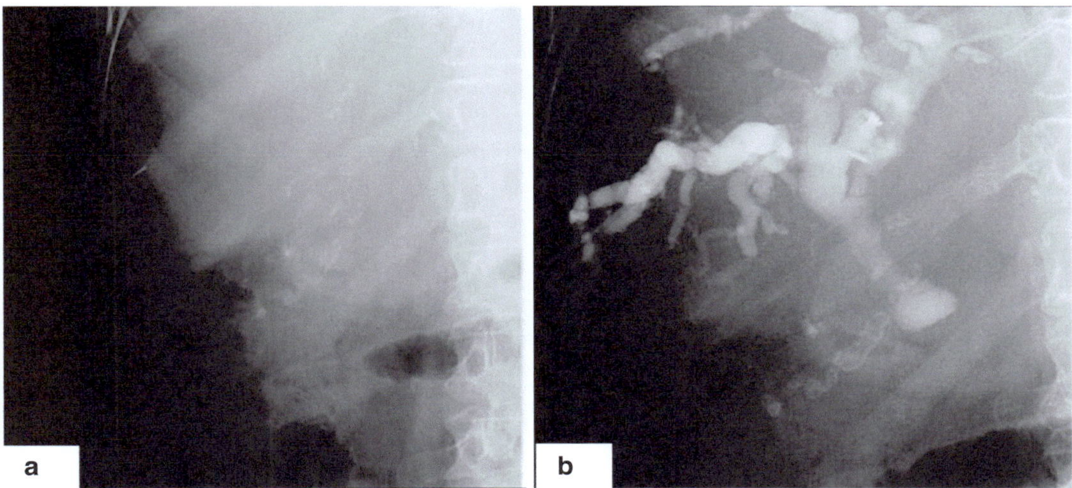

Fig. 7.1 Cholangiography. (**a**) Lateral puncture right hepatic tract. (**b**) Bile duct opacification with distal obstruction

7.5.3 Biliary Drainage

PTBD as external drainage was carried out in 1952 by Leger [26] and subsequently introduced as clinical use by *Molnar W and AE Stockum* in 1974 [27]. In the following decades, more specialized tools have been introduced and improved for use in the bile ducts, which currently allow to overcome the vast majority of biliary stenosis/obstructions.

Once the PTHC has been performed and the location of the stenosis has been established, sometimes the punctured biliary branch is not the most favorable. In this case, the most suitable one is chosen to perform the procedure. Using *Seldinger* technique, we introduce a 0.018 guide caliber through a 5F catheter that allows exchange by thicker guides (0.035/0.038) to insert the Pigtail drainage catheter with calibers between 7 and 10 F (Fig. 7.2).

Access to the bile duct can be done in both right and left branches. It depends on multiple anatomical (absence of left lobe, interposition of digestive tract, presence of prosthetic material in abdominal wall) and tumor factors (presence of metastases or location of biliary stenosis). The right access (Fig. 7.2) is performed intercostal through the axillar midline and is usually the most favorable for biliary navigation to common bile duct; but it has the disadvantage that it is more annoying for the patient. The left access is done through anterior abdominal wall, less uncomfortable for the patient but technically more complex. It is indicated in obstructions of the left ducts with permeability of the right, bilateral drainages with high obstructions, and right tumor lesions that prevent channeling right bile ducts (Fig. 7.3).

Once the external catheter is placed, fixed to the skin, and connected to the pouch, it is left for several days (3–5) to decompress the bile duct, improving the inflammatory or infectious component (cholangitis) and therefore the clinical status and laboratory tests of obstructive jaundice. In the absence of cholangitis and recent jaundice, in the same session we proceed to the passage of stenosis and placement of an external–internal drainage.

The decompression of the bile duct decreases the edematous component and secondarily allows it to overcome stenosis in most cases. The intervention is performed by ensuring biliary access with an introducer of caliber between 8 and 10 F. Then it is accessed with navigation catheters (4–5 F) and guides of 0.18″, which allows to overcome the stenosis. Once the digestive tract is reached with the hydrophilic guide, the navigation catheter is passed and the guide is replaced by another one (Amplatz *Type*) being located in the small intestine. Subsequently, we place an external–internal drainage multiperforated catheter, usually 8.5 F, leaving distal end in the intestinal

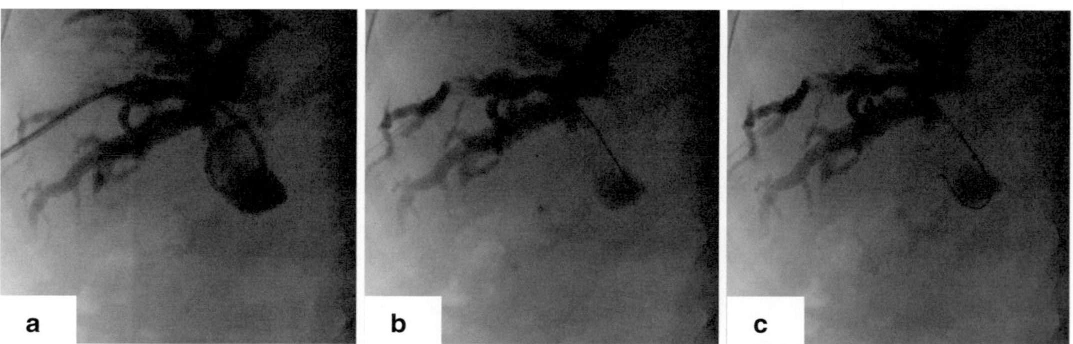

Fig. 7.2 Biliary drainage. (**a**) Navigation catheter in hepatic duct. (**b**) Switch to a high-support guide. (**c**) External drainage catheter placement

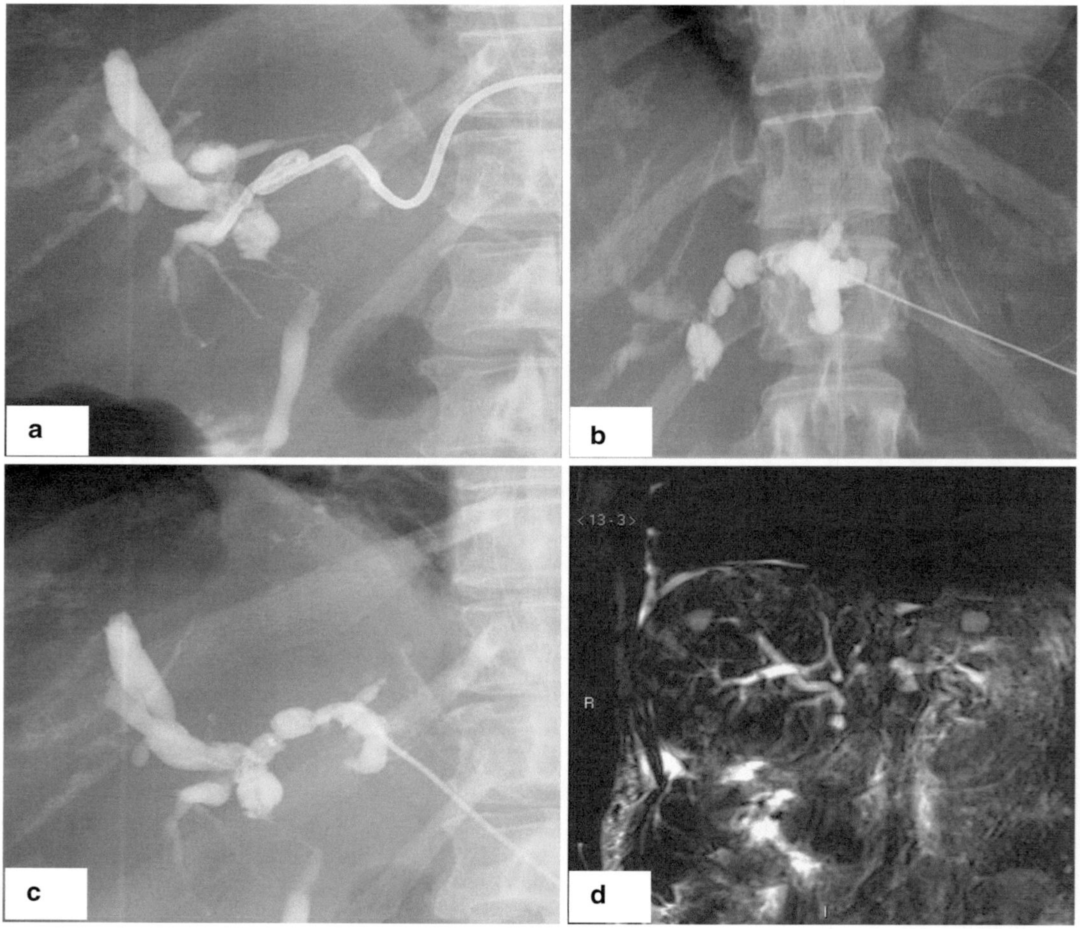

Fig. 7.3 Drainage through left hepatic duct. A 66-year-old woman with colon carcinoma and liver and peritoneal metastases in treatment with chemotherapy. (**a**) Cholangiography. (**b** and **c**) Stenosis in proximal coledocus. (**d**) MRI cholangiography with bile duct dilation and liver metastases

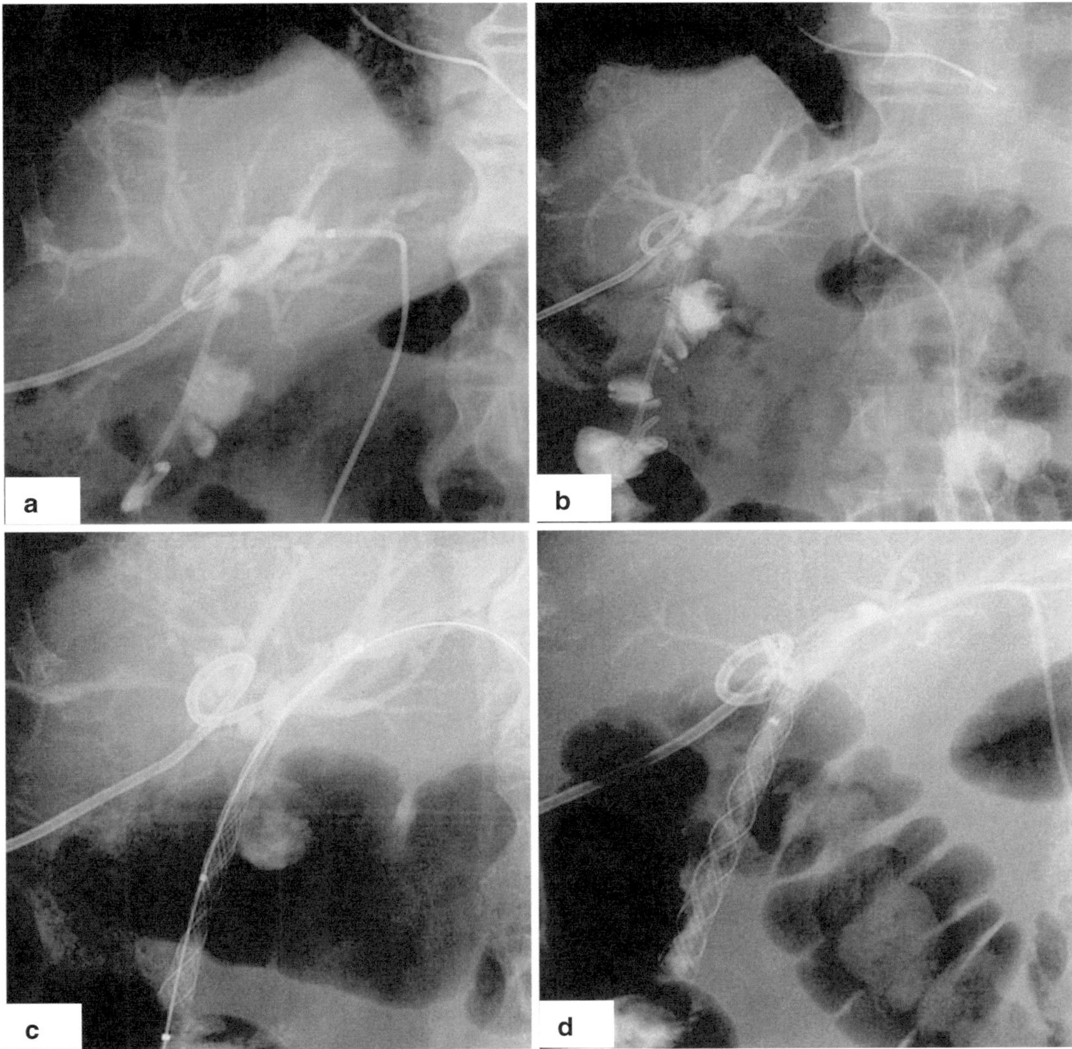

Fig. 7.4 A 72-year-old man underwent hepatojejunal bypass due to adenocarcinoma of the pancreas, with unresectable posterior recurrence. (**a** and **b**) Left external and internal–external drainage. (**c**) Prosthesis is released in common hepatic duct. (**d**) Prosthesis completely expanded

lumen. Cholangiography is performed through the catheter to check the proximal orifices are left in the bile duct above the stenosis and others distal to the stenosis. These drains allow the flow of bile to the intestine avoiding large loss of bile salts and electrolyte alterations (Fig. 7.4).

The technical success of PTDB is defined as the placement of a catheter into the biliary tree with external bile flow or the internal passage to the digestive tract. In the case of cholangitis, the clinical success is the resolution of sepsis with mortality rate reduction. *The Tokyo Guide* recom-

mends early drainage either endoscopic or percutaneous in the treatment of cholangitis [28].

7.5.4 Percutaneous Cholecystostomy

Occasionally in patients with obstructive jaundice, when the common bile duct stenosis is distal to the cystic duct, percutaneous cholecystostomy could be performed to decompress the bile duct as a prior step to other interventional procedures on the bile duct. The procedure is performed with radioscopic or ultrasound control with direct trocar puncture or Seldinger technique, leaving placed external drainage catheter similar to PTBD.

7.6 Indications Percutaneous Biliary Drainage

The main indications for PTBD and percutaneous cholecystostomy in case of obstructions due to malignant neoplasms of the bile ducts are described in Tables 7.1, 7.2, and Table 7.3 describes the main contraindications.

Table 7.1 Biliary drainage indications

– Proximal obstructions of bile ducts not resectable by Surgery.
– Distal obstruction not resectable by Surgery, not being possible retrograde endoscopic drainage.
– Step prior to placement of self-expanding metal prostheses (SEMS).
– Decompression in severe acute cholangitis if endoscopic papillotomy is not possible.
– Preoperative biliary drainage and improvement of jaundice symptoms.
– Optimization of bilirubin level for the administration of chemotherapy.
– Endoscopic percutaneous combination therapy (rendezvous).
– Percutaneous access for brachytherapy and phototherapy treatment.

Table 7.2 Percutaneous cholecystostomy indications

– Management of acute cholecystitis.
– Access to the bile duct when the stenosis is distal to the cystic.
– Access to biliary procedures described in Table 7.1 (5% of cases).

Table 7.3 Percutaneous biliary drainage

Absolute contraindications	Relative contraindications
– Severe bleeding disorders – Critically ill patient with short life expectancy – Presence of vascularized tumors or hydatidic cysts stroke	– Reversible coagulopathy – Hemodynamic instability – Iodized contrasts allergy – Ascites

7.7 Biliary Drainage Complications

Percutaneous and endoscopic biliary drainages in malignant obstructions are associated with a higher risk of complications than in other situations [25, 29]. Published articles suggest similar rates of mortality and complications in both [29, 30]. Most relevant complications include hemorrhage, biliary sepsis, pancreatitis, and cholecystitis [31]. When bleeding occurs in the PTBD, the origin is usually portal, due to its proximity to the bile duct, which is usually solved by mobilizing the catheter or changing it to a thicker one. In case of peripheral portal branches origin, bleeding stops spontaneously. Arterial injury is rare and in case of persistent bleeding through the catheter, selective arteriography is necessary. The risk of pancreatitis is lower in percutaneous drainage (5%) than endoscopic drainage (15%) [25, 32]. Other complications such as pneumothorax or pleural effusion are less common.

When an external drain is maintained due to a failed attempt of internal drainage, electrolyte abnormalities, and malnutrition must be taken into account to correct them, until internal drainage is achieved.

In permanent drains, blockages or malfunctions and infections are frequent, which are solved with periodic catheter replacements and pericatheter care.

Accidental catheter removal can occur between 3 and 9% [33]. Inserting a new catheter is safe and possible when there is a previous fistulous tract, using 4 or 5 F catheters and hydrophilic guides to rechannel the tract.

7.8 Biliary Percutaneous Treatment in Malignant Neoplastic Obstructions

Percutaneous treatment of malignant obstructive jaundices requires a PTBD with passage of tumor stenosis and of self-expanding metal covered or uncoated stents (SEMS) placement. SEMS have become standard palliative treatments in the management of malignant biliary obstruction given the high success rates and long-term permeability. The placement of SEMS should be preceded by imaging studies, especially cholangiopancreatography by MRI [34], to establish the length of stenosis, location of affected bile ducts, and tumor extension. There are controversies in placing SEMS above the papilla or transpapillary in high biliary obstructions.

However, a retrospective review showed no significant differences in permeability duration or occlusion rates [35]. Usually, the stents are placed in a second session, after the PTBD or sometimes it can be implanted in a single act, when the general conditions of the patient and absence of cholangitis allow it (Figs. 7.4, 7.5, and 7.6).

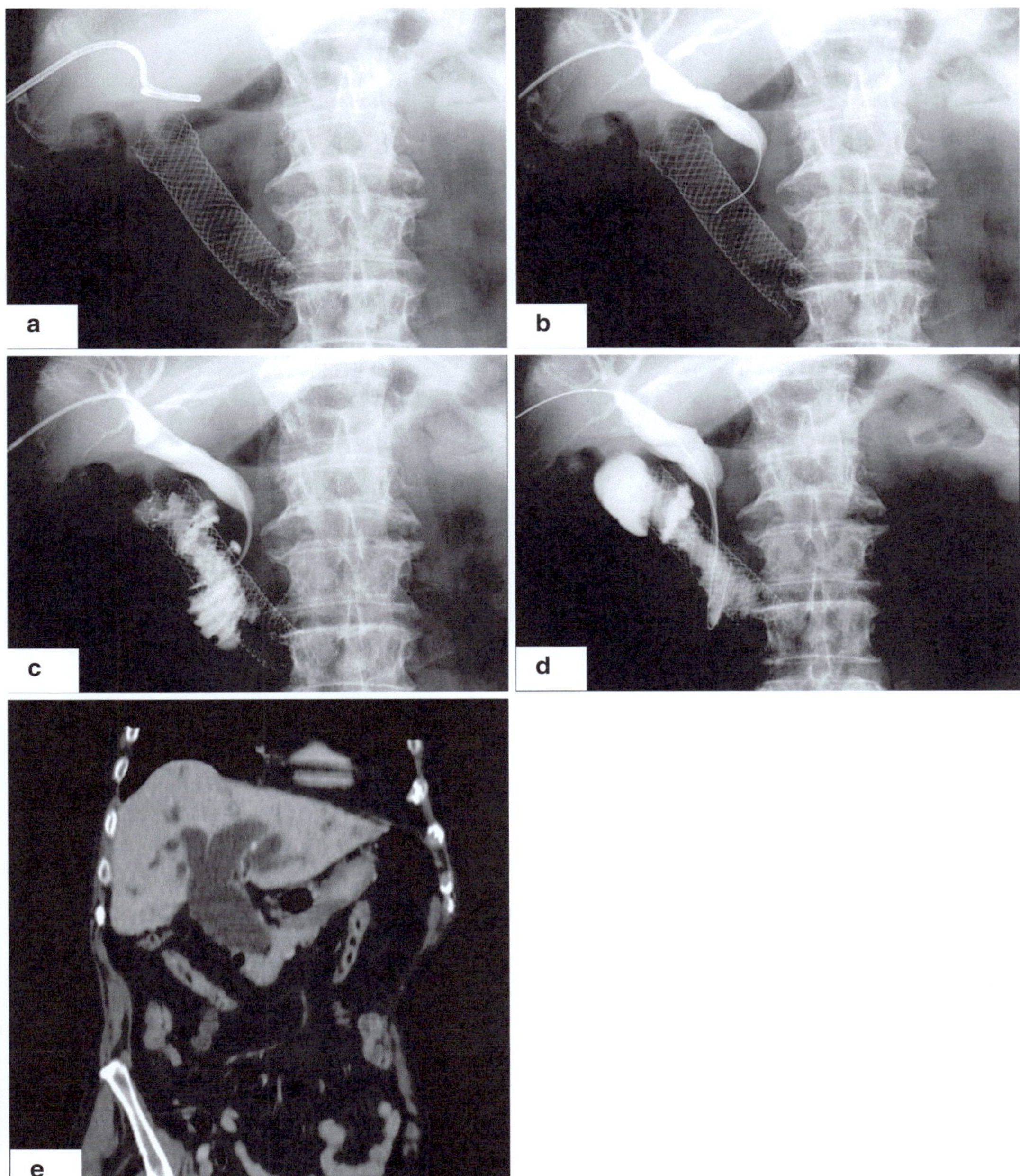

Fig. 7.5 A 80-year-old man with duodenum adenocarcinoma and a previous duodenal prosthesis, presenting with biliary obstruction tumor. Palliative treatment. (**a**) Biliary drainage. (**b**) The guide is passed through the stenosis. (**c**) Catheter crosses the duodenal prosthesis. (**d**) Release of the prosthesis. (**e**) MPR CT scan shows biliary obstruction

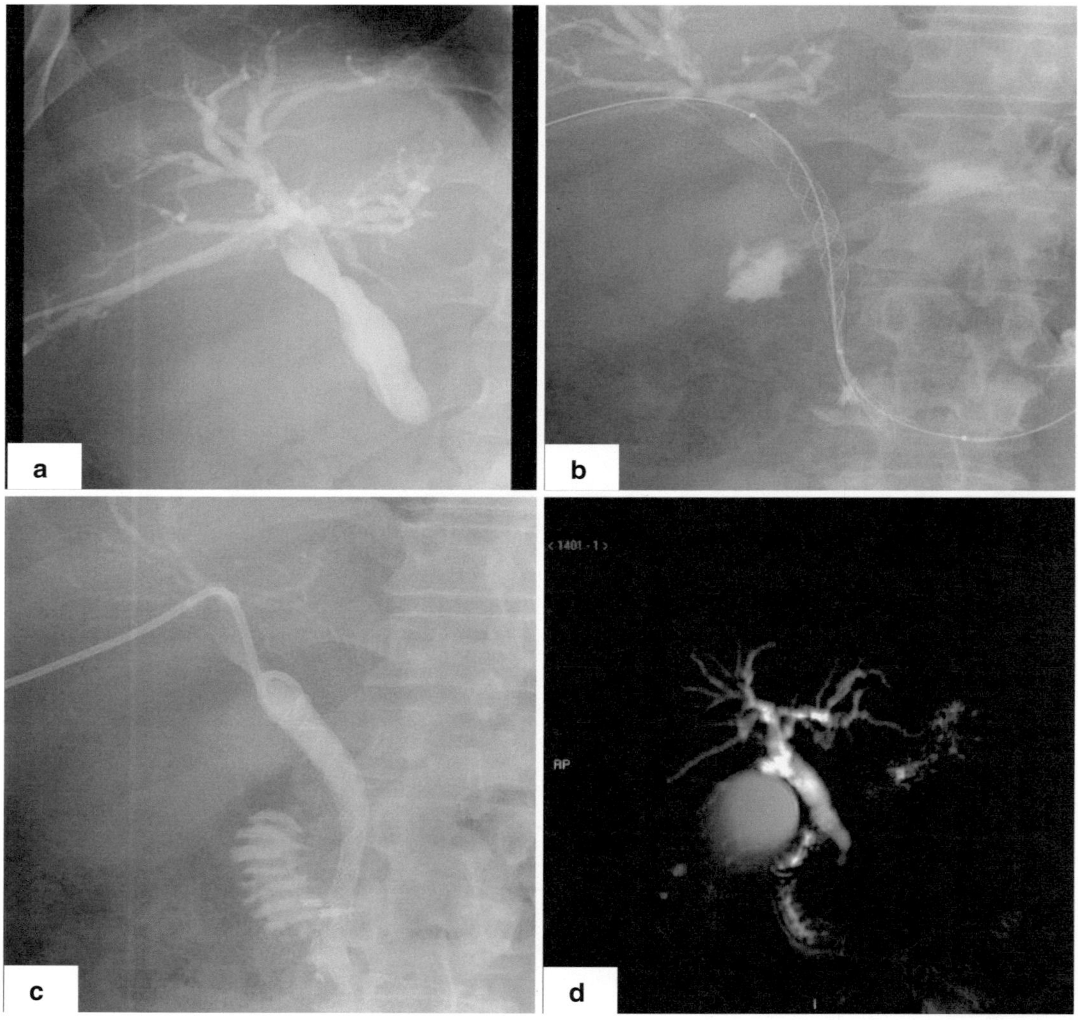

Fig. 7.6 A 64-year-old man with non-resectable pancreas adenocarcinoma. (**a**) Biliary drainage. (**b**) Prosthesis is released on high-support guidance. (**c**) 48-h control with adequate opening of the uncoated metal stent. (**d**) MR cholangiography prior to the biliary procedure

As a rule, it is preferable to leave the biliary prosthesis passing the papilla, which would allow, in case of obstruction, to perform an endoscopic approach. As for the use of balloons for dilation of the stenosis or prosthesis, it is usually preferable to wait for 24–48 h which is when the prostheses reach their maximum diameter (Figs. 7.5 and 7.6). Therefore, we leave an external drainage for 48 h to perform transcatheter cholangiography and check the degree of opening of the prosthesis and permeability of the same, not being necessary in most cases balloon dilations. Currently there are available stents of multiple lengths and calibers 8 and 10 mm…, which allow to select the most appropriate to the length of the stenosis.

In high obstructions that affect the hepatic ducts, it is sometimes necessary to leave two prostheses in place either in "T" or in "Y." One of them preferably the right that reaches the papilla. In these cases, it may be preferable to place uncoated stents to preserve the permeability of the contralateral duct [36]. It is recommended stent placement in the most viable lobe, to drain more than 50% of liver volume with lower cholangitis and greater survival [37]. A randomized multicenter trial in distal biliary malignant obstructions showed no significant differences between covered and uncoated stents [38].

We currently place metal stents in patients, where neoadjuvant therapy is indicated and the patient may be candidates for oncological surgery, using short lengths to allow hepatic derivative surgery.

7.8.1 Indications

The main indication for the placement of the biliary prosthesis is for patients with non-resectable neoplasms. In patients with pancreatic cancer:

- Approximately 50% have advanced metastatic disease (stage IV) and their life expectancy after diagnosis is 6 months. In this group, for those who present poor general conditions and large tumors the indication would be endoscopic plastic stents. For those with a life expectancy greater than 3 months, the placement of a metal stent would be indicated.
- Patients with stage III pancreatic cancer with locally advanced disease, non resectable and with survival rate greater than 12 months, if adequate systemic or local treatment is established, placement of metal stents would be indicated.

7.8.2 Complications of Metallic Stents in Malignant Obstruction of Bile Ducts

The most common complications of stents in malignant biliary obstruction are hemorrhage, cholangitis, cholecystitis, pancreatitis, stent migration, and obstruction [38].

Coated metal stents migrate more often than uncoated metal stents. The risk of bleeding is more related to the point of puncture. The more peripheral it is, the lower the risk of bleeding is [39]. Avoiding balloon dilation of the prosthesis minimizes the risk of bleeding [38]. Cholangitis is the most frequent infectious complication after

stent placement. It is lower in PTBD than in endoscopic drainage [40]. Peri-procedure antibiotic coverage is recommended. Pancreatitis is more common in coated stents and usually determined by the injection of contrast into the pancreatic duct [41]. Cholecystitis is almost always caused by neoplastic involvement of the cystic or uncoated transcystic stent; which is resolved by percutaneous cholecystostomy.

Acute Obstruction is usually caused by hemobilia with clots formation. Chronic obstruction is usually due to tumor overgrowth at the margins of the prosthesis or toward the inside of the prosthesis through the mesh in the uncoated ones [42].

7.9 Conclusions

Palliative treatment of malignant obstruction of the bile ducts remains the main indication of percutaneous and endoscopic treatment. The proper use of covered and uncoated stents on a case-by-case basis allows to offer a clinically effective result and avoids necessary secondary procedures. Since the survival rate in malignant tumor pathology of bile ducts is limited, existing technology such as SEMS, remains adequate permeability in most patients. In malignant obstructions of the bile ducts, the goal is to improve the survival and permeability of the bile duct by eliminating local tumor growth. Among the innovative techniques is intraductal radiofrequency ablation that in pilot studies have demonstrated safety in devices for radiofrequency administration. Pilot studies of drug-releasing SEMS have shown improvements in permeability rates, but studies to demonstrate increased survival are lacking.

References

1. Rossi P, Salvatori FM, Maccioni F, Maradei A, Santoro P, D'Erme M, Gandini R. Percutaneous management in the pathology of the bile ducts. Monogr Diag Imag. 1991;9:23–46.
2. Leng JJ, Zhang N, Dong JH. Percutaneous transhepatic and endoscopic biliary drainage for malignant biliary tract obstruction: a meta-analysis. World J Surg Oncol. 2014;12(1):272.

3. Kalser MH, Barkin J, Macintyre JM. Pancreatic cancer. Assessment of prognosis by clinical presentation. Cancer. 1985;56(2):397–402. https://doi.org/10.1002/1097-0142(19850715)56:2<397::AID-CNCR2820560232>3.0.CO;2-I.

4. Freelove R, Walling AD. Pancreatic cancer: diagnosis and management. Am Fam Physician. 2006;73(3):485–92.

5. Hawes RH, Xiong Q, Waxman I, Chang KJ, Evans DB, Abbruzzese JL. A multispecialty approach to the diagnosis and management of pancreatic cancer. Am J Gastroenterol. 2000;95(1):17–31.

6. Khan SA, Davidson BR, Goldin R, Pereira SP, Rosenberg WM, Taylor-Robinson SD, Thillainayagam AV, Thomas HC, Thursz MR, Wasan H. Guidelines for the diagnosis and treatment of cholangiocarcinoma. Gut. 2002;51:VI1–9.

7. Olnes MJ, Erlich R. A review and update on cholangiocarcinoma. Oncology. 2004;66:167–79.

8. Miller G, Jarnagin WR. Gallbladder carcinoma. Eur J Surg Oncol. 2008;34(3):306–12.

9. Shanbhogue AK, Tirumani SH, Prasad SR, Fasih N, McInnes M. Benign biliary strictures: a current comprehensive clinical and imaging review. AJR Am J Roentgenol. 2011;197(2):W295–306.

10. Feldman MK, Coppa CP. Noninvasive imaging of the biliary tree for the interventional radiologist. Tech Vasc Interv Radiol. 2015;18(4):184–96.

11. Wu XP, Ni JM, Zhang ZY, et al. Preoperative evaluation of malignant perihilar biliary obstruction: negative-contrast CT cholangiopancreatography and CT angiography versus MRCP and MR angiography. AJR Am J Roentgenol. 2015;205(4):780–8.

12. Soto JA, Alvarez O, Lopera JE, Múnera F, Restrepo JC, Correa G. Biliary obstruction: findings at MR cholangiography and cross-sectional MR imaging. RadioGraphics. 2000;20(2):353–66.

13. Canto MI, Hruban RH, Fishman EK, et al. Frequent detection of pancreatic lesions in asymptomatic high-risk individuals. Gastroenterology. 2012;142(4):796–804. quiz e14–e15

14. Kosuge T, Yamamoto J, Shimada K, Yamasaki S, Makuuchi M. Improved surgical results for hilar cholangiocarcinoma with procedures including major hepatic resection. Ann Surg. 1999;230(5):663–71.

15. Nimura Y, Kamiya J, Kondo S, et al. Aggressive preoperative management and extended surgery for hilar cholangiocarcinoma: Nagoya experience. J Hepato-Biliary-Pancreat Surg. 2000;7(2):155–62.

16. Sewnath ME, Birjmohun RS, Rauws EA, Huibregtse K, Obertop H, Gouma DJ. The effect of preoperative biliary drainage on postoperative complications after pancreaticoduodenectomy. J Am Coll Surg. 2001;192(6):726–34.

17. Hatfield AR, Tobias R, Terblanche J, et al. Preoperative external biliary drainage in obstructive jaundice. A prospective controlled clinical trial. Lancet. 1982;2(8304):896–9.

18. Sugiura Y, Nakamura S, Iida S, et al. Extensive resection of the bile ducts combined with liver resection for cancer of the main hepatic duct junction: a cooperative study of the Keio Bile Duct Cancer Study Group. Surgery. 1994;115(4):445–51.

19. Povoski SP, Karpeh MS Jr, Conlon KC, Blumgart LH, Brennan MF. Association of preoperative biliary drainage with postoperative outcome following pancreaticoduodenectomy. Ann Surg. 1999;230(2):131–42.

20. Ferrero A, Lo Tesoriere R, Viganò L, Caggiano L, Sgotto E, Capussotti L. Preoperative biliary drainage increases infectious complications after hepatectomy for proximal bile duct tumor obstruction. World J Surg. 2009;33(2):318–25.

21. Lygidakis NJ, van der Heyde MN, Lubbers MJ. Evaluation of preoperative biliary drainage in the surgical management of pancreatic head carcinoma. Acta Chir Scand. 1987;153(11–12):665–8.

22. Marcus SG, Dobryansky M, Shamamian P, et al. Endoscopic biliary drainage before pancreaticoduodenectomy for periampullary malignancies. J Clin Gastroenterol. 1998;26(2):125–9.

23. Kloek JJ, van der Gaag NA, Aziz Y, et al. Endoscopic and percutaneous preoperative biliary drainage in patients with suspected hilar cholangiocarcinoma. J Gastrointest Surg. 2010;14(1):119–25.

24. Spanish society of Vascular and Interventional Radiology. Interventionism on the bile duct. Work standards. https://servei.org/?mdocs-file=8019.

25. Kapoor BS, Mauri G, Lorenz JM. Management of biliary strictures: state-of-the-art. Radiology. 2018;289:590–603. https://doi.org/10.1148/radiol.2018172424.

26. Leger L, Zara M. Cholangiography and drainage by transhepatic puncture. Press Med. 1952;60(42):936–7.

27. Molnar W, Stockum AE. Relief of obstructive jaundice through percutaneous transhepatic catheter—a new therapeutic method. Am J Roentgenol. 1974;122:356–67.

28. Nilsson U, Evander A, Ihse I, Lunderquist A, Mocibob A. Percutaneous. Transhepatic cholangiography and drainage. Acta Radiol. 1983;24:433–9.

29. Burke DR, Lewis CA, Cardella JF, et al. Quality improvement guidelines for percutaneous transhepatic cholangiography and biliary drainage. J VascInterv Radiol. 2003;14(9 Pt 2):S243–6.

30. Libby ED, Leung JW. Prevention of biliary stent clogging: a clinical review. Am J Gastroenterol. 1996;91(7):1301–8.

31. Born P, Rösch T, Brühl K, et al. Long-term outcome in patients with advanced hilar bile duct tumors undergoing palliative endoscopic or percutaneous drainage. Z Gastroenterol. 2000;38(6):483–9.

32. Wang AY, Strand DS, Shami VM. Prevention of post-endoscopic retrograde cholangiopancreatography pancreatitis: medications and techniques. Clin Gastroenterol Hepatol. 2016;14(11):1521–1532.e3.

33. Hatzidakis A, Krokidis M, Kalbakis K, Romanos J, Petrakis I, Gourtsoyiannis N. ePTFE/FEP-covered

metallic stents for palliation of malignant biliary disease: can tumor ingrowth be prevented? Cardiovasc Intervent Radiol. 2007;30(5):950–8.

34. Freeman ML, Overby C. Selective MRCP and CT-targeted drainage of malignant hilar biliary obstruction with self-expanding metallic stents. Gastrointest Endosc. 2003;58(1):41–9.

35. Cosgrove N, Siddiqui AA, Adler DG, et al. A comparison of bilateral side-by-side metal stents deployed above and across the sphincter of Oddi in the management of malignant hilar biliary obstruction. J Clin Gastroenterol. 2017;51(6):528–33.

36. Moy BT, Birk JW. An update to hepatobiliary stents. J Clin Transl Hepatol. 2015;3(1):67–77.

37. Vienne A, Hobeika E, Gouya H, et al. Prediction of drainage effectiveness during endoscopic stenting of malignant hilar strictures: the role of liver volume assessment. Gastrointest Endosc. 2010;72(4):728–35.

38. Kullman E, Frozanpor F, Söderlund C, et al. Covered versus uncovered self-expandable nitinol stents in the palliative treatment of malignant distal biliary obstruction: results from a randomized, multicenter study. Gastrointest Endosc. 2010;72(5):915–23.

39. Liu YS, Lin CY, Chuang MT, Tsai YS, Wang CK, Ou MC. Success and complications of percutaneous transhepatic biliary drainage are influenced by liver entry segment and level of catheter placement. Abdom Radiol (NY). 2018;43(3):713–22.

40. Lee MJ, Dawson SL, Mueller PR, et al. Failed metallic biliary stents: causes and management of delayed complications. Clin Radiol. 1994;49(12):857–62.

41. Shimizu S, Naitoh I, Nakazawa T, et al. Predictive factors for pancreatitis and cholecystitis in endoscopic covered metal stenting for distal malignant biliary obstruction. J Gastroenterol Hepatol. 2013;28(1):68–72.

42. Lee SH, Park JK, Yoon WJ, et al. Optimal biliary drainage for inoperable Klatskin's tumor based on Bismuth type. World J Gastroenterol. 2007;13(29):3948–55.

Pancreatic Surgical Resections

8

Juan Bellido-Luque,
Inmaculada Sanchez-Matamoros Martin,
Dolores Gonzalez-Fernandez,
and Angel Nogales Muñoz

8.1 Introduction

The standard operation for tumors of the pancreatic head is the pancreaticoduodenectomy (Whipple procedure). Surgical treatment for tumors of the pancreas body or tail is distal pancreatectomy.

Adjuvant chemotherapy has proven advantageous in terms of prolonging overall survival, but different treatment regimens are still controversial [1].

8.2 The Pancreaticoduodenectomy (Kausch–Whipple Procedure)

In 1910, Walter Kausch and Allan Whipple first performed pancreaticoduodenectomy (PD) in a patient with pancreatic tumor located in pancreatic head [2, 3].

For a long time, this surgical procedure was associated with high morbidity and mortality and a poor long-term outcome, causing the surgical community to be against this surgery [4, 5].

During the following years, some changes in the surgical steps used in the operation, with various modifications such as vascular resections and extended lymphadenectomy, PD has become the standard operative procedure for tumors of the pancreatic head.

The PD is divided into three parts:

- Exploration: A complete intra-abdominal examination is performed trying to exclude metastasis disease. Extensive Kocher maneuvers should be done to check retroperitoneum and SMV/SMA infiltration. A tunnel is dissected between the neck of the pancreas anteriorly and the SMV-portal vein posteriorly to exclude infiltration of SMV.
- Resection: The pancreas head-duodenum-common bile duct is removed with lymphadenectomy associated.
- Reconstruction of the gastrointestinal continuity. The gastric stump, pancreas body, and proximal common bile duct are then ensembled into jejunal loop to reconstruct the gastrointestinal continuity.
- The digestive tract reconstruction after first PD consisted of pancreaticoenterostomy and gastroenterostomy via a proximal jejunal loop, with side-to-side anastomosis between the distal jejunum and gallbladder, and side-

J. Bellido-Luque (✉) · I. Sanchez-Matamoros Martin
A. Nogales Muñoz
Biliopancreatic Surgical Division, Gastrointestinal
Surgical Department, Virgen de la Macarena
Hospital, Seville, Spain
e-mail: j_Bellido_1@hotmail.com; macu.san.mat@
gmail.com; anogal@telefonica.net

D. Gonzalez-Fernandez
Fremap Hospital, Seville, Spain
e-mail: gonzalezfernandezd9@gmail.com

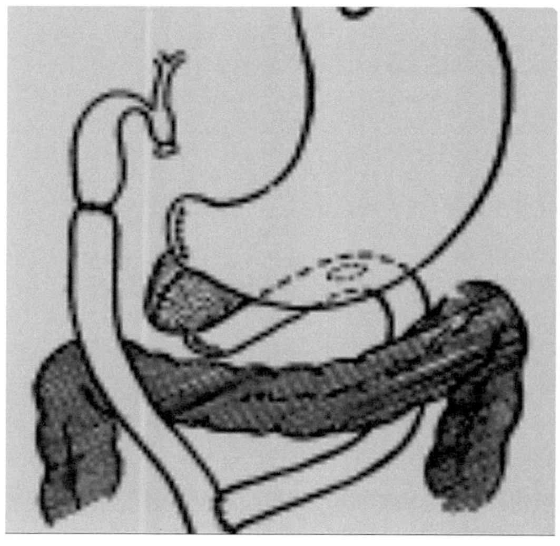

Fig. 8.1 Whipple reconstruction after PD

to-side anastomosis between the proximal and distal jejunum (Fig. 8.1).

During the following years, the reconstruction was made in the order of bile duct, pancreas, stomach, and jejunum.

In 1944, *Charles Child* proposed a new method of reconstruction, namely an anastomosis between the jejunal and pancreatic stump, end-to-side anastomosis of the common bile duct and jejunum, and end-to-side anastomosis of the stomach and jejunum, or in the sequence of pancreas, bile duct, stomach, and jejunum. This has since been known as the Child's operation [6] (Fig. 8.2).

At around the same time, in 1943, *Cattel* designed a refinement of the operation which consisted of an end-to-end anastomosis between the proximal jejunal stump and stomach, end-to-side anastomosis between the pancreas and jejunum, and end-to-side anastomosis between the bile duct and intestine, or the stomach-pancreas-bile duct-jejunum sequence, which is termed the Cattel's method (Fig. 8.3). The Whipple procedure, Child's operation, and Cattel's method are three traditional techniques for digestive tract reconstruction after PD.

Recently, the most commonly used surgical reconstruction worldwide after PD are:

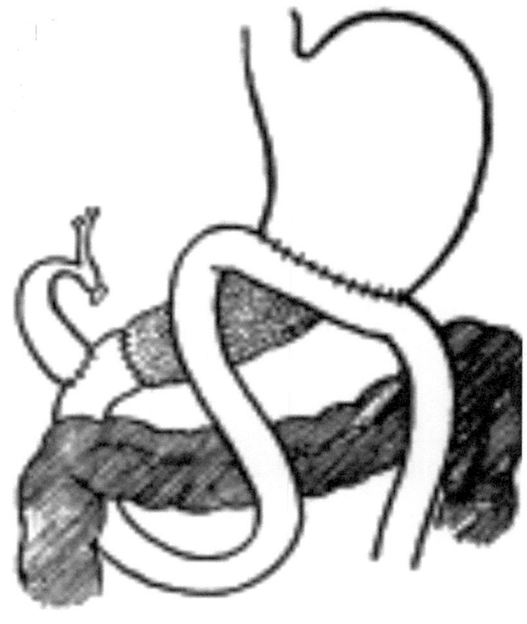

Fig. 8.2 Child's reconstruction after PD

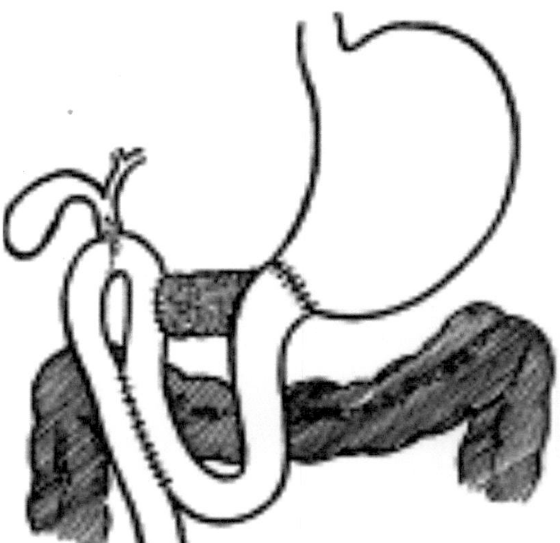

Fig. 8.3 Cattel's reconstruction after PD

1. *Standard Child reconstruction (s-child)* (Fig. 8.4)
2. *Child reconstruction with Braun entero-enterostomy (BE-Child)* (Fig. 8.5)
3. *Isolated-Roux-En-Y reconstruction* (Fig. 8.6)

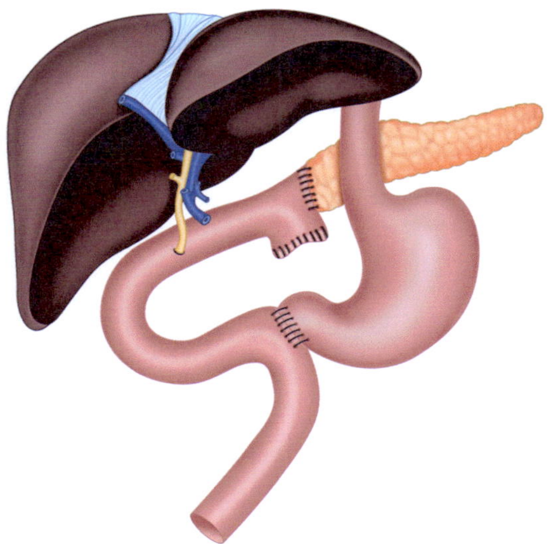

Fig. 8.4 This reconstruction method is defined as pancreaticojejunostomy (PJ) followed by hepaticojejunostomy (HJ) and by gastrojejunostomy (GJ)

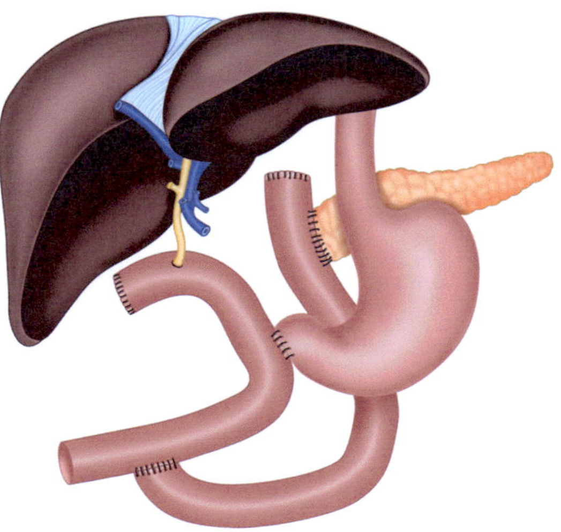

Fig. 8.6 The Isolated-Roux-En-Y reconstruction uses a jejunal loop for the biliary and the gastric anastomosis and an additional isolated jejunal loop to drain the pancreatic juice

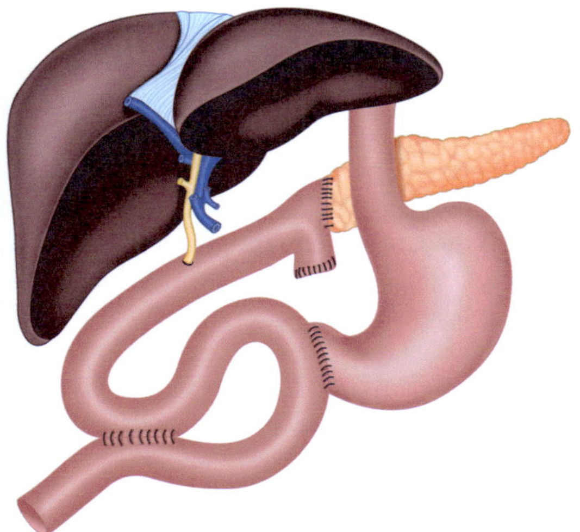

Fig. 8.5 BE-Child is defined as s-Child with an additional entero-enterostomy between the afferent and efferent loop of the GJ to facilitate the drainage of pancreatic juice and bile

Surgical Reconstruction After Pancreatic Surgery and POPF (Postoperative Pancreatic Fistula)

Schorn, S et al. published a systematic review comparing the most common surgical reconstruction after PD [7] in terms of postoperative complications. This paper showed 20.4% POPF grade A/B/C after pancreatic resection with BE-Child and 36.7% after s-Child. Nevertheless, no clinically relevant risk difference could be observed in the overall pooled meta-analysis of POPF grade A/B/C [8] (Table 8.1).

When Iso-Roux-En-Y vs. s-Child were compared, no relevant differences regarding POPF grade A/B/C were identified. However, in the sub-analysis of POPF grade B/C, the meta-analysis showed a twofold increased risk for developing POPF grade B/C in patients with s-Child. The subgroup analysis of RCT was not able to detect any relevant difference for POPF grade A/B/C between BE- and s-Child.

Regarding the rates of the pancreas texture, the main pancreatic duct, and of type of anastomosis, no differences were seen when those three reconstructions were compared.

Surgical Reconstruction After Pancreatoduodenectomy Delayed Gastric Emptying

Schorn, S et al. in their published metanalysis showed that 22.7% patients developed postoperative Delayed Gastric Emptying (DGE) after BE-Child and 36.9% after s-Child reconstruction.

Table 8.1 Postoperative pancreatic fistula grades

	Grade A	Grade B	Grade C
Clinical conditions	Well	Often well	Appearing ill
Specific treatment[a]	No	Yes/no	Yes
US/CT (if obtained)	Negative	Negative/positive	Positive
Persistent drainage (after 3 weeks)	No	Usually yes	Yes
Reoperation	No	No	Yes
Death related to POPF	No	No	Possibly yes
Signs of infections	No	Yes	Yes
Sepsis	No	No	Yes
Readmission	No	Yes/no	Yes/no

[a]Partial (peripheral) or total parenteral nutrition, antibiotics, enteral nutrition, somatostatin analogue and/or minimal invasive drainage. *US* ultrasonography, *CT* computed tomography, *POPF* postoperative pancreatic fistula

The overall pooled RR showed that BE-Child was associated with a slightly decreased, but non-significant risk for DGE compared to s-Child. This protective effect of a BE-Child was even more visible after stratifying patients into clinically relevant DGE grade B/C according to ISGPS [9]. 8.3% of patients showed DGE grade B/C after PD with BE-Child vs. 18.7% of patients after s-Child. The overall RR of 0.40 showed a strongly reduced risk for clinically relevant DGE grade B/C in patients with BE-Child.

No differences were seen when Iso-Roux-En-Y and s-Child for DGE grade A/B/C, were compared [8].

No protective effect was visible in the comparison of Iso-Roux-En-Y vs. s-Child. The overall pooled RR of RCT comparing Iso-Roux-En-Y against s-Child was not able to detect any benefit of Iso-Roux-En-Y for DGE Grade A/B/C.

Reconstruction of the Gastrointestinal Continuity After Classical PD Versus Pylorus-Preserving PD

- Previous meta-analysis showed no effect of BE-Child in patients undergoing classical PD vs. Pylorus-Preserving PD (PPPD) [7].
- The meta-analysis of postoperative complications revealed a strong decreased risk for postoperative complications after classical PD and no effect was detectable in the subgroup analysis of patients undergoing PPPD.
- No differences in the incidence of all kinds of POPF in patients undergoing classical PD or PPPD when BE-Child was performed.

- No effect of BE-Child was detectable for clinically relevant POPF in patients undergoing PPPD.
- PD + BE-Child showed a strongly diminished risk for clinically relevant POPF.
- No effect was visible for all kinds of DGE in classical PD + BE-Child vs. PPPD + BE-Child
- The subgroup analysis of clinically relevant DGE B/C revealed a strongly reduced risk in patients undergoing classical PD + BE-Child and PPPD + BE-Child.
- No effect could be observed of Iso-Roux-En-Y in patients with PD and PPPD for mortality and for overall postoperative complications.
- No relevant differences were detectable in the analysis of overall POPF and clinically relevant POPF, DGE, and clinically relevant DGE in PD + Iso-Roux-En-Y vs. PPPD + Iso-Roux-En-Y [7].

8.3 Methods for Restoration of Pancreatico-Enteric Continuity

During the first PD performed, the main pancreas stump was ligated and sutured without anastomosis. This factor developed gradual atrophy of the pancreas, complete loss of endocrine and exocrine function, postoperative diabetes, and reduced quality of life. When surgeons confirmed those postoperative complications, they decided to abandon this technique.

In 1941, pancreaticojejunostomy (PJ) was first used clinically for the management of pancreatic stump following PD. This new modification preserved pancreatic function and reduced POPF (postoperative pancreatic fistula) [10].

The basic types of PJ are:

8.3.1 Invagination Pancreaticojejunostomy

Invagination Pancreaticojejunostomy (IPJ) is performed by invagination of the pancreatic stump into the intestine in either an end-to-end or an end-to-side manner. This anastomosis does not require main pancreatic duct identification.

Bassi et al. [11], published the incidence of POPF rate ranged between 9.9 and 28.5% after IPJ, and the different definitions used in pancreatic leakage resulted in highly significant differences between them.

Other complications:

- Postoperative due to erosion of peripancreatic vessels by extravasated pancreatic juice, which has been described in 2–8% of cases after POPF [12]. The morbidity rate increased from 6 to 26% when POPF became manifested.

Two fashions of IPJ have been published: End-to-end and end-to-side IPJ. A prospective study involving 295 consecutive patients who underwent PD showed end-to-end PJ resulted in more complications than end-to-side PJ with significant differences [13]. Based on limited evidence, it is still unclear which PJ technique is superior and there is not enough evidence to suggest one over the other.

8.3.2 Binding Pancreaticojejunostomy

Peng et al. described a Binding Pancreaticojejunostomy (BPJ) technique in 2004. The author published a prospective randomized trial comparing conventional pancreaticojejunostomy (CPJ) vs. BPJ. POPF occurred in 7.2%, while none of the 106 patients randomized to the BPJ group developed POPF with significant differences [14]. Postoperative complications developed in 36.9% of the patients in the CPJ group, compared with 24.5% in the BPJ group ($p = 0.048$). The author concluded that BPJ can be safely performed even for cases with a soft pancreatic texture. Three prospective studies indicated that BPJ is a safe and secure technique that decreases the rate of POPF formation (8.9% by Buc [15] 3.0% by Nordback [16] and 0% by Hashimoto [17]). However, no repeatable RCT data about BPJ except Peng's RCT that was reported in other centers which probably results from the technical limitations of BPJ itself.

8.3.3 Duct-to-Mucosa Pancreaticojejunostomy

Duct-to-Mucosa Pancreaticojejunostomy (DmPJ) was first performed by Varco in 1945 [18]. The classical duct-to-mucosa technique can be considered to be a two-layer anastomotic technique, with the inner layer consisting of suturing of Wirsung's duct to jejunal mucosa.

Main advantages of DmPJ are:

- This technique allows for tight adhesion between the pancreatic stump and the jejunum enabling rapid and close adherence due to absence of effusion, and rapid anastomotic patency and exocrine function [19].
- DmPJ does not take into account the size of the residual pancreas, eliminating the problem of too loose or too tight invagination in IPJ.
- Eversion of jejunal mucosa with its accompanying mucosal destruction is not required, as in BPJ.

Due to these benefits, DmPJ is considered to be safe with a low incidence of pancreatic leak [20]. However, DmPJ presents several drawbacks:

- Dead space may exist between the pancreatic stump and jejunal wall, resulting in retention

Table 8.2 RCTs comparing DmPJ and IPJ

References	Pancreatic fistula (%)	Morbidity rate (%)	Mortality rate (%)
Chou et al., 1996	2 vs. 7	13 vs. 21	3 vs. 4
Bassi et al., 2003	13 vs. 15	54 vs. 53	2 vs. 0
Langrehr et al., 2005	2 vs. 2	40 vs. 38	0 vs. 0
Berger et al., 2009	23 vs. 12	53 vs. 49	2 vs. 0
Han et al., 2009	2 vs. 6	9 vs. 15	1 vs. 1

of pancreatic juice from the accessory or tiny pancreatic ducts.

- DmPJ is difficult and the anastomosis is likely to obstruct when the Wirsung's duct has a smaller diameter.

To date, five RCTs have been published to compare DmPJ and IPJ (Table 8.2).

8.4 Pancreaticogastrostomy

Waugh and Clagett in 1946 performed the first Pancreaticogastrostomy (PG) [21].

Benefits associated with PG:

- The stomach has a thick wall and abundant blood flow.
- The pancreatic remnant is located close to the dorsal side of the stomach.
- There is no enterokinase expression in the stomach. This factor is the reason for no pancreatic enzyme activation.

McKay et al. [22] revealed a lower incidence of pancreatic fistula, overall complications, and mortality rate for PG when compared with PJ. However, A recently published multicenter study [23] demonstrated that the overall incidence of postoperative complications did not differ significantly between PJ and PG. However, PG was more efficient than PJ in reducing the incidence of POPF.

During the last years, there have been 7 RCTs that compared complication rates between PG and PJ (Table 8.3).

Three RCTs showed that the incidence of POPF was significantly higher following PJ than PG, as was the severity of pancreatic. The hospital readmission rate for complications was significantly lower after PG, weight loss was lower and exocrine function better. The rate and severity of POPF were significantly lower with the PG technique than with PJ. The remaining four randomized controlled trials revealed a significant difference between PJ and PG with regard to intra-abdominal fluid collections, but without any significant differences in pancreatic fistula, overall postoperative complications, DGE, and mortality rates.

A meta-analysis [24] showed PG had significantly lower rates of postoperative intra-abdominal fluid collection and multiple intra-abdominal complications than PJ in 4 RCTs. Twenty-two observational clinical studies demonstrated significant differences between PG and PJ in frequencies of postoperative biliary fistula, intra-abdominal fluid collection, pancreatic fistula, morbidity, and mortality. The overall analysis revealed significant differences in frequencies of intra-luminal hemorrhage and grade B/C pancreatic fistula between the two groups. However, the authors concluded that the current

Table 8.3 RCTs–PG versus PJ

Study	POPF rate (%) (PG vs. PJ)	Morbidity rate (%)	Mortality rate (%)
Yeo et al., 1995	12 vs. 11	49 vs. 43	0 vs. 0
Duffas et al., 2005	16 vs. 20	46 vs. 47	12 vs. 10
Bassi et al., 2005	13 vs. 16	29 vs. 39	0 vs. 1
Fernández et al., 2008	4 vs. 18	23 vs. 44	—
Wellner et al., 2012	10 vs. 12	N/A	2 vs. 2
Topal et al., 2013	8 vs. 19.8	61.7 vs. 59.3	N/A
Figueras J, 2013	10.4 vs. 34.5	N/A	N/A

literature has no adequate evidence to prove that PG is superior to PJ for patients undergoing PD in postoperative complications.

Main drawbacks of PG:

- Anastomotic bleeding. Fibre et al. [25] reported a 12% preoperative rate due to bleeding at the pancreatic margin.
- Pancreatic duct obstruction, atrophy, and destruction of endocrine and exocrine pancreatic function. Lemaire et al. [26] reported a reduction in pancreatic exocrine function and a worsening of pancreatic atrophy after PG. In another study, PG was more frequently associated with severe steatorrhea compared with PJ (70 vs. 21.7%, $p < 0.025$) suggesting impairment of fat metabolism [27].

In conclusion, both PG and PJ are safe, with no significant difference in complication rates. However, the effect of PG on digestive physiology could lead to long-term complications.

8.5 Ways to Decrease Complications After Pancreatic Anastomosis

- *Use of occlusive substances*: Neoprene injection [28] in the MPD to occlude the duct thus neutralizing exocrine pancreatic secretion is an option that has not reduced the rate of POPF according to a randomized clinical trial. Other studies showed that fibrin glue application does not reduce the incidence of anastomotic leaks [29].
- *Use of somatostatin*: Prophylactic use of somatostatin and octreotide in pancreatic surgery remains controversial and several meta-analyses conclude contradictory conclusions. A current meta-analysis focused on the effects of somatostatin analogues in pancreatic surgery concluded that somatostatin analogues reduce postoperative complications but do not reduce perioperative mortality, and they do shorten hospital stay in patients undergoing pancreatic surgery for malignancy [30].
- *Wrapping*: Use of the omentum or falciform ligament to wrap pancreaticojejunal anastomosis. The main reasons of it are:
  - To avoid the autolytic effect and proteolytic activity of pancreatic juice and infected fluids on surrounding organs, especially the abdominal vessels.
  - To reduce the postoperative bleeding rate.
  - To reduce the rate of PF by avoiding complications arising from it.
  - The literature on wrapping in oncologic pancreatic surgery is rare, and usually consists of retrospective studies with a low level of evidence. Nevertheless, it seems that wrapping decreases postoperative bleeding and POPF, and when this occurs is less severe than when not using wrapping [31].
- *Use of stents*: The benefit of an internal or external stent across pancreatico-enteric anastomosis remains controversial. In the study published by Poon et al., the patients were randomized to have either an external stent inserted across the anastomosis to drain the pancreatic duct or no stent. This trial showed a reduction in the incidence of POPF from 20% in the non-stented group to 6.7% in the stented group [32].

References

1. Neoptolemos JP, Stocken DD, Friess H, Bassi C, Dunn JA, Hickey H, et al. A randomized trial of chemoradiotherapy and chemotherapy after resection of pancreatic cancer. N Engl J Med. 2004;350:1200–10.
2. Whipple AO. Treatment of carcinoma of the ampulla of Vater. Ann Surg. 1935;102:763–8. (abstract)
3. Kausch W. Das Karzinoma der Papilla duodeni and seine radikale Entfernung. Betir Klin Chir. 1912;78:439–86. (abstract)
4. Gudjonsson B. Cancer of the pancreas. 50 years of surgery. Cancer. 1987;60:2284–303.
5. Gudjonsson B. Carcinoma of the pancreas: critical analysis of costs, results of resections, and the need for standardized reporting. J Am Coll Surg. 1995;181:483–503.
6. Büchler MW, Friess H, Wagner M, Kulli C, Wagener V, Z'Graggen K. Pancreatic fistula after pancreatic head resection. Br J Surg. 2000;87(7):883–9.

7. Schorn S, Demir IE, Vogel T, et al. Mortality and postoperative complications after different types of surgical reconstruction following pancreaticoduodenectomy—a systematic review with meta-analysis. Langenbeck's Arch Surg. 2019;404:141–57.

8. Tan WJ, Kow AW, Liau KH. Moving towards the New International Study Group for Pancreatic Surgery (ISGPS) definitions in pancreaticoduodenectomy: a comparison between the old and new. HPB (Oxford). 2011;13:566–72.

9. Wente MN, Bassi C, Dervenis C, Fingerhut A, Gouma DJ, Izbicki JR, Neoptolemos JP, Padbury RT, Sarr MG, Traverso LW, Yeo CJ, Buchler MW. Delayed gastric emptying (DGE) after pancreatic surgery: a suggested definition by the International Study Group of Pancreatic Surgery (ISGPS). Surgery. 2007;142(5):761–8.

10. Hunt VC. Surgical management of carcinoma of the ampulla of vater and of the periampullary portion of the duodenum. Ann Surg. 1941;114(4):570–602.

11. Bassi C, Dervenis C, Butturini G, International Study Group on Pancreatic Fistula Definition, et al. Postoperative pancreatic fistula: an international study group (ISGPF) definition. Surgery. 2005;138(1):8–13.

12. Böttger TC, Junginger T. Factors influencing morbidity and mortality after pancreaticoduodenectomy: critical analysis of 221 resections. World J Surg. 1999;23(2):164–71. discussion 171–2

13. Cheng Q, Zhang B, Zhang Y, Jiang X, Zhang B, Yi B, Luo X, Wu M. Predictive factors for complications after pancreaticoduodenectomy. J Surg Res. 2007;139(1):22–9.

14. Peng SY, Wang JW, Li JT, Mou YP, Liu YB, Cai XJ. Pancreaticojejunostomy—a safe and reliable anastomosis procedure. HPB (Oxford). 2004;6(3):154–60.

15. Buc E, Flamein R, Golffier C, Dubois A, Nagarajan G, Futier E, et al. Peng's binding pancreaticojejunostomy after pancreaticoduodenectomy: a French prospective study. J Gastrointest Surg. 2010;14:705–10.

16. Nordback I, Räty S, Laukkarinen J, Järvinen S, Piironen A, Leppiniemi J, et al. A novel radiopaque biodegradable stent for pancreatobiliary applications—the first human phase I trial in the pancreas. Pancreatology. 2012;12:264–71.

17. Hashimoto D, Hirota M, Yagi Y, H. Baba End-to-side pancreaticojejunostomy without stitches in the pancreatic stump. Surg Today. 2013;43(7):821–4.

18. Varco RL. A method of implanting the pancreatic duct into the jejunum in the Whipple operation for carcinoma of the pancreas: case report. Surgery. 1945;18:569–73.

19. Bassi C, Falconi M, Molinari E, Mantovani W, Butturini G, Gumbs AA, Salvia R, Pederzoli P. Duct-to-mucosa versus end-to-side pancreaticojejunostomy reconstruction after pancreaticoduodenectomy: results of a prospective randomized trial. Surgery. 2003;134(5):766–71.

20. Lee SE, Yang SH, Jang JY, Kim SW. Pancreatic fistula after pancreaticoduodenectomy: a comparison between the two pancreaticojejunostomy methods for approximating the pancreatic parenchyma to the jejunal seromuscular layer: interrupted vs. continuous stitches. World J Gastroenterol. 2007;13(40):5351–6.

21. Waugh JM, Clagett OT. Resection of the duodenum and head of pancreas for carcinoma: an analysis of thirty cases. Surgery. 1946;20:224–32.

22. McKay A, Mackenzie S, Sutherland FR, et al. Meta-analysis of pancreaticojejunostomy versus pancreaticogastrostomy reconstruction after pancreaticoduodenectomy. BJS. 2006;93(8):929–36.

23. Martin RF, Zuberi KA. The evidence for technical considerations in pancreatic resections for malignancy. Surg Clin N Am. 2010;90(2):265–85.

24. He T, Zhao Y, Chen Q, Wang X, Lin H, Han W. Pancreaticojejunostomy versus pancreaticogastrostomy after pancreaticoduodenectomy: a systematic review and meta-analysis. Dig Surg. 2013;30(1):56–9.

25. Fabre JM, Arnaud JP, Navarro F, Bergamaschi R, Cervi C, Marrel E, Domergue J. Results of pancreatogastrostomy after pancreatoduodenectomy in 160 consecutive patients. Br J Surg. 1998;85(6):751–4.

26. Lemaire E, O'Toole D, Sauvanet A, Hammel P, Belghiti J, Ruszniewski P. Functional and morphological changes in the pancreatic remnant following pancreaticoduodenectomy with pancreaticogastric anastomosis. Br J Surg. 2000;87(4):434–8.

27. Rault A, SaCunha A, Klopfenstein D, Larroudé D, Epoy FN, Collet D, Masson B. Pancreaticojejunal anastomosis is preferable to pancreaticogastrostomy after pancreaticoduodenectomy for long-term outcomes of pancreatic exocrine function. J Am Coll Surg. 2005;201(2):239–44.

28. Dubernard JM, Traeger J, Neyra P, Touraine JL, Blanc N, Devonec M. Long-term effect of néoprène injection in the canine pancreatic duct. Transplant Proc. 1979;11:1498–9.

29. Suc B, Msika S, Fingerhut A, Fourtanier G, Hay JM, Holmières F, Sastre B, Fagniez PL. Temporary fibrin glue occlusion of the main pancreatic duct in the prevention of intra-abdominal complications after pancreatic resection: prospective randomized trial. Ann Surg. 2003;237:57–65.

30. Koti RS, Gurusamy KS, Fusai G, Davidson BR. Meta-analysis of randomized controlled trials on the effectiveness of somatostatin analogues for pancreatic surgery: a Cochrane review. HPB (Oxford). 2010;12:155–65.

31. Mimatsu K, Oida T, Kano H, Kawasaki A, Fukino N, Kida K, Kuboi Y, Amano S. Protection of major vessels and pancreaticogastrostomy using the falciform ligament and greater omentum for preventing pancreatic fistula in soft pancreatic texture after pancreaticoduodenectomy. Hepato-Gastroenterology. 2011;58:1782–6.

32. Poon RT, Fan ST, Lo CM, Ng KK, Yuen WK, Yeung C, Wong J. External drainage of pancreatic duct with a stent to reduce leakage rate of pancreaticojejunostomy after pancreaticoduodenectomy: a prospective randomized trial. Ann Surg. 2007;246:425–33. discussion 433–435

Current Status of Vascular Resections in Pancreatic Cancer Surgery

Juan Bellido-Luque,
Inmaculada Sanchez-Matamoros Martin,
Dolores Gonzalez-Fernandez,
and Angel Nogales Muñoz

9.1 Introduction

Radical surgical resection remains the only potentially curative treatment for patients with pancreatic cancer. Pancreatic resection followed by adjuvant chemotherapy is performed in about 20% of all pancreatic ductal adenocarcinoma (PDAC) by the time of diagnosis [1]. Despite this, in the patient group considered unresectable, approximately one-third of the patients can be resected following neoadjuvant therapy [2].

The only option for the long-term survival of a patient with resectable PDAC is R0 radical resection with an average 5-year survival of 20–25% [3].

The major obstacle to improve these poor results is the fact that PDAC diagnosis is made late and in an advanced tumor stage in the majority of patients. As pancreatic surgery is challenging with regard to preoperative diagnostic, surgical procedures as well as postoperative care and complication management, the value of centralization of pancreatic surgery in centers of excellence and high-volume institutions is unquestionable today.

In this setting, implying experience of the individual surgeon who continuously performs pancreatic resections and the environment with an interdisciplinary team of specialists to optimize perioperative care and complication management, mortality rates following major pancreatic resections below 5% are standard today [4, 5].

As a result of the development of surgical techniques and technologies, extended operations, including vascular resections, have become more frequently performed in specialized centers.

Moore et al. performed the first superior mesenteric vein (SMV) resection and reconstruction [6]. Portal vein resection for complete removal of the PDAC was presented systematically by

J. Bellido-Luque (✉) · I. Sanchez-Matamoros Martin
A. Nogales Muñoz
Biliopancreatic Surgical Division, Gastrointestinal
Surgical Department, Virgen de la Macarena
Hospital, Seville, Spain
e-mail: j_Bellido_1@hotmail.com;
macu.san.mat@gmail.com; anogal@telefonica.net

D. Gonzalez-Fernandez
Fremap Hospital, Seville, Spain
e-mail: gonzalezfernandezd9@gmail.com

Fortner [7], who first described a "regional pancreatectomy" involving total pancreatectomy, radical lymph node clearance, combined portal vein resection, and/or combined arterial resection and reconstruction.

These extended surgical interventions carried greater morbidity and mortality than conventional surgery. This was the reason why they were abandoned.

With the improvement of surgical technique, anesthesia, and critical care support, the interest in vascular resection in cases with isolated involvement of the portal vein (PV) and/or superior mesenteric vein (SMV) in locally advanced pancreatic cancer has gradually been renewed during the last decade [8].

Currently, it is accepted that pancreatoduodenectomy with vein resection does not increase the postoperative risk, but there are still no reliable proofs that it significantly improves survival. Porto-mesenteric vein resection is a standard procedure at high-volume pancreatic centers. Nowadays, only arterial resections are still a controversial issue. Nevertheless, attempts at resection involving reconstruction of the main arteries such as the coeliac axis, hepatic artery, and superior mesenteric artery (SMA) have been reported, although in small case series [9].

The present review gives an overview of the development and current state of venous and arterial resections in PDAC surgery.

9.2 Resectability of Pancreatic Ductal Adenocarcinomas

Selection of patients for vascular resection is based on the probability of obtaining complete surgical resection (R0). The presence and extent of vascular involvement are determined on high-quality thin section images, with an anatomical basis for the classification of tumors as "borderline resectable," "locally advanced," or metastatic [10]. Many classifications have been used to define the extent of PDAC, which is based on the relationship between the tumor and the venous or arterial axes. The most common system is the National Comprehensive Cancer Network's (NCCN) classification, updated in November 2018 (Table 9.1).

The notion of a "borderline" tumor has recently changed to take into account the anatomical classification, the probability of histologically incomplete resection (R1), the patient's clinical status (general condition, comorbidities, performance status, "fragility syndrome"), and the "biological" status of the disease. The International Consensus on the definition of "borderline" tumors recommends to use a threshold CA 19-9 rate $\geq$500 units/ml for the latter [11].

Defined patients with borderline resectable PDAC (BR-PDAC) according to the three distinct dimensions, anatomical, biological, and conditional:

1. Anatomic factors include tumor contact with the superior mesenteric artery and/or celiac artery of less than 180° without showing stenosis or deformity, tumor contact with the common hepatic artery without showing tumor contact with the proper hepatic artery and/or celiac artery, and tumor contact with the superior mesenteric vein and/or portal vein including bilateral narrowing or occlusion without extending beyond the inferior border of the duodenum.

2. Biological factors include potentially resectable disease based on anatomic criteria but with clinical findings suspicious for (but unproven) distant metastases or regional lymph node metastases diagnosed by biopsy or positron emission tomography-computed tomography. This also includes a serum carbohydrate antigen (CA) 19-9 level of more than 500 units/ml.

3. Conditional factors include the patients with potentially resectable disease based on anatomic and biologic criteria and with Eastern Cooperative Oncology Group (ECOG) performance status of 2 or more.

   The definition of BR-PDAC requires one or more positive dimensions.

Table 9.1 National Comprehensive Cancer Network's (NCCN) classification

Resectability status	Arterial	Venous
Resectable	No arterial tumor contact (celiac axis [CA], superior mesenteric artery [SMA], or common hepatic artery [CHA])	No tumor contact with the superior mesenteric vein (SMV) or portal vein (PV) or ≤180° contact without vein contour irregularity
Borderline Resectable [2]	*Pancreatic head/uncinate process* • Solid tumor contact with CHA without extension to celiac axis or hepatic artery bifurcation allowing for safe and complete resection and reconstruction • Solid tumor contact with the SMA of ≤180° • Solid tumor contact with variant arterial anatomy (ex: accessory right hepatic artery, replaced right hepatic artery, replaced CHA, and the orgin of replaced or accessory artery) and the presence and degree of tumor contact should be noted if present as it may affect surgical planning *Pancreatic body/tail* • Solid tumor contact with the CA of ≤180° • Solid tumor contact with the CA of >180° without involvement of the aorta and with intact and uninvolved gastroduodenal artery thereby permitting a modified Appleby procedure [some members prefer this criteria to be in the unresectable category]	• Solid tumor contact with the SMV or PV of >180°, contact of ≤180° with contour irregularity of the vein or thrombosis of the vein but with suitable vessel proximal and distal to the site of involvement allowing for safe and complete resection and vein reconstruction • Solid tumor contact with the inferior vena cave (IVC)
Unresectable [2]	• Distant metastasis (including non-regional lymph node metastasis) *Head/uncinate process* • Solid tumor contact with SMA >180° • Solid tumor contact with the CA >180° • Solid tumor contact with the first jejunal SMA branch *Body and tail* • Solid tumor contact of >180° with the SMA or CA • Solid tumor contact with the CA and aortic involvement	*Head/uncinate process* • Unreconstructible SMV/PV due to tumor involvement or occlusion (can be due to tumor or bland thrombus) • Contact with most proximal draining jejunal branch into SMV *Body and tail* • Unreconstructible SMV/PV due to tumor involvement or occlusion (can be due to tumor or bland thrombus)

PDAC resectability status

9.3 Neoadjuvant Therapy and Patient Selection

The purpose of neoadjuvant therapy is to increase the rate of patients candidates for potentially curative secondary resection. A systematic review published in 2017 compared the pathological data in patients who underwent "upfront" surgery to those who underwent surgery after "neoadjuvant treatment." A significant reduction in the relative risk (RR) of R1 resection (RR = 0.66) and other negative predictive factors (tumor size, lymph node metastases, perineural extension,

and lymphatic emboli) was observed after neoadjuvant treatment [12].

For borderline resectable PDAC, several more recent studies including two meta-analyses [13, 14] have confirmed that survival was improved after neoadjuvant therapy followed by surgery than after upfront surgery followed by adjuvant therapy, even in an intent-to-treat analysis.

The NCCN recommendations version 1.2019 (November 8, 2018) state that: "Immediate" resection of borderline tumors is no longer recommended (unlike 2016 recommendations), despite the absence of a randomized trial (neoadjuvant therapy vs. "immediate" surgery) and the definition of the "best therapeutic protocol to use" [15].

On the other hand, in patients with unresectable pancreatic cancer (NCCN definition) that were explored with the intent of pancreatectomy and irreversible electroporation for margin extension after neoadjuvant therapy, R0 resections could be achieved in 80% of the cases in non-metastatic patients [16].

Neoadjuvant therapy was also not related to increased 30-day mortality and postoperative morbidity rates [17].

9.4 Venous Resections and Reconstruction

The classification proposed by the International Study Group of Pancreatic Surgery divided the venous resection into four types depending on the extent of the invasion of the portal vein and superior mesenteric vein and the performed reconstruction [18]:

- I: Venorrhaphy
- II: Patch
- III: Primary anastomosis (Fig. 9.1)
- IV: Interposition conduit

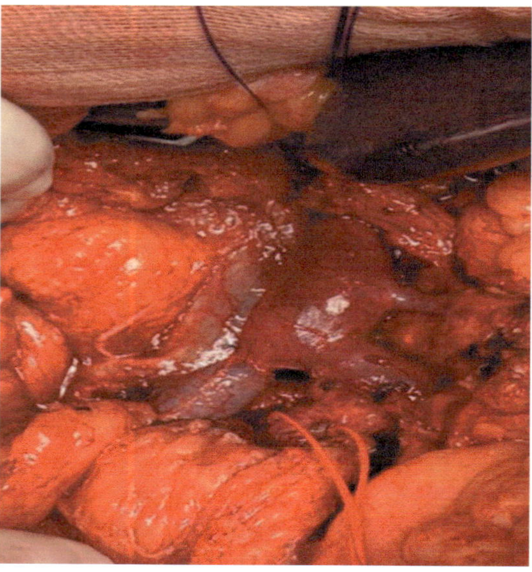

Fig. 9.1 Primary end-end anastomosis after venous resections

An end-end anastomosis is almost always possible with extensive mobilization of the root of the mesentery. Technically, an extensive Kocher maneuver combined with a Cattell–Braasch maneuver is a safe technic to perform pancreatic and venous resection with primary anastomosis (Fig. 9.2).

In type IV venous resection, if mesenteric root mobilization and lowering of the right liver are insufficient to compensate for the length of the vascular resection, interposed graft reconstruction may be used, including an autologous venous or peritoneal, a cryopreserved homologous, a heterologous or a prosthetic graft [19] (Fig. 9.3). This meta-analysis of 14 studies including 257 venous resections with interposition grafts and 570 without, showed that when venous reconstruction was performed with an interposition graft, postoperative morbidity, mortality, and survival at 1, 3, and 5 years were comparable to those observed with other reconstruction techniques. However, the risk of venous axis thrombosis was significantly higher at 6 months (OR = 2.75; 95% CI = 1.32–5.73; $p = 0.007$).

In a large multicenter retrospective review from the United Kingdom that included 1588 Patients with borderline resectable tumors, venous resection in pancreatic cancer surgery was also reported as safe and feasible [20].

Ravikumar et al. published in 2014 a median survival of 18 months for the standard procedure and 18.2 months for patients undergoing venous resection. The in-hospital mortalities were similar in both groups [21].

One meta-analysis published in 2016 (27 studies—9005 patients including 1587 pancreatectomies with venous resections) reported an increased risk of postoperative mortality and resection R1/R2 vs. R0. In addition, survival at 1, 3, and 5 years was significantly reduced. Median overall survival was 14.3 months in the venous resection group vs. 19.5 months in the standard pancreatectomy group. This meta-analysis concluded that neoadjuvant treatment was recommended in the setting of planned venous resection with the level of evidence 2 [22].

Due to previous findings, if pancreatic resection with a tumor negative margin is possible,

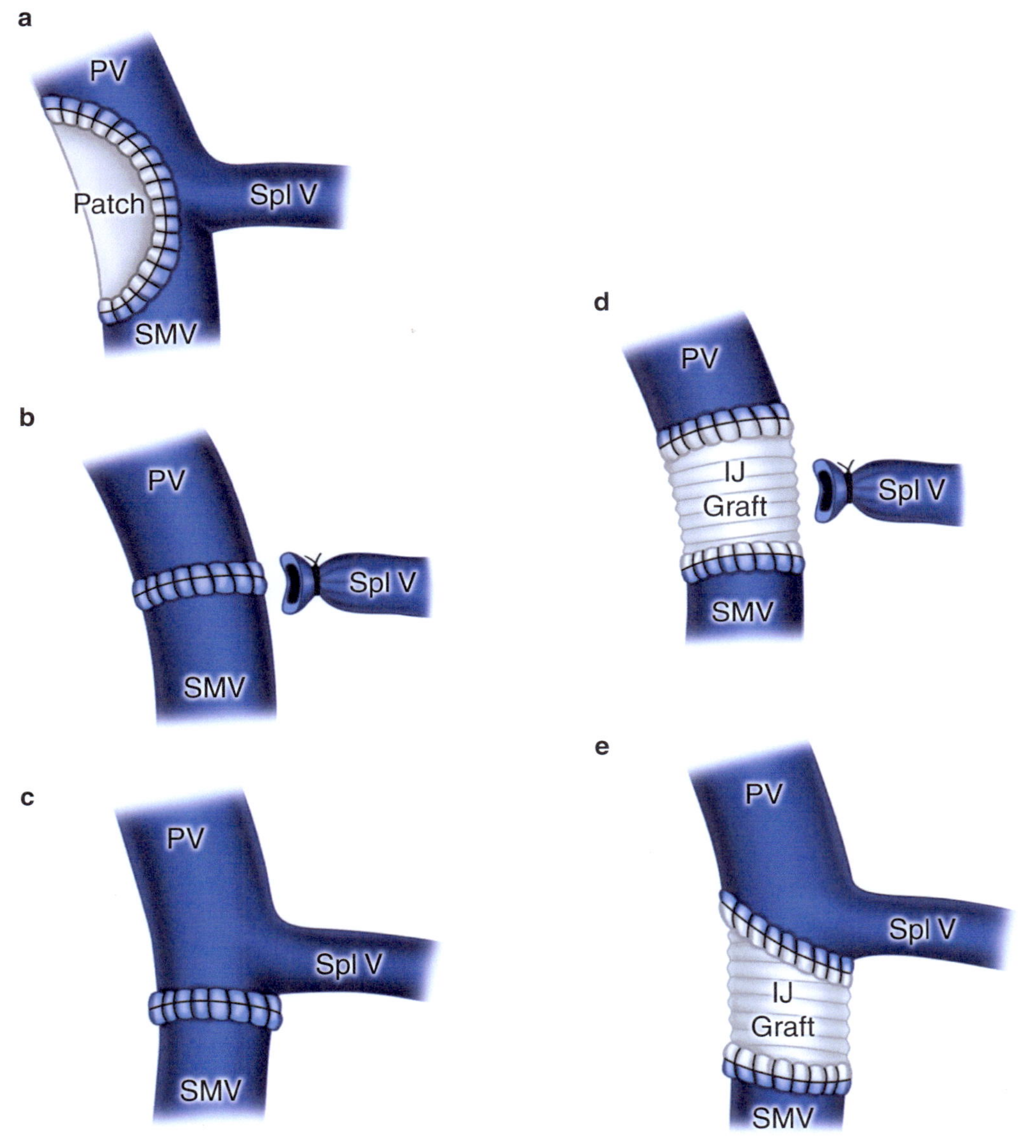

Fig. 9.2 Types of venous reconstruction. (**a**) Patch reconstruction. (**b**) End-end anastomosis. Splenic vein is ligated. (**c**) End-end anastomosis. Splenic vein is preserved. (**d**) Interposition conduit with splenic vein resected. (**e**) Interposition conduit below splenoportal junction

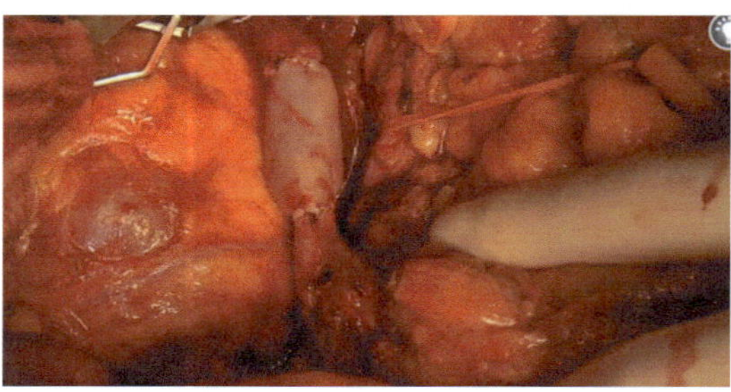

Fig. 9.3 Type IV venous reconstruction below spleno-portal junction, with cryopreserved Homologous prosthetic graft

venous resection should be performed. Currently, this approach is now internationally well-accepted.

9.5 Arterial Resections

Two main procedures have been published with arterial resections:

- Coeliac axis resection in left-sided pancreatic resections.
- Right-sided common hepatic artery or superior mesenteric artery resections.

Actual evidence regarding this topic suggests that arterial resections should only be performed in highly selected patients. The invasion of the common hepatic artery (CHA) or the gastroduodenal artery (GDA) at its origin, of the superior mesenteric artery (SMA), or the celiac axis (CA) is usually considered as a contraindication for resection due to the risks of both morbidity and mortality, and poor oncological results [23].

Nevertheless patients with no progressive or responding disease after neoadjuvant therapy could be the main indications for arterial resections [24].

A meta-analysis published in 2011 selected 26 studies (adding up to 366 arterial resections vs. 2243 non-arterial resection pancreatectomies) including only five studies with SMA resections. This meta-analysis reported [25]:

- Significantly increased risk of morbidity and surgical mortality.
- Significant reduction in survival at 1 year, including after exclusion of post-operative with no survivors at 5 years.
- Significantly higher operative mortality.

In 2018, the Mayo Clinic group reported results in 111 patients who underwent pancreatectomy with AR [26]. Overall 90-day major morbidity and mortality were 54 and 13%, respectively. Post-pancreatectomy hemorrhage was associated with major morbidity, reoperation, and increased mortality. Median survival was 28.5 months.

Three situations can be distinguished and AR must be planned:

1. Anatomical variants of HA:
   (a) Right HA arising from the SMA: This situation increases the rate of common HA resection during PD when this artery is involved.
   (b) The HA could not be the main liver vascular flow artery: Preoperative embolization followed by "en bloc" resection may be performed with no significant risks of liver/biliary ischemia due to development of intrahepatic arterial shunts.
   (c) If the HA perfuses the total liver, it requires reconstruction of any type of anastomosis to ensure vascularization of the biliary tree and the hepaticojejunostomy following PD. HA should be reconstructed before continuing pancreatic resection to avoid any liver ischemia, particularly when an associated venous resection is needed.
2. PD and resection of HA:
   Most PDs with AR reported in the literature included resection of the common HA with posterior reconstruction. Only one Japanese study by Miyazaki et al. [27] reported 20/21 patients who underwent HA resection without reconstruction. Twelve of these patients had received preoperative embolization of the common HA (CHA) for

collateral vessel formation. In this short series there was no relevant specific morbidity.

3. Distal pancreatectomy (DP) with celiac axis resection (DP-CAR), for pancreatic carcinomas of the body and tail with invasion of the CA or the origin of the CHA: The "Appleby" procedure was initially described for the resection of gastric cancers invading the celiac area. Nimura et al. [28] described this technique for body and tail pancreatic adenocarcinomas and showed improved survival compared to standard DP.

The principles of the intervention are:

(a) Increase the rate of R0 resectability.

(b) Ensure lymphatic clearance around the CA and its branches.

(c) Preserve the collateral circulation from the SMA and pancreaticoduodenal arcades (PDA) to the liver, the biliary tract, and the stomach.

(d) Avoid any arterial reconstruction with subsequent anastomotic complications.

This procedure is contraindicated when the CA is invaded at its origin on the aorta or if the GDA is invaded. Many authors are in favor of the use of preoperative occlusion of CHA of the three branches of the CA to ensure the development of arterial collaterals thus reducing the risk of bile ducts and gastric ischemia Embolization should be performed 1–2 weeks before resection. This procedure, which avoids any arterial reconstruction, remains controversial.

ARs are currently rarely indicated, and should always begin with an "artery first" approach to accurately evaluate any persistent arterial involvement confirmed by frozen section examination.

9.6 Conclusions

PD with venous resection improves survival compared to no resection, especially after neoadjuvant treatment. PD with arterial resection is associated with increased morbidity and mortality and has not been shown to be beneficial. A DP-CAR is associated with increased morbidity and mortality and the oncological benefit of this approach has not been clearly demonstrated.

References

1. Hartwig W, Hackert T, Hinz U, et al. Pancreatic cancer surgery in the new millennium: better prediction of outcome. Ann Surg. 2011;254(2):311–9.
2. Gillen S, Schuster T, Büschenfelde CM, et al. Preoperative/neoadjuvant therapy in pancreatic cancer: a systematic review and meta-analysis of response and resection percentages. PLoS Med. 2010;7:1–15.
3. Schnelldorfer T, Ware A, Sarr M, et al. Long-term survival after pancreatoduodenectomy for pancreatic adenocarcinoma is cure possible. Ann Surg. 2008;247(3):456–62.
4. Birkmeyer JD, Siewers AE, Finlayson EVA, et al. Hospital volume and surgical mortality in the United States. N Engl J Med. 2002;346(15):1128–37.
5. McPhee JT, Hill JS, Whalen GF, et al. Perioperative mortality for pancreatectomy: a national perspective. Ann Surg. 2007;246(2):246–53.
6. Moore G, Sako Y, Thomas L. Radical pancreaticoduodenectomy with resection and reanastomosis of the superior mesenteric vein. Surgery. 1951;30:550–3.
7. Fortner J. Regional resection of cancer of the pancreas: a new surgical approach. Surgery. 1973;73(2):307–20.
8. Hartwig W, Werner J, Jäger D, Debus J, Büchler MW. Improvement of surgical results for pancreatic cancer. Lancet Oncol. 2013;14:e476–85.
9. Mollberg N, Rahbari N, Koch M, Hartwig W, Hoeger Y, Büchler MW, Weitz J. Arterial resection during pancreatectomy for pancreatic cancer: a systematic review and metaanalysis. Ann Surg. 2011;254:882–93.
10. Beleù A, Calabrese A, Rizzo G, Capelli P, Bellini N, Caloggero S, et al. Preoperative imaging evaluation after downstaging of pancreatic ductal adenocarcinoma: a multi-center study. Cancers. 2019;11:E267. https://doi.org/10.3390/cancers11020267.
11. Isaji S, et al. International consensus on definition and criteria of borderline resectable pancreatic ductal adenocarcinoma. Pancreatology. 2018;18:2–11.
12. Schorn S, Demir IE, Reyes CM, Saricaoglu C, Samm N, Schirren R, et al. The impact of neoadjuvant therapy on the histopathological features of pancreatic ductal adenocarcinoma—a systematic review and meta-analysis. Cancer Treat Rev. 2017;55:96–106.
13. Versteijne E, Vogel JA, Besselink MG, Busch ORC, Wilmink JW, Daams JG, et al. Meta-analysis comparing upfront surgery with neoadjuvant treatment in patients with resectable or borderline resectable pancreatic cancer. Br J Surg. 2018;105:946–58.
14. Unno M, Hata T, Motoi F. Long-term outcome following neoadjuvant therapy for resectable and borderline resectable pancreatic cancer compared to

upfront surgery: a meta-analysis of comparative studies by intention-to-treat analysis. Surg Today. 2019;49:295–9.

15. Khorana AA, Mangu PB, Berlin J, Engebretson A, Hong TS, Maitra A, et al. Potentially curable pancreatic cancer: American society of clinical oncology clinical practice guideline update. J Clin Oncol. 2017;35:2324–8.

16. Kluger MD, Rashid MF, Rosario VL, et al. Resection of locally advanced pancreatic cancer without regression of arterial encasement after modern-era neoadjuvant therapy. J Gastrointest Surg. 2018;22:235–41.

17. Cooper AB, Parmar AD, Riall TS, et al. Does the use of neoadjuvant therapy for pancreatic adenocarcinoma increase postoperative morbidity and mortality rates? J Gastrointest Surg. 2015;19:80–7.

18. Dunne DFJ, Kleeff J, Yip VS, Neoptolemos JP, Urrutia R, Abbruzzese J, et al. Arterial resection in pancreatic cancer. In: Pancreatic cancer. New York, NY: Springer New York; 2017. p. 1–16.

19. Song W, Yang Q, Chen L, Sun Q, Zhou D, Ye S, et al. Pancreatoduodenectomy combined with portal-superior mesenteric vein resection and reconstruction with interposition grafts for cancer: a meta-analysis. Oncotarget. 2017;8:81520–8.

20. Allema JH, Reinders ME, Van Gulik TM, et al. Portal vein resection in patients undergoing pancreatoduodenectomy for carcinoma of the pancreatic head. Br J Surg. 1994;81:1642–6.

21. Ravikumar R, Sabin C, Hilal MA, et al. Portal vein resection in borderline resectable pancreatic cancer: a United Kingdom multicenter study. J Am Coll Surg. 2014;218:401–11.

22. Giovinazzo F, Turri G, Katz MH, Heaton N, Ahmed I. Meta-analysis of benefits of portal-superior mesenteric vein resection in pancreatic resection for ductal adenocarcinoma. Br J Surg. 2016;103:179–91.

23. Bockhorn M, Uzunoglu FG, Adham M, Imrie C, Milicevic M, Sandberg AA, et al. Borderline resectable pancreatic cancer: a consensus statement by the international study group of pancreatic surgery (ISGPS). Surgery. 2014;155:977–88.

24. Del Chiaro M, Segersvärd R, Rangelova E, et al. Cattell–Braasch maneuver combined with artery-first approach for superior mesenteric-portal vein resection during pancreatectomy. J Gastrointest Surg. 2015;19:2264–8.

25. Mollberg N, Rahbari NN, Koch M, Hartwig W, Hoeger Y, Büchler MW, et al. Arterial resection during pancreatectomy for pancreatic cancer: a systematic review and meta-analysis. Ann Surg. 2011;254:882–93.

26. Tee MC, Krajewski AC, Groeschl RT, Farnell MB, Nagorney DM, Kendrick ML, et al. Indications and perioperative outcomes for pancreatectomy with arterial resection. J Am Coll Surg. 2018;227:255–69.

27. Miyazaki M, Yoshitomi H, Takano S, Shimizu H, Kato A, Yoshidome H, et al. Combined hepatic arterial resection in pancreatic resections for locally advanced pancreatic cancer. Langenbeck's Arch Surg. 2017;402:447–56.

28. Nimura Y, Hattori T, Miura K, Nakashima N, Hibi M. Resection of advanced pancreatic body-tail carcinoma by Appleby's operation. Shujutu. 1976;30:885–9.

Juan Bellido-Luque,
Inmaculada Sanchez-Matamoros Martin,
Dolores Gonzalez-Fernandez,
and Angel Nogales Muñoz

10.1 Introduction

Laparoscopic pancreaticoduodenectomy (LPD) was first reported by Gagner in 1994 [1].

Since then, more centers have performed this procedure in malignant and benign diseases or low-grade malignant neoplasms.

LPD is still considered to be a technically demanding procedure due to its wide dissection around critical anatomical structures, that why this procedure has not gained uniform acceptance [2, 3].

Distal pancreatectomy is the fundamental surgery for the treatment of body-tail tumors of the pancreas. Since Cuscheri et al. reported the first laparoscopic distal pancreatectomy (LDP) in 1996 [4], LDP has been applied to the surgical treatment of pancreatic tumors have increased over the last decade.

10.2 Laparoscopic Distal Pancreatectomy

Distal pancreatectomy is relatively suitable as a laparoscopic procedure because, in principle, it does not necessitate reconstruction. LDP has become common as a treatment method for not only benign tumors but also pancreatic ductal adenocarcinoma (PDAC) due to the development of relevant surgical instruments and techniques.

There are different surgical options for LDP (Table 10.1).

Laparoscopic distal pancreatectomy is usually performed for benign conditions, borderline tumors, and other conditions such as pancreatitis and islet cell tumors. The indications for laparoscopic left distal pancreatectomy are summarized in Table 10.2.

J. Bellido-Luque (✉) · I. Sanchez-Matamoros Martin
A. Nogales Muñoz
Biliopancreatic Surgical Division, Gastrointestinal
Surgical Department, Virgen de la Macarena
Hospital, Seville, Spain
e-mail: j_Bellido_1@hotmail.com;
macu.san.mat@gmail.com; anogal@telefonica.net

D. Gonzalez-Fernandez
Fremap Hospital, Seville, Spain
e-mail: gonzalezfernandezd9@gmail.com

Table 10.1 Surgical procedures for LDP

Laparoscopic distal pancreatectomy with splenectomy	LDP
Laparoscopic spleen preserving distal pancreatectomy (Warshaw technique) [5]	LSpDP
Laparoscopic spleen and vessel preserving distal pancreatectomy	LSVpDP
Laparoscopic-assisted distal pancreatectomy	LADP
Single incision distal pancreatectomy	SIDP
Robotic distal pancreatectomy	RDP

Table 10.2 Indications for laparoscopic distal pancreatectomy

Benign	Borderline	Malignant
Acute/chronic pancreatitis	Neuroendocrine tumors	Invasive carcinoma
Trauma	Mucinous cystic neoplasia	Metastatic renal cell carcinoma
Serous cystic neoplasia	IPMN (intraductal mucinous neoplasm)	
Transplantation for the live donor		

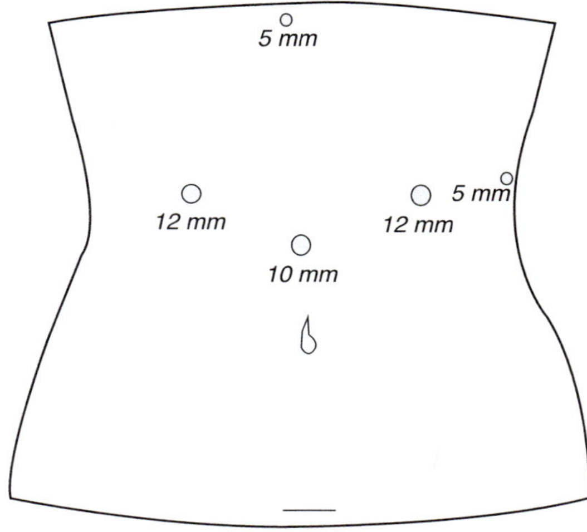

Fig. 10.1 Trocar placement in LDP. Suprapubic incision for specimen retrieval

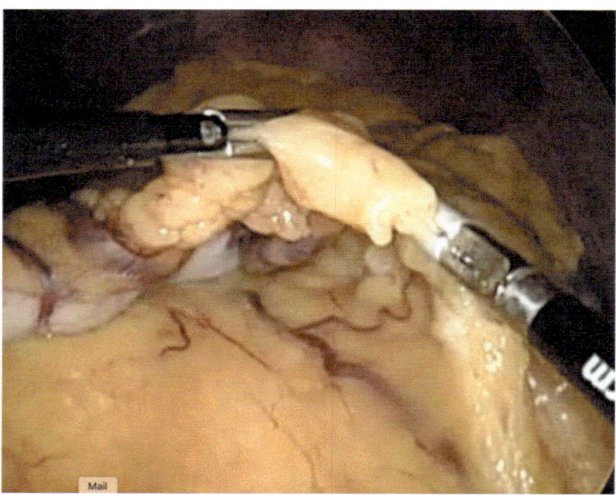

Fig. 10.2 Gastrocolic ligament division using Ligasure® 5 mm

10.3 Laparoscopic Distal Pancreatectomy (LDP) with Splenectomy

1. Patient position and trocar placement:

    The patient is positioned either in supine or left lateral decubitus position, depending on where the tumor is located. The pneumoperitoneum is performed using a Veress needle in the left hypochondrium. Once 14 mm Hg intraabdominal pressure is achieved, one 10 mm trocar in supraumbilical position for 10 mm/30° scope and two 12 mm trocars in left and right vacium are placed respectively. Two 5 mm trocars are placed in epigastric and left hypochondrium (Fig. 10.1).

2. Division of gastrocolic and gastrosplenic ligaments (Fig. 10.2).

    The liver is retracted by a grasper through the epigastric 5 mm trocar. The gastrocolic ligament is opened using a vessel sealer and posterior aspect of the stomach is exposed.

    Short gastric vessels are sectioned in the same fashion (Short gastric vessels are preserved if the Warshaw procedure is going to be performed).

3. Dissection of inferior pancreatic margin (Fig. 10.3).

    The inferior margin of the pancreas is dissected medially and the anterior aspect of the superior mesenteric vein is identified and exposed. A tunnel is created above this vein

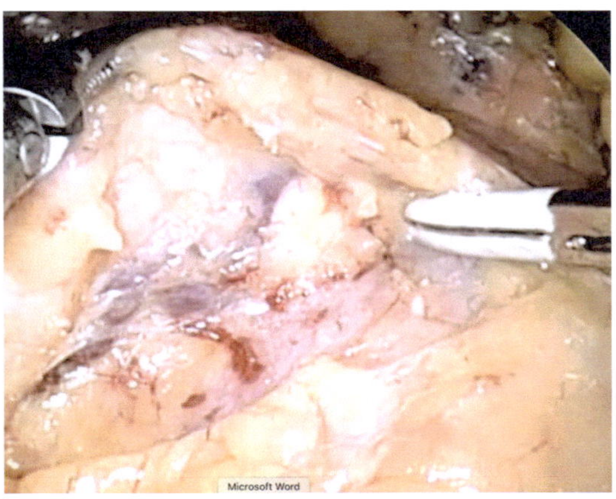

Fig. 10.3 Inferior pancreatic margin is identified and dissected

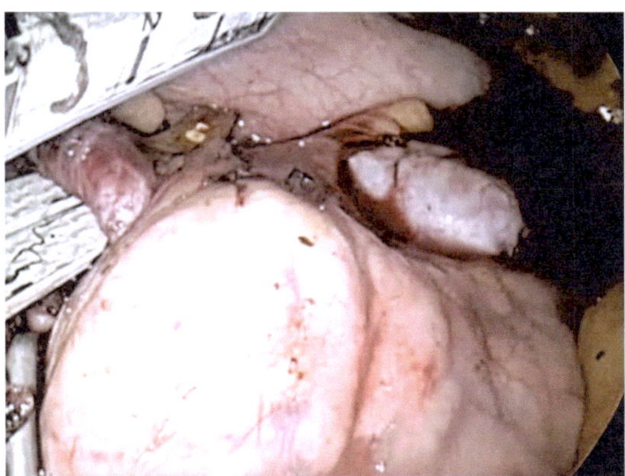

Fig. 10.5 Splenic artery is dissected and transected using a vascular endostapler

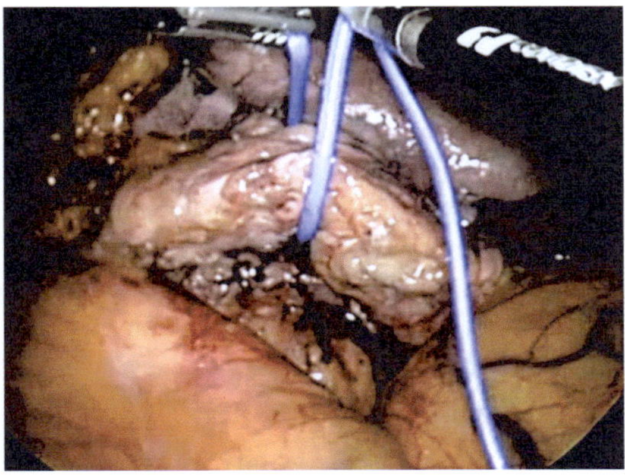

Fig. 10.4 The body of the pancreas is lifted using a vaseloop

and a tape is placed through the tunnel and the pancreas is completely encircled and lifted using the tape (Fig. 10.4).

4. Transection Splenic artery and vein (Figs. 10.5 and 10.6).

Splenic artery is transected previously using a vascular endostapler, clips, or hemolooks. After the first vascular control of the artery, the splenic vein is progressively dissected. The lack of arterial vascularization of the spleen will quickly decrease the flow of the splenic vein, enabling safe dissection and vein transection. When it is performed, its diameter is only 1 or 2 mm and it can be controlled easily with clips. Completeness of the spleen's vascular control can then be checked as the ischemic nature of the splenic tissue is easy to identify.

5. Pancreas transection (Fig. 10.7).

After dissection of the inferior margin of the pancreas and splenic vessels ligation, pancreatic parenchyma is transected. The transection is usually done by a stapler with a staple height of 3.8–3.5 mm. However, in very thick cases, it can be transected by an energy device instead.

6. Specimen retrieval.

The specimen is removed from suprapubic incision due to its good aesthetic results and low incisional hernia rates.

Several meta-analyses and review articles have been published comparing open distal pancreatectomy (ODP) to LDP [6–9]. They concluded that LDP is safe, feasible, and associated with less blood loss, fewer overall complications, a shorter time to oral intake, and a shorter postoperative hospital stay compared with ODP.

LDP in PDAC is still under debate, especially the R0 resection rate and long-term survival outcome. Ricci et al. [10] reported in their meta-analysis that the R0 resection rates of LDP and ODP were similar (86.3 vs. 80.7%), and there was no statistical difference regarding the number of harvested lymph nodes (12.9 vs. 12.8%). Finally, no difference was found in terms of overall survival.

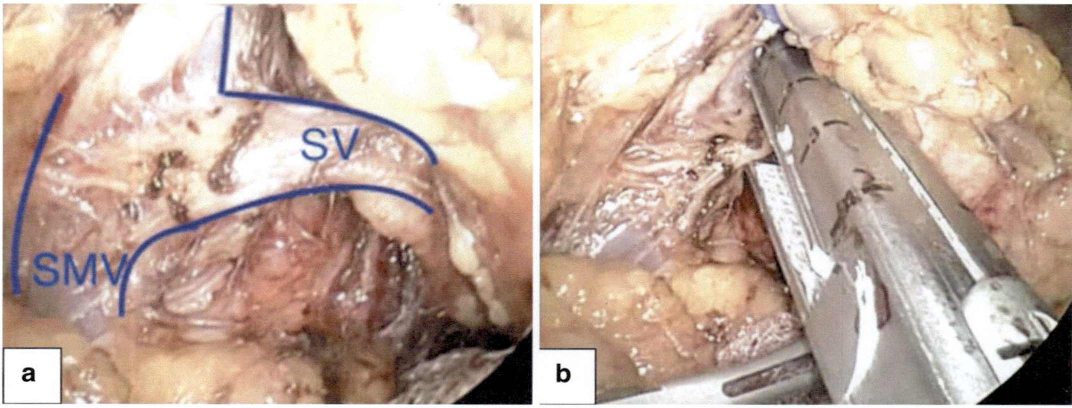

Fig. 10.6 (**a**) Splenomesenteric axis. (**b**) Splenic vein is transected at the origin using a vascular endostapler

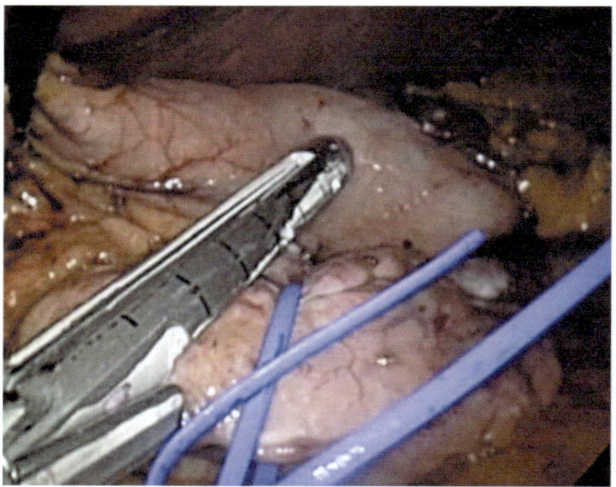

Fig. 10.7 Pancreas body is transected with violet cartridge endostapler

10.4 Laparoscopic Pancreaticoduodenectomy (LPD)

Pancreaticoduodenectomy is a highly demanding procedure even in the hands of skilled surgeons with specific training. Gagner and Pomp [1] first reported on LPD in 1994; during the following years, this procedure has not been widespread due to its complexity. Recent advances in laparoscopic procedures and technological innovations, LPD have all contributed to the increased popularity and acceptance.

10.4.1 Indications for LPD

The main contraindications of LPD are patients who require concomitant vessel reconstruction because these cases are presumed to have high complication and mortality rates. At the beginning of the LPD, best indications were small, benign, or low-grade tumors of the pancreatic head, duodenal ampulla, and distal common bile duct. Recently, the indications have been expanded to carcinomas located at the pancreatic head and uncinate process of the pancreas, duodenum, and duodenal ampulla. Patients with Mucinous cystic neoplasms and intraductal papillary mucinous neoplasms (IPMN) located in the pancreatic head are also good candidates for LPD [11].

1. Patient position and trocar placement.

   The patient is positioned in supine with legs and arms opened. The surgeon stands between the legs. Once the pneumoperitoneum is performed, one 10 mm trocar in supraumbilical position for 10 mm/30° scope and two 12 mm trocars in left and right vacium are placed, respectively. Two 5 mm trocars are placed in the epigastric and right hypochondrium, and one 12 mm in left hypochondrium (Fig. 10.8).

2. Lesser sac opening.

   The lesser sac is entered by creating a window into the gastrocolic omentum using

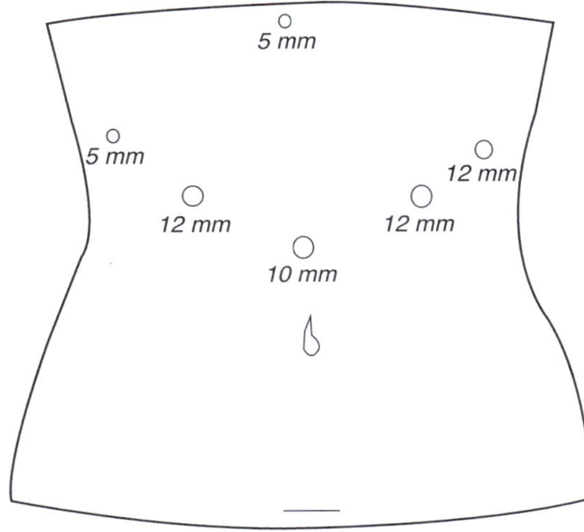

Fig. 10.8 Trocar placement in LPD

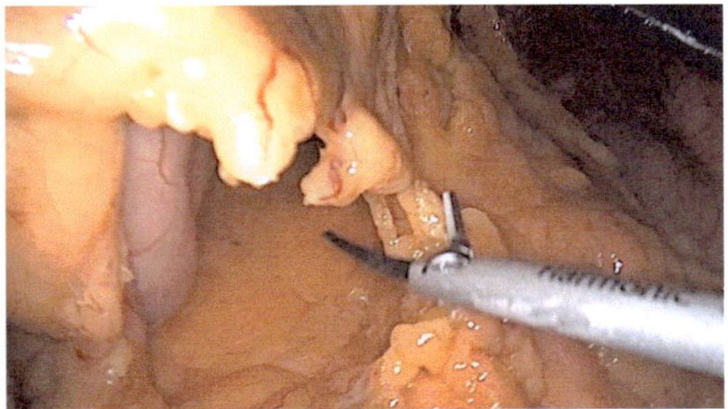

Fig. 10.9 Gastrocolic ligament is sectioned using a sealing device

a vessel sealer. The gastrocolic ligament is completely transected, avoiding injury to the gastroepiploic vessels (Fig. 10.9).

The right gastroepiploic vessels are stapled or clipped. The gastric antrum is transected using an Endostapler 60 mm.

3. Colon hepatic flexure mobilization.

The dissection is continued by mobilizing the hepatic flexure of the colon and part of the right colon to achieve appropriate exposure of the pancreatic head and the duodenum (Fig. 10.10).

4. Kocher maneuver.

The duodenum is completely freed from the retroperitoneal attachments (Fig. 10.11).

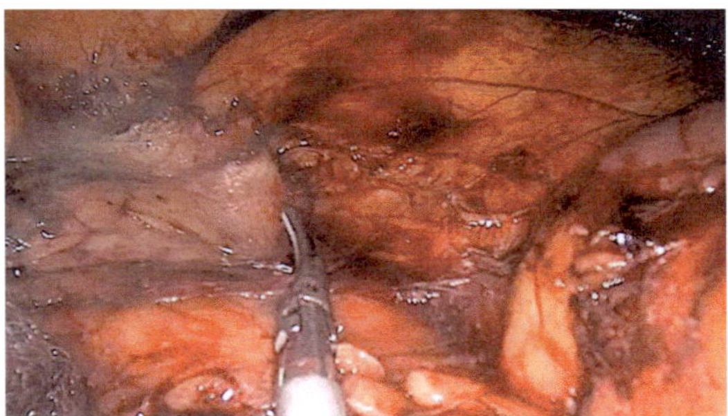

Fig. 10.10 Hepatic flexure is taken down, exposing the duodenum

The cava vein and aorta are exposed. Interaortocava limph nodes are removed.

5. Division of pyloric and gastroduodenal arteries.

The hepatic and gastroduodenal arteries are exposed. Excision of lymph node 8 A facilitates the exposure of the hepatic artery. The gastroduodenal artery is carefully dissected free and ligated and divided (Fig. 10.12).

6. Common bile duct transection:

The common bile duct is identified in hepatoduodenal ligament, dissected at 360°, and is transected sharply, leaving the posterior wall slightly longer than the anterior wall to facilitate later reconstruction (Fig. 10.13a, b). A Bulldog clamp is used to decrease bile spillage.

7. Retropancreatic window.

The inferior aspect of the pancreas is retracted upward and downward pressure on the transverse mesocolon is placed. An avascular plane is identified between the anterior superior mesenteric vein (SMV) and the posterior aspect of the pancreatic neck, creating a window (Fig. 10.14).

8. Treitz Ligament dissection and division of the distal bowel:

The ligament of Treitz is divided from the right side, the jejunum is divided with a laparoscopic stapler and the proximal jejunum is brought back behind the superior mesenteric vessels. By maintaining the dissection close to the bowel and opening the peritoneal window widely.

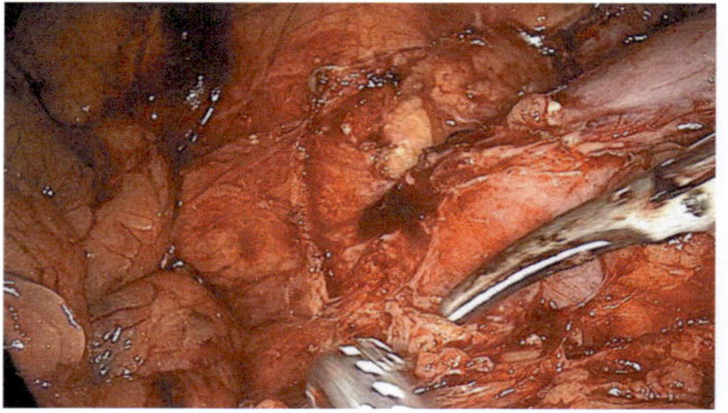

Fig. 10.11 Duodenum full medial mobilization

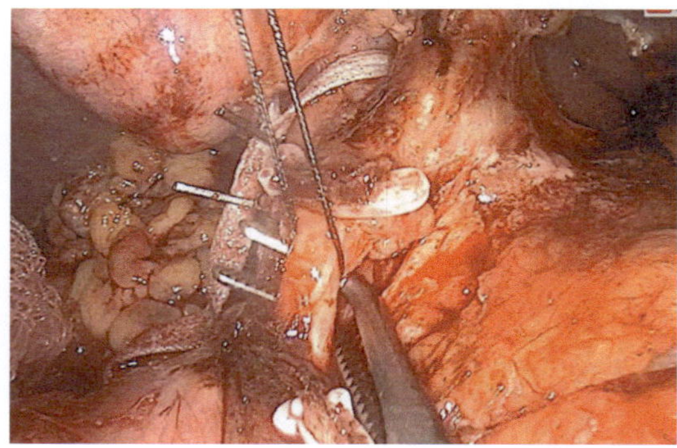

Fig. 10.12 Pyloric artery is clipped and transected. Gastroduodenal artery is identified

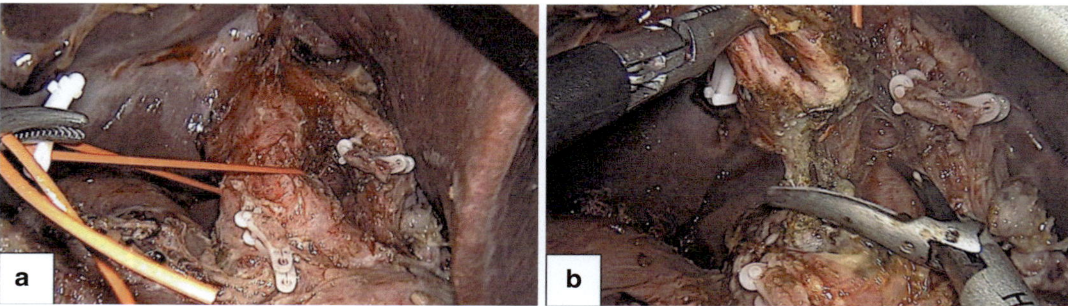

Fig. 10.13 (**a**) Common bile duct is identified and encircled. (**b**) Common bile duct is transected and the lymphatic tissue is resected

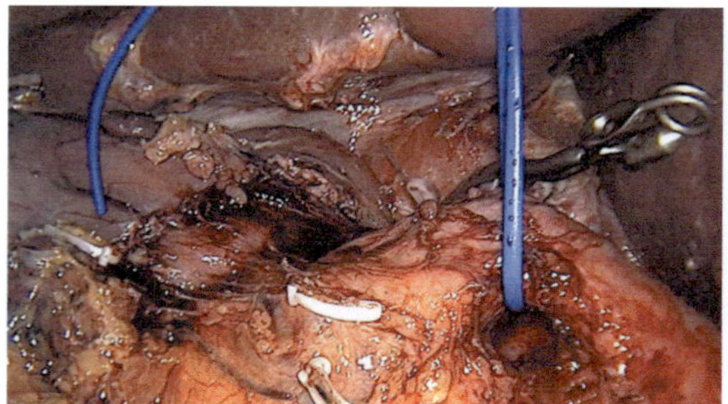

Fig. 10.14 Window is created between the pancreas neck and SMV. The pancreas is lifted using a vaseloop

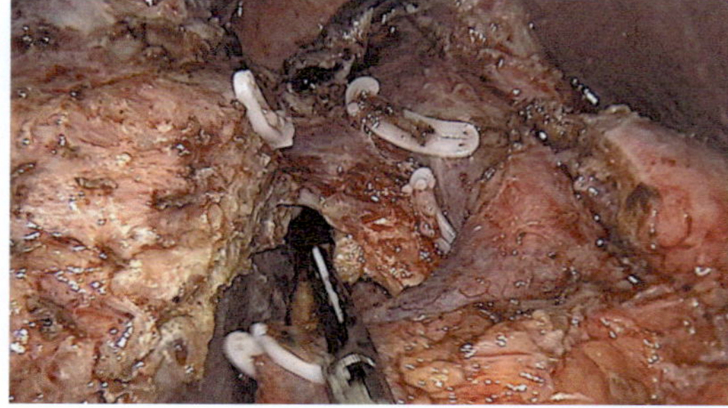

Fig. 10.15 Uncinate process dissection. Mesopancreas is excised using vessel sealer

9. Uncinate process dissection and mesopancreas excision:

   The uncinate process is carefully dissected from the lateral aspect of the SMV while clipping small vessels. The SMV is retracted medially. The SMA dissection is carried out using a vessel-sealing device. The inferior pancreaticoduodenal artery is usually clipped and divided. A complete, en bloc excision of the uncinate process and mesopancreas is confirmed (Fig. 10.15).

10. Pancreatic transection:

   It is performed with ultrasonic shears. The duct is then transected sharply with cold scis-

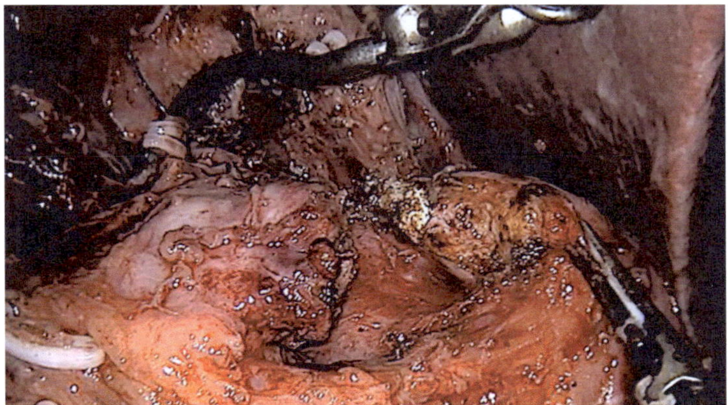

Fig. 10.16 Pancreas neck transection with vessel sealer

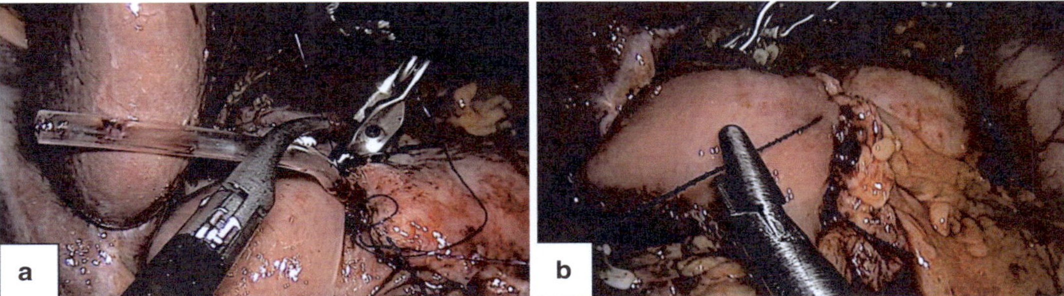

Fig. 10.17 (**a**) Tutor placed through the pancreaticojejunal anastomosis. (**b**) Running suture between anterior aspect of the pancreas and the jejunum

sors 2–3 mm to the right of the parenchymal transection line to leave a stump that will facilitate the future duct-to-mucosa reconstruction (Fig. 10.16).

11. Specimen removal.

The specimen is placed inside a bag and extracted through a suprapubic incision. It is retrieved and sent for pathological analysis.

12. Reconstruction.

10.4.2 Pancreaticoyeyunostomy (Duc-to-Mucosa Anastomosis)

A running suture is carried out between the posterior aspect of the pancreas and the seromuscular layer of the jejunum using a barbed suture 4.0. An opening is created in the jejunum with cautery. One or two interrupted sutures are placed using absorbable 4.0 monofilament suture performing the posterior face of the anastomosis. A tutor is placed from the pancreas duct to the jejunum and the anterior face of the anastomosis is done with other 3–4 sutures (Fig. 10.17a, b).

A running suture with long absorbable barbed suture 4.0 is placed between the anterior aspect of the pancreas and the seromuscular layer of the jejunum.

10.4.3 Hepaticojejunostomy

An end-to-side hepaticojejunostomy is performed using running barbed suture. The surgeon moves to the left side of the patient. Posterior and anterior wall anastomosis are done with two running sutures from the right side to the left side of the patient (Fig. 10.18).

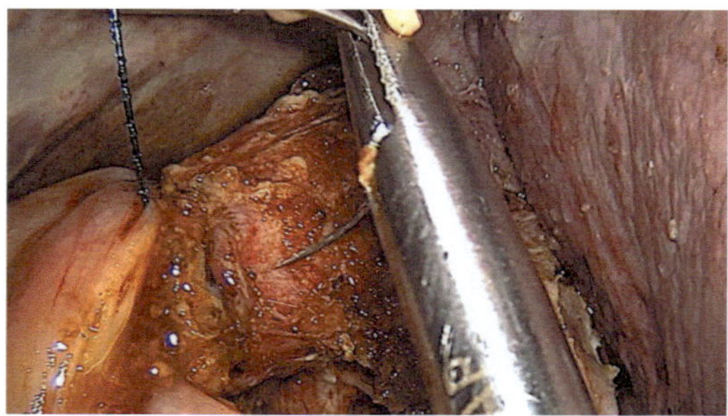

Fig. 10.18 Hepaticojejunostomy with running barbed 4.0 suture

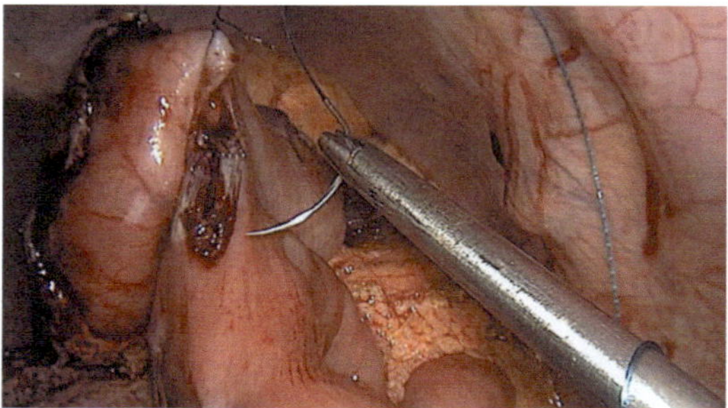

Fig. 10.19 Mechanical Gastrojejunal anastomosis

10.4.4 Gastrojejunostomy

An antecolic side-to-side gastrojejunostomy is constructed using an EndoGIA 60 blue cartridge. The orifice is closed with a running barbed 4.0 suture (Fig. 10.19). The Endogia orifice is closed using a running barbed suture.

Two 19-Fr Blake drains are placed in proximity of the hepaticojejunostomy/pancreaticojejunostomy and treitz ligament.

At present, the evidence is conflicting as regards the safety and reproducibility of LPD. The majority of retrospective studies and three of the published RCTs have reported equivalent short-term outcomes with LPD as compared to the OPD (open pancreaticoduodenectomy).

Palanivelu et al. showed that LPD was associated with longer operative time but reduced intraoperative blood loss. Hospital stay was shorter with LPD (7 vs. 13 days; $P = 0.001$) as compared with OPD. Short-term perioperative outcomes, including major morbidity, mortality, rates of postoperative pancreatic fistula, delayed gastric emptying, and postoperative hemorrhage were comparable [12].

Poves et al. (2018) confirmed that longer operative time and shorter hospital stays were observed in the LPD arm (13.5 vs. 17 days; $P = 0.024$). Fewer Clavien-Dindo grade III or higher complications were reported in the LPD Group; however, pancreas-specific complications were comparable between both groups. The lymph node yield and R0 resection rates were similar [3].

van Hilst J et al. evaluated LPD versus OPD. The study was prematurely terminated by the data and safety monitoring board because of a difference in 90-day complication-related mortality. The mortality in the LPD group was 10% ($n = 5/50$) as compared to 2% ($n = 1/49$) in the OPD group. Causes of mortality included bowel ischemia from intraoperative vascular damage, post-pancreatectomy hemorrhage, and POPF. The authors concluded that these safety concerns were unexpected and worrisome, especially in the setting of trained surgeons working in centers performing 20 or more PDs annually [13].

Wang M et al. compared LPD and OPD performed by experienced surgeons who had already done at least 104 LPD procedures individually. Two hundred ninety-seven patients in each arm were compared. The postoperative length of stay was significantly shorter for patients in the LPD group (median 15 vs. 16 days; $P = 0.02$) and 90-day mortality was similar in both groups (2%). The authors concluded that LPD offers equal perioperative safety with a reduction in the length of hospital stay in experienced hands. However, the clinical benefit of LPD over OPD was marginal, despite extensive procedural expertise and future research should focus to identify patient groups who would benefit most from LPD [14].

10.5 Robotic Pancreaticoduodenectomy

Due to the inherent advantages of the robotic platforms over laparoscopy, Robotic Pancreaticoduodenectomy (RPD) became increasingly popular since its first description in 2003 [15]. In general, the available retrospective data thus far shows comparable perioperative and short-term oncological outcomes with RPD, LPD, and OPD.

Zureikat et al. compared 211 RPDs with 817 OPDs for perioperative outcomes. The study demonstrated that post-learning curve, RPD, and OPD are comparable in safety and short-term oncologic efficacy. However, OPD patients had a higher percentage of PDAC cases and a greater proportion of non-dilated (<3 mm) pancreatic ducts. RPD was associated with longer operative times, reduced blood loss, and a smaller number of major complications [16].

Torphy RJ et al. compared OPD with LPD/RPD for short and long-term outcomes over 5 years (2010–2015). The 90-day mortality and unplanned 30-day readmissions were equivalent between MIPD and OPD. Mortality, despite being comparable in the groups, was high (6.7% in OPD and 5% in the LPD). A high conversion rate of 15% with RPD and 25% with LPD was noted. RPD cases that required conversion had a significantly increased odds of 90-day mortality (OR, 3.99; 95% CI: 1.27–12.51) as compared to the completed RPD cases. LPD cases that required conversion to open did not show any higher odds for mortality. Of concern, 38.6% of OPDs and 35.6% of MIPDs were performed at low-volume centers, despite a known inverse PD hospital volume and mortality association, which was also confirmed in this study. R0 resection, lymph nodes yield, and receipt of adjuvant chemotherapy were equivalent between the groups [17].

References

1. Gagner M, Pomp A. Laparoscopic pylorus-preserving pancreatoduodenectomy. Surg Endosc. 1994;8:408–10.
2. Nickel F, Haney CM, Kowalewski KF, et al. Laparoscopic versus open pancreaticoduodenectomy: a systematic review and meta-analysis of randomized controlled trials. Ann Surg. 2020;271:54–66.
3. Poves I, Burdio F, Morato O, et al. Comparison of perioperative outcomes between laparoscopic and open approach for pancreatoduodenectomy: the PADULAP randomized controlled trial. Ann Surg. 2018;268:731–9.
4. Cuschieri A, Jakimowicz JJ, van Spreeuwel J. Laparoscopic distal 70% pancreatectomy and splenectomy for chronic pancreatitis. Ann Surg. 1996;223(3):280–5.
5. Warshaw AL. Conservation of the spleen with distal pancreatectomy. Arch Surg. 1988;123:550–3.
6. Nigri GR, Rosman AS, Petrucciani N, et al. Metaanalysis of trials comparing minimally invasive and open distal pancreatectomies. Surg Endosc. 2011;25:1642–51.
7. Xie K, Zhu YP, Xu XW, Chen K, Yan JF, Mou YP. Laparoscopic distal pancreatectomy is as safe and feasible as open procedure: a meta-analysis. World J Gastroenterol. 2012;18:1959–67.
8. Jusoh AC, Ammori BJ. Laparoscopic versus open distal pancreatectomy: a systematic review of comparative studies. Surg Endosc. 2012;26:904–13.
9. Venkat R, Edil BH, Schulick RD, Lidor AO, Makary MA, Wolfgang CL. Laparoscopic distal pancreatectomy is associated with significantly less overall morbidity compared to the open technique: a systematic review and meta-analysis. Ann Surg. 2012;255:1048–59.
10. Ricci C, Casadei R, Taffurelli G, et al. Laparoscopic versus open distal pancreatectomy for ductal adenocarcinoma: a systematic review and meta-analysis. J Gastrointest Surg. 2015;19:770–81.
11. Song KB, Kim SC, Hwang DW, et al. Matched case-control analysis comparing laparoscopic and open pylorus-preserving pancreaticoduodenectomy in patients with periampullary tumors. Ann Surg. 2015;262:146–55.
12. Palanivelu C, Senthilnathan P, Sabnis SC, et al. Randomized clinical trial of laparoscopic versus open pancreatoduodenectomy for periampullary tumours. Br J Surg. 2017;104:1443–50.
13. van Hilst J, de Rooij T, Bosscha K, et al. Laparoscopic versus open pancreatoduodenectomy for pancreatic or periampullary tumours (LEOPARD-2): a multicentre, patient-blinded, randomised controlled phase 2/3 trial. Lancet Gastroenterol Hepatol. 2019;4:199–207.
14. Wang M, Li D, Chen R, et al. Laparoscopic versus open pancreatoduodenectomy for pancreatic or periampullary tumours: a multicentre, open-label, randomised controlled trial. Lancet Gastroenterol Hepatol. 2021;6:438–47.
15. Giulianotti PC, Coratti A, Angelini M, et al. Robotics in general surgery: personal experience in a large community hospital. Arch Surg. 2003;138:777–84.
16. Zureikat AH, Postlewait LM, Liu Y, et al. A multi-institutional comparison of perioperative outcomes of robotic and open pancreaticoduodenectomy. Ann Surg. 2016;264:640–9.
17. Torphy RJ, Friedman C, Halpern A, et al. Comparing short-term and oncologic outcomes of minimally invasive versus open pancreaticoduodenectomy across low and high volume centers. Ann Surg. 2019;270:1147–55.

Quality Standards in Pancreatic Surgery

11

Jose-María Álamo, Miguel-Angel Gómez-Bravo, Carmen Bernal-Bellido, Gonzalo Suárez-Artacho, and Javier Padillo-Ruiz

11.1 Introduction

With the advent of super-specialization and centralization of surgical procedures, the need to define quality standards in the different surgical techniques and processes has become a fundamental objective to improve health outcomes. In the area of general surgery, the treatment of colorectal cancer [1] or breast cancer [2]. They have published in recent years numerous studies focused on unifying these quality standards. However, pancreatic cancer has not been able to promote these studies, with very few articles published in this regard.

The main objectives of major pancreatic resections for pancreatic cancer should be, in principle, not to cause the death of the patient and to achieve the longest disease-free time if not its cure. To do this, the radical nature of the resection must be as complete as possible, depending on how advanced the tumor is, and the choice of the reconstruction technique must be the most correct. Obviously, in achieving these two objectives, factors that are beyond the surgeon come into play. On the one hand, regarding the curative efficacy of resection, oncological factors such as the biology and kinetics of the excised cancer (vascular, lymphatic and perineural invasion, histological pathway, etc.) and the response to chemotherapy treatment. On the other hand, regarding the morbidity and mortality of the surgical intervention, the patient's comorbidity is a factor to take into account when indicating resection, and it is a well-analyzed fact with different morbidity scores (ASA, POSSUM, etc.).

In this chapter, we will focus on those factors associated with surgery that could have an impact on both previously described objectives: postoperative survival of the patient and long-term survival in cancer terms. Regarding postoperative morbidity, the terms used should be described according to well-defined and agreed standards [3–5].

The selection of quality indicators is based on clinical practice guidelines [6–12], consensus conferences [13–16], and review papers on the quality of pancreatic cancer surgery and the development of indicators [17–22].

J. M. Álamo (✉)
Biliopancreatic Surgical Division, Virgen del Rocío Hospital, Seville, Spain

HPB Division, General Surgery Department, Virgen del Rocío Hospital, Seville, Spain

M. A. G. Bravo · C. B. Bellido · G. S. Artacho
Biliopancreatic Surgical Division, Virgen del Rocío Hospital, Seville, Spain

J. P. Ruiz
Gastrointestinal Surgical Department, Biliopancreatic Surgery Unit, Virgen del Rocio Hospital, Seville, Spain

11.2 Mortality

Mortality is considered by far one of the most important indicators of quality in surgery, and this holds true for pancreatic surgery. Postoperative

© The Author(s), under exclusive license to Springer Nature Switzerland AG 2023
J. Bellido Luque, A. Nogales Muñoz (eds.), *Recent Innovations in Surgical Procedures of Pancreatic Neoplasms*, https://doi.org/10.1007/978-3-031-21351-9_11

mortality must be minimized regardless of the surgical technique. A recent meta-analysis exploring volume–outcome relationship in pancreatic surgery reported a strong inverse association between hospital volume and postoperative mortality is considered by far one of the most important indicators of quality in surgery, and this holds true for pancreatic surgery. Postoperative mortality must be minimized regardless of the surgical technique. A meta-analysis exploring volume–outcome relationship [23] in pancreatic surgery reported a strong inverse association between hospital volume and postoperative mortality.

Depending on the extent of pancreatic resection, mortality is subject to variations. In a recent complete survey of pancreatic resections in Germany [24], in-hospital mortality differs between 7 and 23% depending on the extent of pancreatic resections. This confirms the meta-analysis of the current international literature. As already outlined, there is also a strong volume–outcome relationship in pancreatic surgery. This effect is stronger than in all other areas of surgery.

In the published Spanish series, mortality ranges from 0.0% of Fernández-Cruz et al. [25] to 14.35% of Balsells-Valls et al. [26]. The acceptable quality indicator should be <10%.

11.3 Postoperative Bleeding

Postoperative bleeding is a relatively common complication in major pancreatic cancer surgery. The most common is undoubtedly gastrointestinal bleeding associated with the gastrojejunal anastomosis line, and in most cases it can be solved by hemostatic endoscopic treatment. Gastrointestinal bleeding sequential to intestinal anastomosis is less frequent and usually resolves with conservative treatment. The most lethal, however, is usually intra-abdominal hemorrhage secondary to a gastroduodenal artery pseudoaneurysm. In our experience, treatment by percutaneous embolization is the treatment of choice, and if it is not possible, it is a surgical emergency, although, in both cases, hepatic artery thrombosis may be the side effect.

Table 11.1 Associated factors in recurrence of pancreatic cancer

Indicator	Tumoral recurrence (p)
Diabetes	0.001
Smoking	0.033
Alcoholism	0.737
Vascular resection	0.999
R1 resection	0.002
Lymph metastasis	0.000
Pancreatic fistula	0.647
Postoperatory bleeding	0.345

Multivariant analysis

In the published series, the incidence of postoperative bleeding, without specifying the origin, ranges between 2% in Fernández-Cruz et al. and 16% in Figueras et al. The acceptable quality indicator should be <10%. We must take into account that postoperative bleeding will influence the postoperative survival of the patient, but not long-term survival according to a study carried out by our group with 220 analyzed patients (Table 11.1).

11.4 Pancreatic Fistula

Unlike hemorrhage, the appearance of a pancreatic fistula does not usually compromise the life of the patient except in the few cases of grade C fistula following the International Study Group of Pancreatic Fistula (*ISGPF classification*), which is usually avoided with the correct placement of intra-abdominal drains. In our series, its appearance is not associated with long-term survival in relation to the appearance of distant metastasis or recurrence (Table 11.1). That is why, despite being a frequently used indicator in pancreatic surgery, its real relevance should be questioned, since it is only indicative of a longer hospital stay. And this, as we discussed in the introduction, is not part of the two main objectives of major pancreatic resections for cancer, that is, guaranteeing the life of the patient and prolonging the disease-free time if not its cure.

However, it is an indicator to take into account regarding the technical quality of pancreatic flow reconstruction. The published series offer percentages of postsurgical fistula that range from 6.25% of Sabaté et al. to 34.8% of Sánchez Cabú et al. There is consensus that the desired quality indicator is between 10 and 18% and always less than 30% [27, 28].

Logically, this indicator should be composed mostly of grade A and B fistulas, although this subclassification has not been analyzed in any study or meta-analysis.

11.5 Surgical Reintervention

The surgical reintervention rate is highly variable. The most frequent cause of early reoperation is sepsis due to suture dehiscence and intra-abdominal or gastrointestinal bleeding. Spanish series ranges between 1.85% of Fernández-Cruz et al. [25] and 14.53% of Domínguez Comesaña et al. [29]. The desirable indicator should be around 10% and should not go beyond 20%.

11.6 Quality of Oncological Resection

Indicators of quality of radical resection comprise nodal retrieval and resection margin status. These can be effectively understood only after proper preoperative staging and accurate pathological examination. Accurate lymphadenectomy provides a high nodal retrieval that is associated with better disease staging and prognostic stratification and must always be carried out to a high standard. Equally important is to obtain maximum clearance at the resection margins since margin positivity has been recognized universally as a prognostic factor, especially by applying the 1-mm clearance to define a radical resection.

In our series analyzed, the presence of metastatic lymphadenopathy and R1 resection is clearly associated with lower survival, so an R0 resection that prevents recurrence and a correct lymphadenectomy that serves as oncological staging are essential (Fig. 11.1).

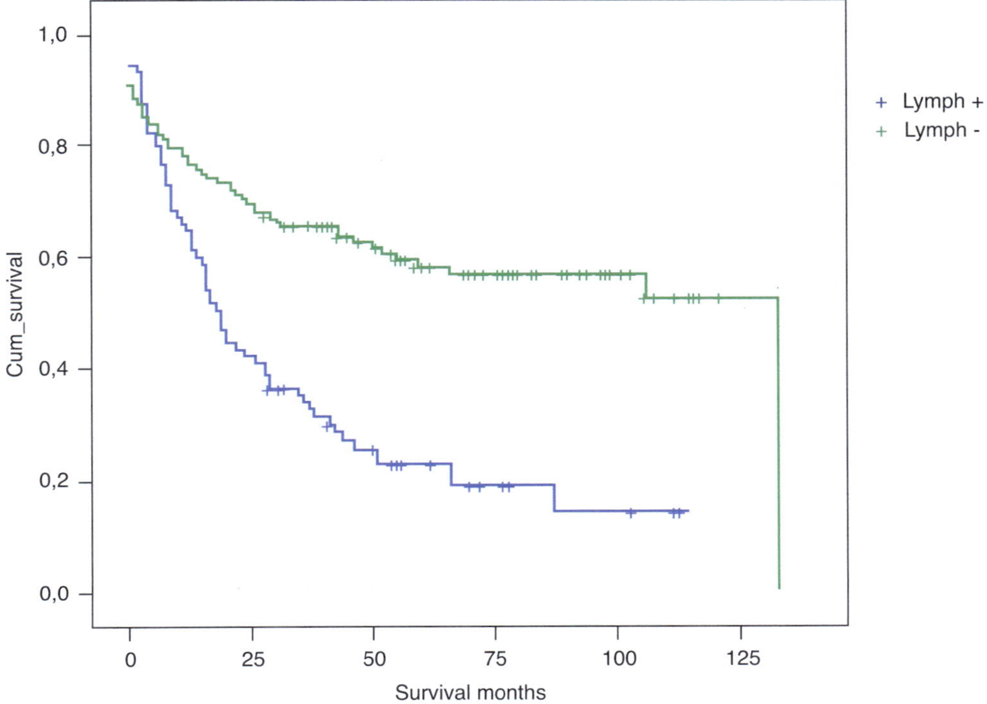

Fig. 11.1 Kaplan Meyer survival curve. Lymphatic node metastasis in resection block

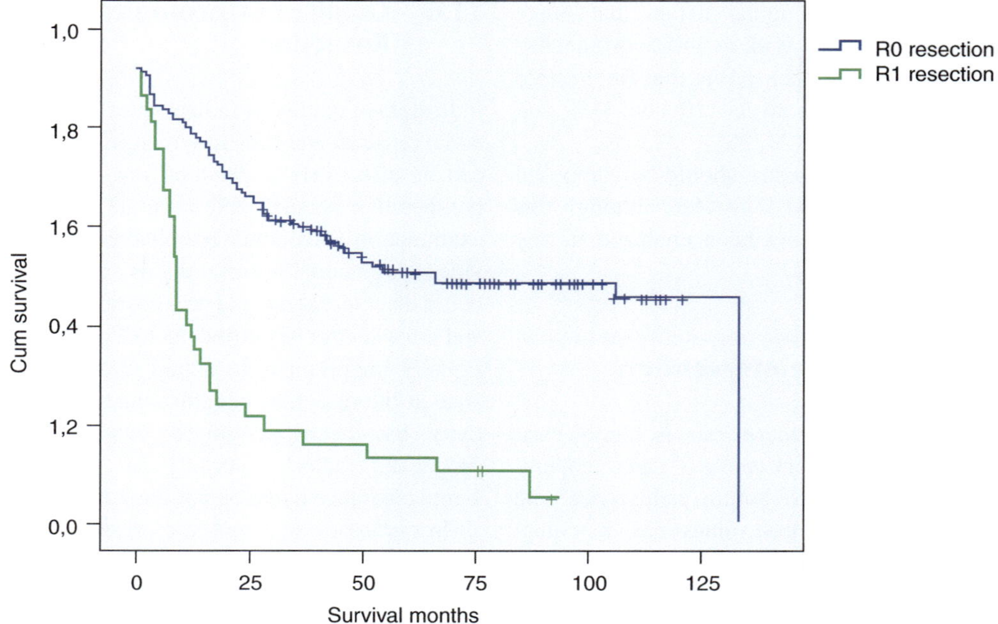

Fig. 11.2 Kaplan Meyer survival curve. Margin of resection

To achieve R0 resection, it is essential to have an adequate rate of venous resections of the mesenteric-portal trunk. This fact is not clearly defined in the scientific literature, but what is clear is that the rate of vascular resections should never be 0. A higher rate is a quality indicator of a correct oncological resection of pancreatic cancer (Fig. 11.2).

11.7 Other Indicators

The surgical waiting list should be of a maximum of 30 days (but preferably much shorter), with strict scheduling of patients based on surgical indication. Of note, those requiring restaging after neoadjuvant therapy should follow a dedicated, structured pathway. Every patient should undergo an elective preoperative multidisciplinary evaluation underlining and managing all possible factors that might decrease the surgical risk and improve outcome.

Radiologists should have expertise in all pancreatic imaging procedures including contrast-enhanced ultrasound, computed tomography, magnetic resonance imaging, interventional angiography, and percutaneous intervention.

The gastrointestinal endoscopy service should ensure both diagnostic and operative procedures. All such diagnostic and interventional services should be available at the hospital with adequate staff, to ensure rapid on-site evaluation and treatment.

Finally, it has been shown that the mortality rate, long-term survival, and resectability rates are directly related to the volume of pancreatic surgery performed at the hospital. That is why a quality indicator should be a volume of no less than 20 major pancreatectomies per year [30, 31].

References

1. van Hoeve J, de Munck L, Otter R, de Vries J, Siesling S. Quality improvement by implementing an integrated oncological care pathway for breast cancer patients. Breast. 2014;23:364–70.
2. Gooiker GA, Kolfschoten NE, Bastiaannet E, van de Velde CJH, Eddes EH, van der Harst E, et al. Evaluating the validity of quality indicators for colorectal cancer care. J Surg Oncol. 2013;108:465–71.

3. Bassi C, Dervenis C, Butturini G, Fingerhut A, Yeo C, Izbicki J, et al. Postoperative pancreatic fistula: an International Study Group (ISGPF) definition. Surgery. 2005;138:8–13.

4. Wente MN, Bassi C, Dervenis C, Fingerhut A, Gouma DJ, Izbicki JR, et al. Delayed gastric emptying (DGE) after pancreatic surgery: a suggested definition by the International Study Group of Pancreatic Surgery (ISGPS). Surgery. 2007;142:761–8.

5. Wente MN, Veit JA, Bassi C, Dervenis C, Fingerhut A, Gouma DJ, et al. Postpancreatectomy hemorrhage (PPH): an International Study Group of Pancreatic Surgery (ISGPS) definition. Surgery. 2007;142:20–5.

6. Evans DB, Jessup JM, Colacchio T. Pancreatic cancer surgical practice guidelines. Pancreatic Cancer Practice Guideline Committee. Oncology. 1997;11:1074–9.

7. Tempero MA, Behrman S, Ben-Josef E, Benson AB 3rd, Cameron JL, Casper ES, et al. Pancreatic adenocarcinoma: clinical practice guidelines in oncology. J Natl Compr Cancer Netw. 2005;3:598–626.

8. Tempero MA, Malafa MP, Behrman SW, Benson AB 3rd, Casper ES, Chiorean EG, et al. Pancreatic adenocarcinoma, version 2.2014: featured updates to the NCCN guidelines. J Natl Compr Canc Netw. 2014;12:1083–93.

9. Cascinu S, Falconi M, Valentini V, Jelic S, ESMO Guidelines Working Group. Pancreatic cancer: ESMO Clinical Practice Guidelines for diagnosis, treatment and follow-up. Ann Oncol. 2010;21 Suppl 5:v55–8.

10. Yamaguchi K, Tanaka M, Committee for Revision of Clinical Guidelines for Pancreatic Cancer of Japan Pancreas Society. EBM-based clinical guidelines for pancreatic cancer 2009 from the Japan Pancreas Society: a synopsis. Jpn J Clin Oncol. 2011;41:836–40.

11. Ujiki MB, Talamonti MS. Guidelines for the surgical management of pancreatic adenocarcinoma. Semin Oncol. 2007;34:311–20.

12. Pancreatic Section, British Society of Gastroenterology, Pancreatic Society of Great Britain and Ireland, Association of Upper Gastrointestinal Surgeons of Great Britain and Ireland, Royal College of Pathologists, Special Interest Group for Gastro-Intestinal Radiology. Guidelines for the management of patients with pancreatic cancer periampullary and ampullary carcinomas. Gut. 2005;54(Suppl 5):v1–6.

13. Takaori K, Bassi C, Biankin A, Brunner TB, Cataldo I, Campbell F, et al. International Association of Pancreatology (IAP)/European Pancreatic Club (EPC) consensus review of guidelines for the treatment of pancreatic cancer. Pancreatology. 2016;16:14–27.

14. Van Laethem JL, Verslype C, Iovanna JL, Michl P, Conroy T, Louvet C, et al. New strategies and designs in pancreatic cancer research: consensus guidelines report from a European expert panel. Ann Oncol. 2012;23:570–6.

15. Martin-Richard M, Ginés A, Ayuso JR, Sabater L, Fabregat J, Mendez R, et al. Recomendaciones para el diagnóstico, la estadificación y el tratamiento de las lesiones premalignas y el adenocarcinoma de páncreas. Med Clin (Barc). 2016;147:465.e1–8.

16. Navarro S, Vaquero E, Maurel J, Bombi JA, de Juan C, Feliu J, et al. Recomendaciones para el diagnóstico, estadificación y tratamiento del cáncer de páncreas (parte II). Med Clin (Barc). 2010;134:692–702.

17. Bilimoria KY, Bentrem DJ, Lillemoe KD, Talamonti MS, Ko CY. Assessment of pancreatic cancer care in the United States based on formally developed quality indicators. J Natl Cancer Inst. 2009;101:848–59.

18. Riall TS, Nealon WH, Goodwin JS, Townsend CM, Freeman JL. Outcomes following pancreatic resection: variability among high-volume providers. Surgery. 2008;144:133–40.

19. Dimick JB, Welch HG, Birkmeyer JD. Surgical mortality as an indicator of hospital quality. The problem with small sample size. JAMA. 2004;292:847–51.

20. Tempero MA, Berlin J, Ducreux M, Haller D, Harper P, Khayat D, et al. Pancreatic cancer treatment and research: an international expert panel discussion. Ann Oncol. 2011;22:1500–6.

21. McGory ML, Shekelle PG, Rubenstein LZ, Fink A, Ko CY. Developing quality indicators for elderly patients undergoing abdominal operations. J Am Coll Surg. 2005;201:870–83.

22. Vollmer CM Jr, Pratt W, Vanounou T, Maithel SK, Callery MP. Quality assessment in high-acuity surgery: volume and mortality are not enough. Arch Surg. 2007;142:371–80.

23. Gooiker GA, van Gijn W, Wouters MWJM, Post PN, van de Velde CJH, Tollenaar RAEM, et al. Systematic review and meta-analysis of the volume-outcome relationship in pancreatic surgery. Br J Surg. 2011;98:485–94.

24. Nimptsch U, Krautz C, Weber GF, Mansky T, Grützmann R. Nationwide in-hospital mortality following pancreatic surgery in Germany is higher than anticipated. Ann Surg. 2016;264:1082–90.

25. Fernández-Cruz L, Cosa R, Blanco L, López-Boado MA, Astudillo E. Pancreatogastrostomy with gastric partition after pylorus-preserving pancreatoduodenectomy versus conventional pancreatojejunostomy. A prospective randomized study. Ann Surg. 2008;248:930–8.

26. Balsells-Valls J, Olsina-Kissler JJ, Bilbao-Aguirre I, Solans-Domenech A, Margarit-Creixell C, Armengol-Carrasco M. Tratamiento quirúrgico de la neoplasia de páncreas y región periampular en una unidad especializada: una década después. Gastroenterol Hepatol. 2006;29:66–70.

27. Ärztliches Zentrum für Qualität in der Medizin (ÄZQ). Manual Qualitätsindikatoren. (äzqSchriftenreihe.) Neukirchen. 2009. www.aezq.de/mdb/literatur/manual-qualitaetsindikatoren

28. Sabater L, Mora I, Gámez JM. Estándares de calidad en la cirugía oncológica pancreática en España. Cir Esp. 2018;96(6):342–51.

29. Dominguez-Comesaña E, Gonzalez-Rodriguez FJ, Ulla-Rocha JL, Lede-Fernandez A, Portela-Serra JL,

Piñón-Cimadevila MA. Morbimortalidad de la resección pancreática. Cir Esp. 2013;91:551–8.

30. Balzano G, Zerbi A, Capretti G, Rocchetti S, Apitanio V, Di Carlo V. Effect of hospital volume on outcome of pancreaticoduodenectomy in Italy. Br J Surg. 2008;95:357–62.

31. Hackert T, Hinz U, Pausch T, Fesenbeck I, Strobel O, Schneider L, et al. Postoperative pancreatic fistula: we need to redefine grades B and C. Surgery. 2016;159:872–7.

Pablo Parra-Membrives, Darío Martínez-Baena,
José Manuel Lorente-Herce,
and Granada Jiménez-Riera

12.1 Introduction

Despite the remarkable scientific advances of the last century, a high incidence of surgical complications is invariably associated with pancreatic surgery. Allen Whipple performed his first pancreatic resection in 1934 on a patient who died 2 days later from a pancreatic fistula. He came to perform only 37 of the procedures that bear his name. Almost a century after this first procedure, pancreatic surgery still presents a not negligible morbidity rate of 58% and a mortality rate of 4% in best hands. The acceptable quality limit of complications has been established in around 73% of operated patients and tolerable mortality extends to 10% [1, 2].

The surgeon facing a pancreatic resection must assume the potential appearance of four immediate complications (pancreatic fistula, postoperative bleeding, delayed gastric emptying, and remnant pancreatitis) and four late complications (exocrine and endocrine pancreatic insufficiency, long-term cholangitis, and again acute pancreatitis). The incidence and severity of all of them vary according to the characteristics of each group of patients, the experience of the surgeon, and depending on the location of the resection (head, body, or pancreatic tail). The definition of each complication and the available evidence about its diagnosis and the best treatment option will be analyzed below.

12.2 Pancreatic Fistula

A fistula is defined as any abnormal communication between a pancreatic duct and another epithelial surface with the extravasation of fluid rich in pancreatic enzymes. In 2005, an international expert panel (International Study Group for Pancreatic Fistula—ISGPF) established the first consensus criteria to diagnose and classify them. These criteria have been universally accepted and have been used since then in most publications [3]. An updated version of these criteria has been recently published [4].

Thus, a pancreatic fistula is defined as the exit through a surgical or percutaneous drainage of a measurable volume of fluid containing levels of amylase three times higher than the normal plasma values when it appears on the third post-

P. Parra-Membrives (✉) · D. Martínez-Baena
G. Jiménez-Riera
Department of Surgery, University of Seville,
Seville, Spain

Hepatobiliary and Pancreatic Surgery Unit, General
and Digestive Surgery Department, Valme University
Hospital, Seville, Spain
e-mail: pabloparra@aecirujanos.es;
dariobaena@gmail.com; granadajimenez@gmail.com

J. M. Lorente-Herce
Hepatobiliary and Pancreatic Surgery Unit, General
and Digestive Surgery Department, Valme University
Hospital, Seville, Spain
e-mail: lorente82@gmail.com

operative day or thereafter. Prior to biochemical measurement, the experienced pancreatic surgeon will be able to suspect the oncoming of this feared complication if the fluid discharged through the drain is transparent or rather rusty. At this point, the appearance of clinical symptoms related to the appearance of a pancreatic fistula as abdominal pain, fever, delayed gastric emptying, and decline of general appearance must be closely supervised. Common biochemical findings include leukocytosis and elevation of inflammatory markers, especially C-reactive protein and procalcitonin. The onset of symptoms is often insidious, and the patient goes from being in perfect condition to alert the surgeon to feel that something is wrong. Finally, some of these patients end up offering a sensation of being severely ill in the following hours or days with the development of a septic shock, particularly in cases of wide dehiscence of the pancreatoenteric suture.

Although the diagnosis of a pancreatic fistula is made by biochemical determination of abdominal drainage, confirmation of the leak and its severity is established after the patient underwent any abdominal imaging test, usually by CT scan with intravenous contrast [1]. Current technology allows detecting of even slight anastomotic leaks with anatomical precision. The finding of juxta-anastomotic fluid collections should point out the possibility of extravasated pancreatic fluid (Fig. 12.1). The updated classification of severity and clinical impact of pancreatic fistulas established three degrees of pancreatic fistulas. Grade A has been defined as a biochemical fistula and is not referred to as a true pancreatic fistula. It exclusively involves the detection of high amylase levels in drain output fluid in the setting of an asymptomatic patient with no need for therapeutic intervention. A persistent drainage exceeding 3 weeks, the presence of relevant clinical changes (e.g., signs of infection without organ failure) or the need for endoscopic, radiological, or angiographic therapeutic intervention determine the existence of a grade B fistula. Finally, those patients who require a surgical reintervention or those who develop organ failure or die are classified as grade C pancreatic fistula patients. Grades B and C are collectively called clinically relevant pancreatic fistulas (Fig. 12.2).

The risk of suffering a pancreatic fistula varies clearly depending on the pancreatic resection

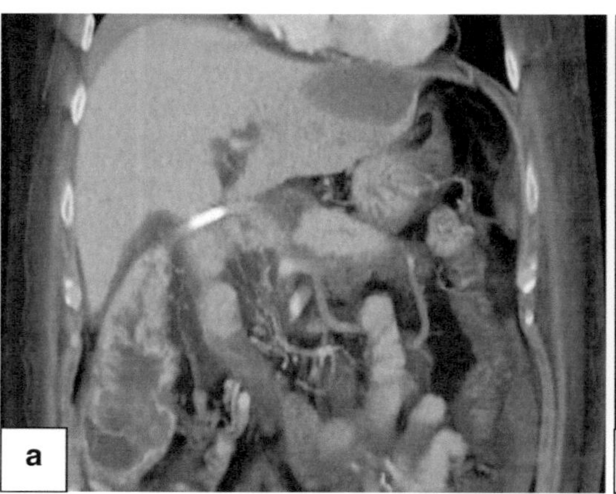

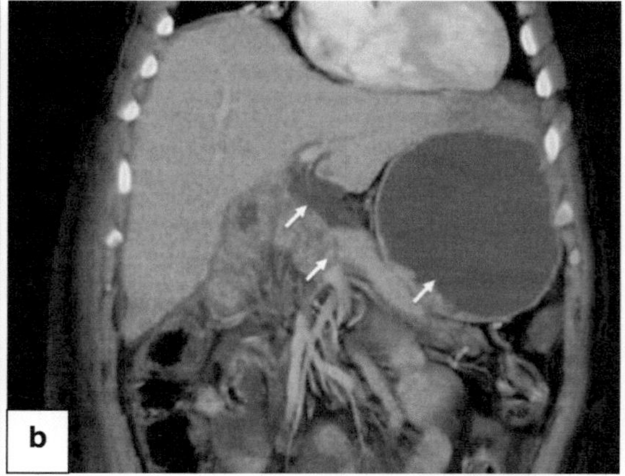

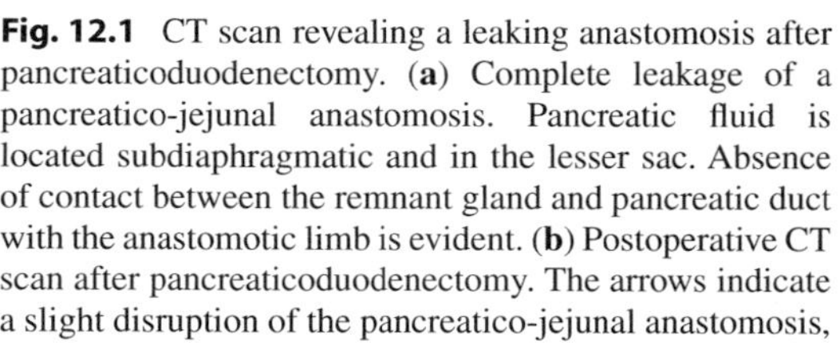

Fig. 12.1 CT scan revealing a leaking anastomosis after pancreaticoduodenectomy. (**a**) Complete leakage of a pancreatico-jejunal anastomosis. Pancreatic fluid is located subdiaphragmatic and in the lesser sac. Absence of contact between the remnant gland and pancreatic duct with the anastomotic limb is evident. (**b**) Postoperative CT scan after pancreaticoduodenectomy. The arrows indicate a slight disruption of the pancreatico-jejunal anastomosis, a collection of peripancreatic fluid and a gastric dilation reactive to the inflammatory process, leading to delayed gastric emptying. From Parra Membrives P, Martínez Baena D, Lorente Herce J, Jiménez Riera G, Sánchez Gálvez MÁ, Martín Balbuena R, et al. Diagnóstico y tratamiento de las complicaciones y secuelas de la cirugía pancreática. Evidencias y desavenencias. Cir Andal. 2019;30(2):186–94

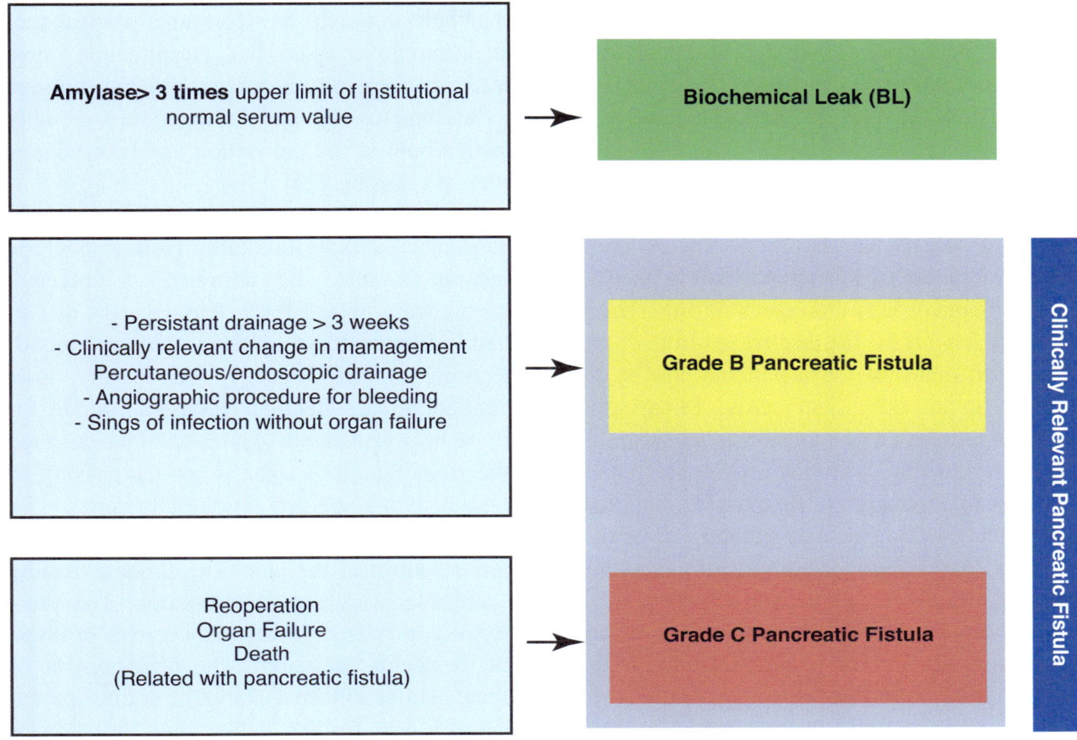

Fig. 12.2 Modified ISGPF classification for pancreatic fistulas (2016)

procedure that is performed. The overall incidence of fistulas, including biochemical leaks, is more elevated after distal pancreatectomy. However, the clinical impact is higher when a fistula develops following pancreatic head resections. Since pancreaticoduodenectomy involves the opening of a jejunal loop for reconstruction, pancreatic fluid spillage throughout a leaking anastomosis is almost always infected. The incidence of clinically relevant fistulas after distal pancreatectomy is 23%. Carrying out a pancreaticoduodenectomy increases this risk to a little over 27%. More than half of the patients who undergo enucleation of a pancreatic lesion will present a pancreatic fistula, 37% of them clinically relevant (grades B and C). Finally, patients who undergo central pancreatectomy have the summative risk of a double pancreatic remnant with enteric anastomosis and will develop a grade B or C fistula in 60% of cases [5].

The benefit of leaving abdominal drains following pancreatic surgery has been extensively analyzed. On the one hand, the suction effect of the drainage and the inflammatory process induced by a perianastomotic foreign body that is placed for a prolonged period could facilitate, rather than prevent, the development of a pancreatic fistula. On the other hand, avoiding abdominal drain placement following pancreatic resection has been shown to increase morbidity and quadruple postoperative mortality [6].

Thus, early withdrawal of the drain has been suggested as an intermediate approach. Many efforts have been made to predict which patients will develop a pancreatic fistula and which will not. The rationale behind this approach is to keep the drains in those patients who will really need them to extract leaking fluid but early remove any foreign body to avoid favoring fistula development. The detection of elevated amylase in the drainage fluid on the first postoperative day has shown to have a high positive predictive value for the prediction of pancreatic fistula occurrence. Several studies have tried to determine the optimal cut-off point, establishing that values of amylase higher than 2000–5000 u/l represent a high risk of developing a pancreatic fistula [6, 7]. A value of 600 u/l on the first postoperative day may have a sufficient negative predictive value to allow the removal of the drain [8]. In addition to amylase, the early elevation of C-reactive protein following surgery has also been shown to predict the development of a pancreatic fistula [9, 10].

Biochemical leak management only requires patience to wait for the discharge of the drain to cease and many of these patients can be controlled on an outpatient basis. Symptomatic patients require close monitoring and usually a long hospital stay. As noted previously, patients developing a pancreatic fistula after pancreaticoduodenectomy present greater severity, a higher rate of infectious complications, a longer hospital stay, and a greater requirement for intensive care support than those whose index procedure was a distal pancreatectomy. In general, patients who develop pancreatic fistula enter a hypercatabolic state and require supplementary nutritional support. The nutrient demand is considerably increased by the surgical healing process itself, the significant protein loss through the enzyme-rich fistula output, and the resource consumption in response to a local or systemic septic process [11]. The enteral nutrition is the preferred way to deliver nutritional support whenever the gastrointestinal tract is functional. Enteral feeding increases the probability of closure of the fistula twice, diminishes the closure time, and allows a shorter hospital stay with fewer complications [12].

Somatostatin and somatostatin analogues have been routinely employed to prevent fistula formation following pancreatic surgery and to accelerate fistula closure after development. However, there is no solid evidence that somatostatin analogues result in a higher closure rate of pancreatic fistula compared with other treatments. Evidence about the beneficial effect on the reduction in the volume of the debit or over the fistula closure time is also lacking [13]. Conversely, a recent study reveals that somatostatin analogues may even favor fistulas formation instead of preventing them, by reducing

splanchnic flow and therefore also perfusion of the anastomotic ends [14]. Despite this, most centers performing pancreatic surgery continue to use somatostatin and its analogues in daily practice both in the prevention and treatment of pancreatic fistulas [15].

Adequate antibiotic coverage is of paramount importance. Leaking fluid after pancreatoenteric anastomosis must be assumed as infected. Patients who present fever, leukocytosis, or elevated inflammatory markers require broad-spectrum antibiotic therapy. As in any other intra-abdominal infectious focus, a sample for culture by percutaneous aspiration of the detected collections should be taken as soon as possible to de-escalate to a targeted antibiotic therapy [11].

The most frequent indication for reoperation is poor control of the infectious process leading to progressive clinical deterioration. The presence of generalized peritonitis, necrosis of intestinal segments, or simply the development of infected collections that cannot be drained percutaneously are further indications for surgery. There is no single or standard surgical procedure that can be recommended for the time of the second surgery. Each patient may require a different technique. However, there is a growing trend to perform what has come to be called pancreatic conservative surgery. When operative findings are limited to undrained infected fluid collections or minimal leakage of pancreatoenteric anastomosis, then debridement, lavage of the collections, and new drain placement may be sufficient. Generally, attempting to repair an anastomosis with a partial disruption may seem tempting, but it is not recommended. Any efforts to suture the leakage point lead more often to increase it than to close it. The application of liquid or sheet sealants is more part of a ritual or a surgical superstition than an intervention with real efficacy [8].

When a major anastomotic leakage is stated, assure the postoperative drainage of the intestinal and pancreatic effluent is more complex. The surgeon should consider undoing the anastomosis. In this case, there are at least five possible technical available procedures, which ordered in increasing complexity are (a) close the jejunal anastomotic end with a mechanical stapler and ensure drainage of the gland by intubating the pancreatic duct or placing a proximity drain, (b) Closure of the jejunal loop in addition to sealing of the pancreatic duct, (c) complete a new pancreatico-enterostomy, (d) reconvert the anastomosis to a pancreatico-gastrostomy, and (e) complete the remnant pancreatectomy [11]. This last procedure counts to be the most aggressive of all and carries a morbidity rate of about 80%, reoperation in one in three patients, and a mortality of more than 40%. As a result, at present less than 5% of patients who require reoperation end up with a total pancreatectomy. Pancreas-preserving surgery is not free of complications, which appear in up to 75% of cases, with one out of every four patients being reoperated. However, its mortality is much lower, estimated at around 17% [16]. Simple drainage of the pancreatic fistula may lead to closure over time even in the case of a complete disruption of the anastomosis, favored by progressive atrophy of the exocrine portion of the gland during the healing process. However, if the fistula persists, elective redo surgery of the failed anastomosis may be necessary once the septic process has overcome and the fistula tract is formed, several weeks after relaparotomy [17]. In any case, the pancreatic surgeon must be aware, when indicating a pancreatectomy, that surgery is only beneficial for patients with pancreatic cancer if they achieve a postoperative period with minor complications. About 35% of patients with grade C fistulas die. Further 26% of them experience a delay in the complementary chemotherapy treatment onset, and up to 67% will never receive it due to a complicated postoperative period [11].

12.3 Postoperative Bleeding

Bleeding is an often fatal surgical complication that occurs in just under 4% of patients. The IGSPF has classified postoperative hemorrhages based on three criteria: (a) the *moment of onset*, which may be early if bleeding presents within the first 24 h after surgery or late if evidenced following the first postoperative day; (b) *the location of bleeding*, which may be intraluminal if

discharged into the gastrointestinal tract or extraluminal if bleeding has an intra-abdominal location and (c) the *severity of the ble*eding. The borderline between mild and severe bleeding is established based on whether there is a three-point drop in hemoglobin levels, a requirement for transfusion of three or more packed red blood cells, or the need for endoscopic, angiographic, or surgical therapeutic intervention [18]. The occurrence of an early hemorrhage is generally due to a technical defect or complication, while late hemorrhages are related to the rupture of a pseudoaneurysm in more than 60% of cases. The infectious, inflammatory, and self-digestion process caused by a pancreatic fistula may lead to the development of a pseudoaneurysm of any of the juxtapancreatic digestive arteries, generally, the common hepatic, splenic, gastroduodenal, or superior mesenteric arteries [8]. The leak of pancreatic juice causes enzymatic degradation of the adjacent arterial walls which in addition to skeletonization of vessels during surgery favors this pseudoaneurysm formation [19].

The diagnosis of postoperative bleeding is not difficult for the experienced surgeon. The clinical evaluation of a sweaty, tachycardic, drowsy, pale, and hypotensive patient practically establishes the diagnosis even without demonstrating an externalization of the bleeding through the gastrointestinal tract or abdominal drainage. As in other causes of bleeding, the evaluation of the blood count is of little use. The decrease in hemoglobin levels is shown late and leukocytosis is often the only laboratory abnormality. Clinical suspicion is confirmed by angio-CT examination for extraluminal bleeding and by endoscopy for intraluminal location. If available, arteriography may add information as well as enable a therapeutic intervention.

Management of bleeding following pancreatic surgery is based on the three parameters of the classification of the IGSPF (Fig. 12.3). Mild and early bleeding only requires observation and conservative management. When bleeding is mild, but of late onset, a diagnostic and therapeutic endoscopy should be performed in cases of intraluminal discharge and an angio-CT scan and eventually an arteriography with embolization in

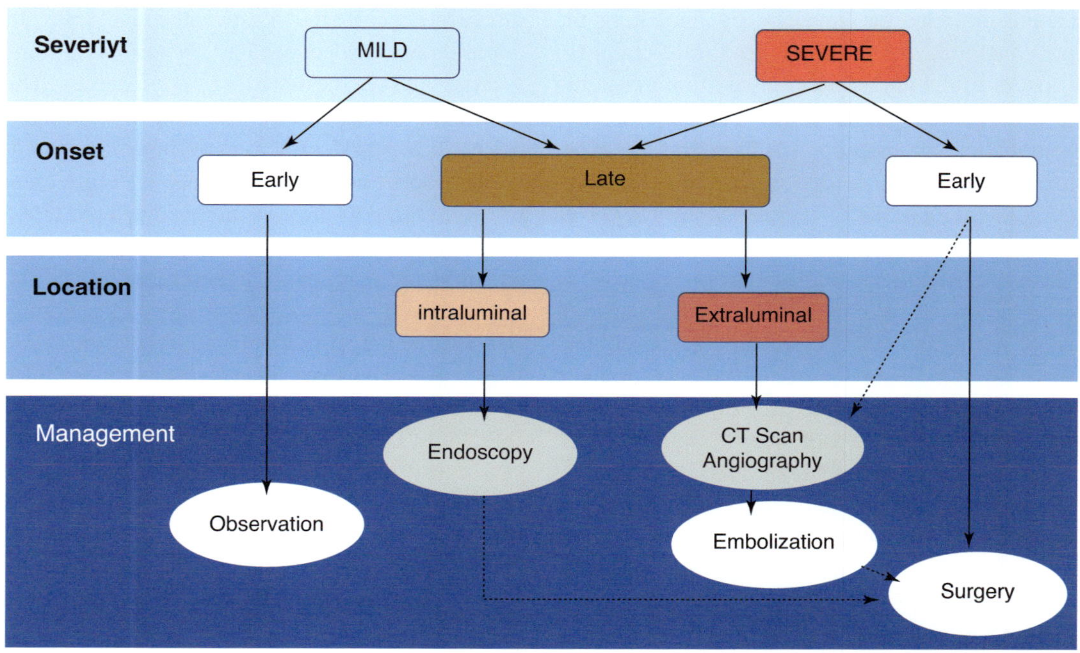

Fig. 12.3 ISGPF classification and management of postoperative hemorrhage following pancreatectomy

cases of intra-abdominal hemorrhage. The pancreatic surgeon must be particularly alert to this variety of delayed hemorrhages, even if they are mild, since they sometimes correspond to an incipient sentinel hemorrhage of massive posterior bleeding. Remarkably, sentinel hemorrhage precedes massive hemorrhage in up to 45% of cases [19]. Sentinel bleeding has been defined as an intermittent and obvious hemorrhage from abdominal drains or gastrointestinal tract, manifesting in this case as hematemesis or melena, that causes a drop in hemoglobin of more than 1.5 g/dl, and that experiences spontaneous stopping without transfusion or re-bleeding within an interval of at least 12 h [20, 21]. Sentinel bleeding ceases due to hypotension of the patient but may precede severe life-threatening bleeding, usually presented at late night and of very difficult surgical control. Therefore, once the pseudoaneurysm has been diagnosed, prompt management is recommended. Embolization of the damaged vessel or covered vascular stent placement should be carried out as soon as possible (Fig. 12.4).

Severe bleeding requires immediate attention. If the hemorrhage presents early, a surgical pitfall must be discarded, and reoperation is the best therapeutic option since the abdominal cavity is relatively virgin and free of inflammatory adhesions. Late onset, as described above, suggests an arterial lesion caused by a pancreatic fistula. Surgical control of bleeding in the context of a hostile operative field caused by the postoperative reparative process in addition to the inflammatory response associated with anastomotic leakage can be extremely difficult and reaches a mortality rate of about 50%. In this setting, surgical access to the bleeding vessel is often only granted after causing several visceral injuries. Thenceforward, vascular repair may be very difficult or even impossible. Due to this, an arteriography and embolization of the bleeding vessel by percutaneous endovascular access should be attempted whenever possible. This approach has shown non-inferiority with respect to surgery and a lower mortality rate of around 20% [19].

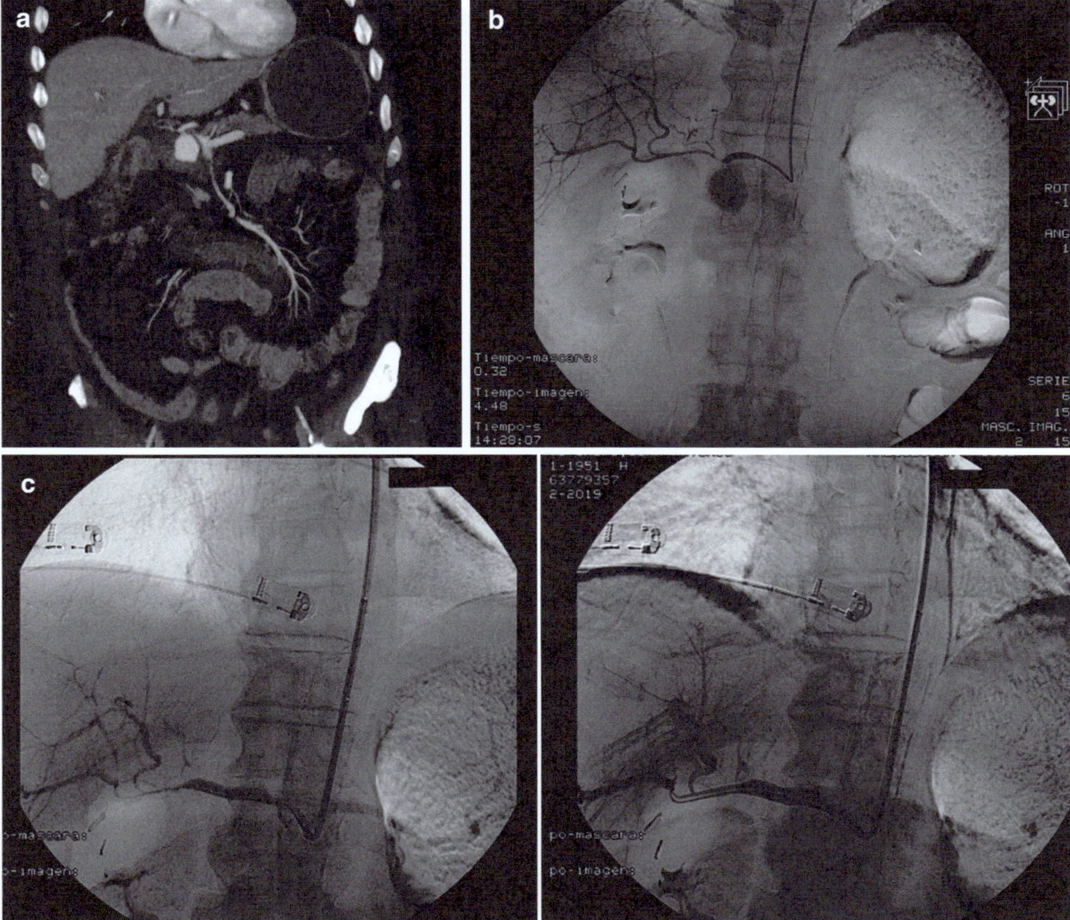

Fig. 12.4 Postoperative bleeding caused by a pseudoaneurysm after pancreaticoduodenectomy. (**a**) Coronal CT scan showing a pseudoaneurysm of the stump of the gastroduodenal artery. (**b**) Arteriographic image showing pseudoaneurysm of the gastroduodenal artery. (**c**) Covered Stent Placement for gastroduodenal artery pseudoaneu-rysm occlusion. From Parra Membrives P, Martínez Baena D, Lorente Herce J, Jiménez Riera G, Sánchez Gálvez MÁ, Martín Balbuena R, et al. Diagnóstico y trata-miento de las complicaciones y secuelas de la cirugía pan-creática. Evidencias y desavenencias. Cir Andal. 2019;30(2):186–94

12.4 Delayed Gastric Emptying

Accomplishment of a consensus definition of delayed gastric emptying is difficult. Food intol-erance during the immediate postoperative period of a pancreatectomy may have different origins and includes invariably a subjective appraisal of both the patient and the surgeon. However, the IGSPF issued in 2007 the most accepted classifi-cation of this complication. The expert panel divided delayed gastric emptying into three grades based on the duration of nasogastric tube insertion or the need for tube replacement [22] (Table 12.1).

The pathogenesis of delayed gastric emptying following pancreaticoduodenectomy is not well known and several theories have emerged. A decrease in serum motilin due to duodenal resec-tion has been proposed as a causal factor. In addi-tion, the existence of a pylorospasm due to denervation and devascularization during the sur-gical procedure has been suggested when delayed

Table 12.1 Consensus definition of delayed gastric emptying after pancreatic surgery

Grade of DGE	Need for nasogastric tube	Inability for oral intake to POD	Vomiting/gastric dilation	Use of prokinetic agents
A	4–7 days or reinsertion after POD >3°	7	±	±
B	8–14 days or reinsertion after POD >7°	14	+	+
C	>14 days or reinsertion after POD >14	21	+	+

DGE Delayed gastric emptying, *POD* Postoperative day

gastric emptying occurs after a pylorus-preserving pancreaticoduodenectomy. However, in most cases delayed emptying is the result of inflammation of the gastric wall remnant in contact with a surgical site collection secondary to pancreatic fistula development [11].

Three different diagnostic tests are available to confirm clinical suspicion of delayed gastric emptying and clarify its origin. A water-soluble contrast radiogram reveals delayed contrast passage and an adequate anastomotic caliber without stenosis. On occasion, an extreme passage delay may not show contrast at the jejunum, mimicking a complete obstruction. In these cases, oral endoscopy will assure a viable anastomosis.

In addition, endoscopy may also be used for the placement of an enteral tube for feeding. Finally, an abdominal CT scan will rule out the presence of retro and perigastric collections as a cause of delayed tolerance of oral intake.

There are no magic therapeutic interventions to manage delayed gastric emptying. First, the correct nutritional status of the patients must be guaranteed by parenteral or enteral tube feeding if available. Second, maintenance of the nasogastric tube until resolution of the condition is generally mandatory. Erythromycin is the only drug that has been revealed to accelerate the recovery of normal gastric emptying. As a motilin agonist, it has been employed in doses similar to or lower than those used as an antibiotic [23, 24]. Any other prokinetic agent has proven to be beneficial. If fluid collections secondary to pancreatic fistulas have already been ruled out or treated, only the patience of the surgeon can be added to the treatment, bearing in mind that only 5% of patients require a prolonged hospital stay due to delayed gastric emptying [11, 25].

12.5 Early Postoperative Pancreatitis

The concept of postoperative acute pancreatitis (POAP) following partial pancreatectomy has gained popularity in recent years. The inflammatory process and potential ischemic injury of the pancreatic stump may impair anastomotic healing and has been suggested as one of the triggers of pancreatic fistula developments [26–28] and was also associated to delayed gastric emptying [29]. However, pancreatic resection involves direct trauma to the pancreas and hyperamylasemia is extremely frequent after pancreatectomy. Thus, considering this the only parameter to define POAP may overestimate the real incidence of the inflammatory process. In addition, postoperative fistula without pancreatitis does exist and most authors agree that despite its close association it represents actually a separate phenomenon [30]. According to this a modification of the ISSGPS definition of postoperative pancreatic fistula was proposed by Connor, assessing the presence of pancreatitis. He proposed a standardized definition of POAP as an increase in serum amylase activity greater than the upper limit of normal range of serum amylase activity on postoperative day 1. The rise in serum levels of amylase in the postoperative period would be significantly less than that traditionally associated with the diagnosis of pancreatitis. In these patients, pancreatic fluid leak would be rather a consequence of pancreatitis than a true pancreatic fistula [31]. With these criteria, over 60% of the patients undergoing pancreatectomy of any type suffer an episode of POAP of any severity, with or without the appearance of a pancreatic fistula [32, 33]. Furthermore, postoperative pancreatic fistula occurred in 37% of patients who develop POAP and over 90% of diagnosed pancreatic fistulas would actually not be true fistula but episodes of acute pancreatitis [26, 28, 30]. Notably, patients who develop pancreatitis following pancreaticoduodenectomy experience a higher increase in the rate of morbidity and a prolonged hospital stay while patients who present POAP succeeding distal pancreatectomy result not in a different postoperative course. Fortunately, the incidence of severe or clinically relevant postoperative pancreatitis does not exceed 8–10%, remarkably concurring with the incidence of grade C fistulas [34]. Despite this, it should be stated that postoperative pancreatitis is an emerging concept and no definition or agreed threshold for its definition is available. The inevitable association between postoperative hyperamylasemia and postoperative is still controversial among pancreatic surgeons [35, 36].

Evidence about any intervention preventing POAP occurrence or progression is lacking. Attempts employing somatostatin have not shown to be useful. Improving pancreatic transection and/or stapling technique to minimize parenchymal injury may be advisable but there are no studies demonstrating the benefit of these measures in reducing the rate of POAP. To conclude, the management of POAP is not different from any other case of pancreatitis [25, 28].

12.6 Diabetes Mellitus

An obvious consequence of the resection of the pancreas is the potential deficiency or inability of the remnant stump to perform its functions as endocrine and exocrine glands. Some studies have unexpectedly shown an improvement in glycemic control after resection of pancreatic cancer in a high percentage of patients, demonstrating the diabetogenic effect of the tumor itself [37]. The risk of developing de novo diabetes following pancreaticoduodenectomy is 15% [38]. In our experience, over 60% of the patients who undergo pancreaticoduodenectomy due to a primary disease of the gland (pancreatic cancer, chronic pancreatitis, or cystic tumors of the pancreas) and 35% of those who were operated on by reason of other extra-pancreatic conditions (distal cholangiocarcinoma, duodenal cancer or ampuloma) progress in their diabetic state requiring a higher level of treatment, either with diet, oral antidiabetics, or insulinization [39]. Diagnosis of diabetes mellitus after resection of the pancreas is made following the conventional WHO criteria. Postoperative levels of glycated hemoglobin should be determined during hospital stay and regularly included as part of the assessment of the correct glycemic control of the patient. Special attention should be paid to patients undergoing total pancreatectomy. The complete absence of pancreatic hormones including insulin, glucagon, and other islet regulation peptides leads to difficult management of diabetes and dangerous episodes of hypoglycemia [40]. It takes several months for the patient to adapt to the new diabetic status and tight glycemic control will be required lifelong. Some studies have suggested better control of postoperative diabetes through the use of continuous insulin infusion devices [41]. Improvement in glycemic control and nutritional status after total pancreatectomy has been revealed to be of paramount importance in preventing tumor recurrence and, more importantly, improving survival [42].

12.7 Exocrine Pancreatic Insufficiency

The nutritional effect of inadequate pancreatic enzyme delivery following pancreatic resections has been historically underweighted but has emerged at present as a major concern. The rate of exocrine pancreatic insufficiency development (EPI) in patients operated on because of chronic pancreatitis is 35–100% following pancreaticoduodenectomy and over 65% if distal resections are performed. Furthermore, despite surgery for pancreatic cancer reduces the incidence to 40% after distal pancreatectomies, EPI occurrence rate remains practically the same if patients undergo pancreatic head resections [43]. The exocrine pancreas has a large functional reserve.

Thus, many patients remain initially asymptomatic despite a decrease in daily enzymatic production. However, enzymatic shortage leads eventually to maldigestion, food malabsorption and finally sarcopenia, osteopenia, and fat-soluble vitamin deficiencies. Symptomatic patients present with diarrhea and fatty stools as well as flatulence and weight loss. The importance of correcting the exocrine deficiency has been stated in a recent study revealing that pancreatic enzyme replacement is an independent factor associated with increased survival after pancreatectomy for periampullary neoplasia [44]. In addition, EPI is postulated as the main cause of non-alcoholic fatty liver disease (NAFLD) after pancreaticoduodenectomy which develops in 8–37% of the patients [45–47].

Accurate diagnosis of EPI requires complex test performance. Detection of more than 7 g of fat in stools per day confirms steatorrhea and pancreatic enzyme shortage but involves collecting a sample on three consecutive days after a diet rich in fat during the previous 3 days. Fetal elastase measurement, which is reduced in EPI, has also been used. However, the test is not widely available and is therefore predominantly employed to confirm diagnosis in doubtful cases. Hence, according to a recent evidence-based practice guideline, all patients who have undergone pancreatic resection in whom exocrine pancreatic insufficiency is clinically suspected should receive treatment without the need for diagnostic confirmation. The recommended dose is 75,000 units of pancreatin at each main meal and 35,000–50,000 after eating snacks [43]. In addition, replacement treatment with pancrelipase has been shown to have significant efficacy in the treatment of postoperative NAFLD [48, 49].

12.8 Cholangitis

The risk of developing cholangitis is inherent to the hepaticojejunostomy procedure. Around 16% of patients undergoing pancreaticoduodenectomy will develop ascending cholangitis over time. In our experience, one-third of them are due to obstruction following local tumor recurrence, a further third is caused by benign scarring resulting in stricture of the bilioenteric anastomosis, and the last third is consecutive to poor emptying of the jejunal loop without occlusion in a new variant of the afferent loop syndrome [50]. A small bile duct size at surgery or the occurrence of postoperative biliary fistula are the main causes of long-term benign anastomotic strictures. However, interpretation of recurrent cholangitis in the absence of bilioenteric anastomotic occlusion is more complex. The anastomosed jejunal loop may retain colonized bile leading to ascending infection due to several reasons. Obstruction by twisting or scaring of the afferent limb to the stomach in Child type reconstruction or at the foot of the Roux-en-Y limb may occur. In addition, duodenal "C" shape reconstruction by passing the jejunal loop behind the mesenteric axis may favor Markedly angulated or excessively fixed afferent limb and adhesion development also contribute to luminal obstruction. However, in the absence of any obstructive cause, a functional disorder characterized by delayed emptying of the afferent loop must be suspected. A paretic limb would lead to bile stasis and bacterial overgrowth favoring ascending cholangitis. This functional afferent limb syndrome may emerge in the setting of radiation enteropathy or relative limb ischemia [51].

Our diagnostic protocol in patients suffering from cholangitis following pancreaticoduodenectomy includes performing magnetic cholangioresonance, hepatobiliary iminodiacetic acid (HIDA) scintigraphy, and a barium gastrointestinal X-ray study [50]. Patients with stenosis of the bilioenteric anastomosis, of benign or malignant origin, show dilatation of the bile duct in cholangioresonance with a sharpening of the passage to the intestinal limb, a delayed emptying of the tracer that is retained in a dilated bile duct in the HIDA scintigraphy and poor or absent barium reflux into the biliary tree. Distinguishing between benign and malignant stenosis is not always easy, even with the addition of a CT scan to the diagnostic protocol. Sometimes only repeated failure of percutaneous anastomotic dilation or operative findings during a planned redo surgery clarifies the diagnosis. The diagnosis of cholangitis due to a functional limb disorder or afferent loop syndrome is made by exclusion. In these patients no dilation of the biliary tree is stated on cholangioresonance, revealing a normal anastomosis. If the patient had undergone a single loop—Child type—reconstruction, the barium X-ray study usually shows a correct reflux of the contrast media to the bile duct that fills and empties without obstacles, also revealing a normal anastomosis. Finally, in these patients the tracer retention is observed in the intestinal loop and not in the bile duct when HIDA scintigraphy is performed (Fig. 12.5).

Percutaneous transhepatic anastomotic balloon dilation results in lasted patency in over 75% of the patients if a benign stricture occurred. However, several attempts may be necessary [52]. Hence, the inability to dilate a bilioenteric anastomosis percutaneously should make mistrust the diagnosis of benignity. However, if percutaneous approach fails, redo surgery of hepaticojejunostomy is necessary. Malignant strictures should be managed by percutaneous self-expandable metallic stent placement for palliative purposes. Finally, patients developing an afferent loop syndrome may benefit from surgical treatment as long as an obstructive cause is identified. Performing a jejuno-jejunal bypass or Roux-en-Y foot revision may be helpful. However, there is no defined treatment for patients with non-obstructive delayed limb emptying. Only the use of cycles of antibiotics with quinolones has been carried out with some success in cases of recurrent cholangitis, although there is no scientific evidence about the real benefit of this intervention [53].

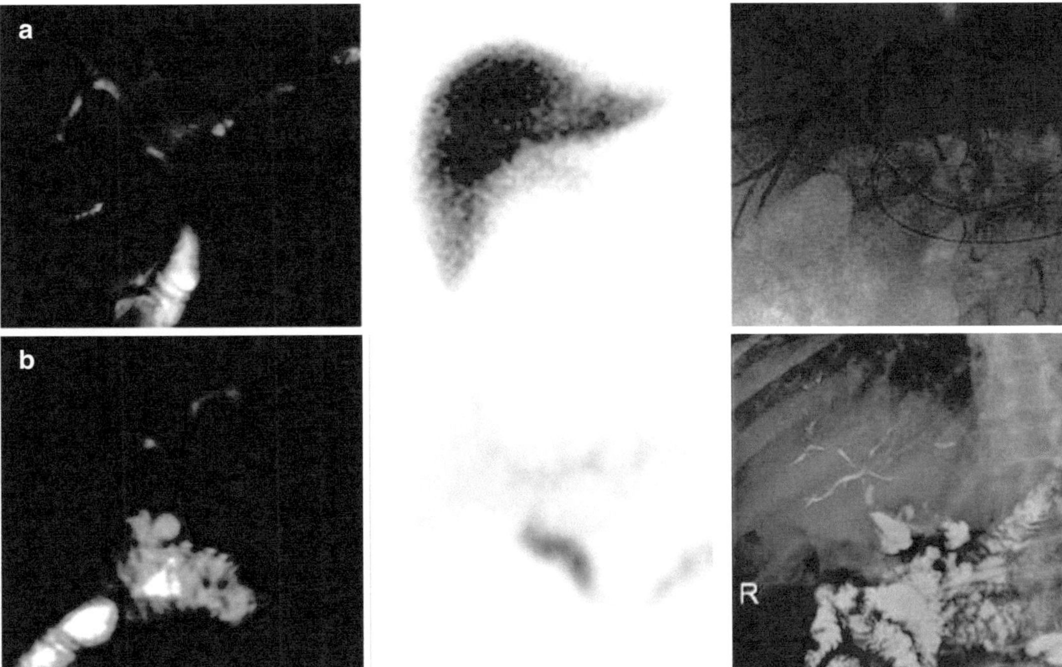

Fig. 12.5 Diagnostic imaging tests for the study of acute cholangitis after pancreaticoduodenectomy. (**a**) Sequence of imaging studies of a bile duct stenosis after pancreaticoduodenectomy: intrahepatic bile duct dilation and distal sharpening with stenosis of the anastomosis in magnetic cholangioresonance, liver tracer retention in HIDA scintigraphy and abrupt stenosis in transhepatic cholangiography (during balloon dilation). (**b**) Sequence of imaging studies in a patient with functional afferent loop syndrome: non-dilated bile duct in magnetic cholangioresonance, tracer retention in jejunal loop, normal contrast reflux to the bile duct with patent anastomosis in the radiological study with barium oral contrast

12.9 Late Acute Pancreatitis

The current improvement in long-term survival of patients undergoing pancreaticoduodenectomy has made surgeons aware of the ocurrence of previously unknown late-onset biliary and pancreatic complications. Late postoperative pancreatitis following pancreaticoduodenectomy is rare with an estimated incidence of 5% in the first 5 postoperative years. In general, acute pancreatitis prior to index surgery is a risk factor for long-term pancreatitis onset, suggesting a certain glandular predisposition [54]. However, impaired drainage of pancreatic enzyme secretion throughout the anastomosis secondary to occlusion of the pancreatico-jejonostomy seems to be associated with this condition. Despite this, anastomotic stricture is only revealed in two-thirds of patients suffering late postoperative pancreatitis.

About 1.4–11% of the pancreatico-jejunal anastomoses develop stenosis in the third postoperative year. Secretin-stimulated magnetic resonance cholangiopancreatography (MRCP) is the preferred method for detection of pancreatic anastomotic stricture, which a sensitivity ranging from 56 to 100% [55]. Risk factors associated with stricture occurrence have not been identified.

It is difficult, if not impossible, to determine which symptoms are associated with anastomotic malfunction, since postprandial abdominal pain development in a patient undergoing a pancreatico-duodenectomy may have multiple origins. In addition, exocrine pancreatic insufficiency may be a consequence of both anastomotic malfunction and pancreatic gland deficiency following resection.

The diagnosis of late postoperative pancreatitis is made by determining high serum amylase levels and performing a CT imaging test (Fig. 12.6). Most patients follow a benign course, and require only fluid replacement, pain control, and nutritional support. Endoscopic dilation of the pancreatico-jejunostomy should be attempted in patients with repeated episodes of pancreatitis secondary to pancreatic secretion outflow occlusion. However, identifying the pancreatic ductal orifice by endoscopic retrograde pancreatography can be challenging and its success rate does not exceed 12.5–28.6%. The use of echoendoscopy with direct ultrasound-guided puncture of the Wirsung to reversely access the anastomotic limb has improved outcomes. However, this procedure is operator dependent and its success rate varies between 33 and 100% in published series. Endoscopic dilation results in morbidity ranging from 16.5 to 33% achieving clinical improvement in 28–100% of the treated patients.

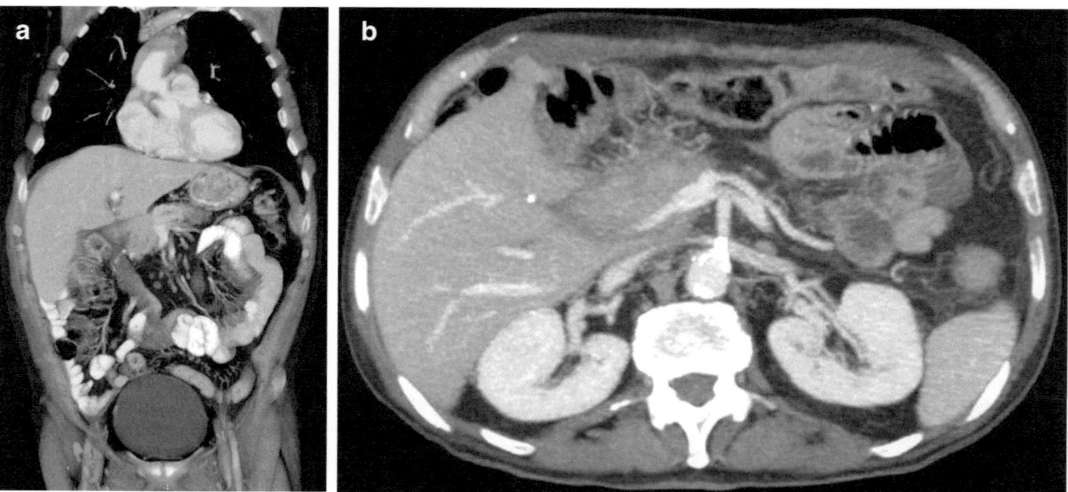

Fig. 12.6 Coronal (**a**) and axial (**b**) view of the CT scan of a patient with pancreatitis of the pancreatic remnant that developed following pancreatic head resection. The effacement of pancreato-jejunal perianastomotic fat is observed

Finally, a few patients suffering chronic pancreatic pain and repeated episodes of pancreatitis due to anastomotic stenosis may require surgery. A recent systematic review of the literature showed only six studies referring to surgical treatment of pancreatico-jejunostomy stenosis, most of them collecting only very few cases. The proposed surgical procedures vary from longitudinal pancreatico-jejunostomy (modified Puestow), to resection of the pancreatic tail and retrograde drainage of the pancreatic duct via a distal pancreatico-jejunostomy, or pancreatico-jejunal redo surgery and finally total pancreatectomy. However, the limited experience and scientific evidence do not allow one to favor one procedure over the other.

References

1. Sabater L, Mora I, Gámez Del Castillo JM, Escrig-Sos J, Muñoz-Forner E, Garcés-Albir M, et al. Outcome quality standards in pancreatic oncologic surgery in Spain. Cir Esp. 2018;96(6):342–51.
2. Sabater L, García-Granero A, Escrig-Sos J, MeC G-M, Sastre J, Ferrández A, et al. Outcome quality standards in pancreatic oncologic surgery. Ann Surg Oncol. 2014;21(4):1138–46.
3. Bassi C, Dervenis C, Butturini G, Fingerhut A, Yeo C, Izbicki J, et al. Postoperative pancreatic fistula: an international study group (ISGPF) definition. Surgery. 2005;138(1):8–13.
4. Bassi C, Marchegiani G, Dervenis C, Sarr M, Abu Hilal M, Adham M, et al. The 2016 update of the International Study Group (ISGPS) definition and grading of postoperative pancreatic fistula: 11 Years After. Surgery. 2017;161(3):584–91.
5. Pulvirenti A, Marchegiani G, Pea A, Allegrini V, Esposito A, Casetti L, et al. Clinical implications of the 2016 international study group on pancreatic surgery definition and grading of postoperative pancreatic fistula on 775 consecutive pancreatic resections. Ann Surg. 2018;268(6):1069–75.
6. Van Buren G, Bloomston M, Hughes SJ, Winter J, Behrman SW, Zyromski NJ, et al. A randomized prospective multicenter trial of pancreaticoduodenectomy with and without routine intraperitoneal drainage. Ann Surg. 2014;259(4):605–12.
7. Maggino L, Malleo G, Bassi C, Allegrini V, Beane JD, Beckman RM, et al. Identification of an optimal cut-off for drain fluid amylase on postoperative day 1 for predicting clinically relevant fistula after distal pancreatectomy: a multi-institutional analysis and external validation. Ann Surg. 2019;269(2):337–43.
8. Nahm CB, Connor SJ, Samra JS, Mittal A. Postoperative pancreatic fistula: a review of traditional and emerging concepts. Clin Exp Gastroenterol. 2018;11:105–18.
9. Partelli S, Pecorelli N, Muffatti F, Belfiori G, Crippa S, Piazzai F, et al. Early postoperative prediction of clinically relevant pancreatic fistula after pancreaticoduodenectomy: usefulness of C-reactive protein. HPB (Oxford). 2017;19(7):580–6.
10. Solaini L, Atmaja BT, Watt J, Arumugam P, Hutchins RR, Abraham AT, et al. Limited utility of inflammatory markers in the early detection of postoperative inflammatory complications after pancreatic resection: Cohort study and meta-analyses. Int J Surg. 2015;17:41–7.
11. Malleo G, Vollmer CM. Postpancreatectomy complications and management. Surg Clin North Am. 2016;96(6):1313–36.
12. Klek S, Sierzega M, Turczynowski L, Szybinski P, Szczepanek K, Kulig J. Enteral and parenteral nutrition in the conservative treatment of pancreatic fistula: a randomized clinical trial. Gastroenterology. 2011;141(1):157–63, 63.e1.
13. Gans SL, van Westreenen HL, Kiewiet JJ, Rauws EA, Gouma DJ, Boermeester MA. Systematic review and meta-analysis of somatostatin analogues for the treatment of pancreatic fistula. Br J Surg. 2012;99(6):754–60.
14. Ecker BL, McMillan MT, Asbun HJ, Ball CG, Bassi C, Beane JD, et al. Characterization and optimal management of high-risk pancreatic anastomoses during pancreatoduodenectomy. Ann Surg. 2018;267(4):608–16.
15. Volk A, Nitschke P, Johnscher F, Rahbari N, Welsch T, Reißfelder C, et al. Perioperative application of somatostatin analogs for pancreatic surgery-current status in Germany. Langenbeck's Arch Surg. 2016;401(7):1037–44.
16. Bressan AK, Wahba M, Dixon E, Ball CG. Completion pancreatectomy in the acute management of pancreatic fistula after pancreaticoduodenectomy: a systematic review and qualitative synthesis of the literature. HPB (Oxford). 2018;20(1):20–7.
17. Ma T, Bai X, Chen W, Li G, Lao M, Liang T. Pancreas-preserving management of grade-C pancreatic fistula and a novel bridging technique for repeat pancreaticojejunostomy: an observational study. Int J Surg. 2018;52:243–7.
18. Wente MN, Veit JA, Bassi C, Dervenis C, Fingerhut A, Gouma DJ, et al. Postpancreatectomy hemorrhage (PPH): an International Study Group of Pancreatic Surgery (ISGPS) definition. Surgery. 2007;142(1):20–5.
19. Roulin D, Cerantola Y, Demartines N, Schäfer M. Systematic review of delayed postoperative hemorrhage after pancreatic resection. J Gastrointest Surg. 2011;15(6):1055–62.

20. Chen JF, Xu SF, Zhao W, Tian YH, Gong L, Yuan WS, et al. Diagnostic and therapeutic strategies to manage post-pancreaticoduodenectomy hemorrhage. World J Surg. 2015;39(2):509–15.
21. Mohsin N, Mohamed E, Gaber M, Obaidani I, Budruddin M, Al BS. Acute tubular necrosis associated with non-hemorrhagic Dengue fever: a case report. Ren Fail. 2009;31(8):736–9.
22. Wente MN, Bassi C, Dervenis C, Fingerhut A, Gouma DJ, Izbicki JR, et al. Delayed gastric emptying (DGE) after pancreatic surgery: a suggested definition by the International Study Group of Pancreatic Surgery (ISGPS). Surgery. 2007;142(5):761–8.
23. Ohwada S, Satoh Y, Kawate S, Yamada T, Kawamura O, Koyama T, et al. Low-dose erythromycin reduces delayed gastric emptying and improves gastric motility after Billroth I pylorus-preserving pancreaticoduodenectomy. Ann Surg. 2001;234(5):668–74.
24. Matsunaga H, Tanaka M, Takahata S, Ogawa Y, Naritomi G, Yokohata K, et al. Manometric evidence of improved early gastric stasis by erythromycin after pylorus-preserving pancreatoduodenectomy. World J Surg. 2000;24(10):1236–41. discussion 42
25. Lytras D, Paraskevas KI, Avgerinos C, Manes C, Touloumis Z, Paraskeva KD, et al. Therapeutic strategies for the management of delayed gastric emptying after pancreatic resection. Langenbeck's Arch Surg. 2007;392(1):1–12.
26. Bannone E, Andrianello S, Marchegiani G, Masini G, Malleo G, Bassi C, et al. Postoperative acute pancreatitis following pancreaticoduodenectomy: a determinant of fistula potentially driven by the intraoperative fluid management. Ann Surg. 2018;268(5):815–22.
27. Nahm CB, Brown KM, Townend PJ, Colvin E, Howell VM, Gill AJ, et al. Acinar cell density at the pancreatic resection margin is associated with post-pancreatectomy pancreatitis and the development of postoperative pancreatic fistula. HPB (Oxford). 2018;20(5):432–40.
28. Kühlbrey CM, Samiei N, Sick O, Makowiec F, Hopt UT, Wittel UA. Pancreatitis after pancreatoduodenectomy predicts clinically relevant postoperative pancreatic fistula. J Gastrointest Surg. 2017;21(2):330–8.
29. Räty S, Sand J, Lantto E, Nordback I. Postoperative acute pancreatitis as a major determinant of postoperative delayed gastric emptying after pancreaticoduodenectomy. J Gastrointest Surg. 2006;10(8):1131–9.
30. Andrianello S, Bannone E, Marchegiani G, Malleo G, Paiella S, Esposito A, et al. Characterization of postoperative acute pancreatitis (POAP) after distal pancreatectomy. Surgery. 2020;169(4):724–31.
31. Connor S. Defining post-operative pancreatitis as a new pancreatic specific complication following pancreatic resection. HPB (Oxford). 2016;18(8):642–51.
32. Birgin E, Reeg A, Téoule P, Rahbari NN, Post S, Reissfelder C, et al. Early postoperative pancreatitis following pancreaticoduodenectomy: what is clinically relevant postoperative pancreatitis? HPB (Oxford). 2018;21(8):972–80.
33. Ikenaga N, Ohtsuka T, Nakata K, Watanabe Y, Mori Y, Nakamura M. Clinical significance of postoperative acute pancreatitis after pancreatoduodenectomy and distal pancreatectomy. Surgery. 2020;169(4):732–7.
34. Ryska M, Rudis J. Pancreatic fistula and postoperative pancreatitis after pancreatoduodenectomy for pancreatic cancer. Hepatobiliary Surg Nutr. 2014;3(5):268–75.
35. Bannone E, Andrianello S, Marchegiani G, Malleo G, Paiella S, Salvia R, et al. Postoperative hyperamylasemia (POH) and acute pancreatitis after pancreatoduodenectomy (POAP): state of the art and systematic review. Surgery. 2021;169(2):377–87.
36. Loos M, Strobel O, Dietrich M, Mehrabi A, Ramouz A, Al-Saeedi M, et al. Hyperamylasemia and acute pancreatitis after pancreatoduodenectomy: two different entities. Surgery. 2021;169(2):369–76.
37. Roeyen G, Jansen M, Hartman V, Chapelle T, Bracke B, Ysebaert D, et al. The impact of pancreaticoduodenectomy on endocrine and exocrine pancreatic function: a prospective cohort study based on pre- and postoperative function tests. Pancreatology. 2017;17(6):974–82.
38. Beger HG, Poch B, Mayer B, Siech M. New onset of diabetes and pancreatic exocrine insufficiency after pancreaticoduodenectomy for benign and malignant tumors: a systematic review and meta-analysis of long-term results. Ann Surg. 2018;267(2):259–70.
39. Parra Membrives P, Díaz Gómez D, Martínez Baena D, Lorente Herce JM. Blood glucose control and risk of progressing to a diabetic state during clinical follow up after cephalic duodenopancreatectomy|Control glucémico y riesgo de progresión del estado diabetológico durante el seguimiento clínico tras duodenopancreatectomía cefálica. Cir Esp. 2011;89(4):218–22.
40. Dresler CM, Fortner JG, McDermott K, Bajorunas DR. Metabolic consequences of (regional) total pancreatectomy. Ann Surg. 1991;214(2):131–40.
41. Struyvenberg MR, Fong ZV, Martin CR, Tseng JF, Clancy TE, Fernández-Del Castillo C, et al. Impact of treatments on diabetic control and gastrointestinal symptoms after total pancreatectomy. Pancreas. 2017;46(9):1188–95.
42. Shi HJ, Jin C, Fu DL. Impact of postoperative glycemic control and nutritional status on clinical outcomes after total pancreatectomy. World J Gastroenterol. 2017;23(2):265–74.
43. Sabater L, Ausania F, Bakker OJ, Boadas J, Domínguez-Muñoz JE, Falconi M, et al. Evidence-based guidelines for the management of exocrine pancreatic insufficiency after pancreatic surgery. Ann Surg. 2016;264(6):949–58.
44. Roberts KJ, Schrem H, Hodson J, Angelico R, Dasari BVM, Coldham CA, et al. Pancreas exocrine replacement therapy is associated with increased survival following pancreatoduodenectomy for periampullary malignancy. HPB (Oxford). 2017;19(10):859–67.
45. Kato H, Isaji S, Azumi Y, Kishiwada M, Hamada T, Mizuno S, et al. Development of nonalcoholic fatty

liver disease (NAFLD) and nonalcoholic steato-hepatitis (NASH) after pancreaticoduodenectomy: proposal of a postoperative NAFLD scoring system. J Hepatobiliary Pancreat Sci. 2010;17(3):296–304.

46. Nomura R, Ishizaki Y, Suzuki K, Kawasaki S. Development of hepatic steatosis after pancreatoduodenectomy. AJR Am J Roentgenol. 2007;189(6):1484–8.

47. Song SC, Choi SH, Choi DW, Heo JS, Kim WS, Kim MJ. Potential risk factors for nonalcoholic steato-hepatitis related to pancreatic secretions following pancreaticoduodenectomy. World J Gastroenterol. 2011;17(32):3716–23.

48. Nagai M, Sho M, Satoi S, Toyokawa H, Akahori T, Yanagimoto H, et al. Effects of pancrelipase on non-alcoholic fatty liver disease after pancreaticoduodenectomy. J Hepatobiliary Pancreat Sci. 2014;21(3):186–92.

49. Yamazaki S, Takayama T, Higaki T, Moriguchi M, Yoshida N, Miyazaki T, et al. Pancrelipase with branched-chain amino acids for preventing nonalcoholic fatty liver disease after pancreaticoduodenectomy. J Gastroenterol. 2016;51(1):55–62.

50. Parra-Membrives P, Martínez-Baena D, Sánchez-Sánchez F. Late biliary complications after pancreaticoduodenectomy. Am Surg. 2016;82(5):456–61.

51. Pannala R, Brandabur JJ, Gan SI, Gluck M, Irani S, Patterson DJ, et al. Afferent limb syndrome and delayed GI problems after pancreaticoduodenectomy for pancreatic cancer: single-center, 14-year experience. Gastrointest Endosc. 2011;74(2):295–302.

52. Okabayashi T, Shima Y, Sumiyoshi T, Sui K, Iwata J, Morita S, et al. Incidence and risk factors of cholangitis after hepaticojejunostomy. J Gastrointest Surg. 2018;22(4):676–83.

53. Pérez-Calvo JI, Olivera-González S, Amores-Arriaga B, Torralba-Cabeza MA. [Cyclic antibiotics in non-surgical patients with recurrent acute bacterial cholangitis]. Rev Clin Esp. 2009;209(4):204–5.

54. Yen HH, Ho TW, Wu CH, Kuo TC, Wu JM, Yang CY, et al. Late acute pancreatitis after pancreaticoduodenectomy: incidence, outcome, and risk factors. J Hepatobiliary Pancreat Sci. 2019;26(3):109–16.

55. Zarzavadjian Le Bian A, Cesaretti M, Tabchouri N, Wind P, Fuks D. Late pancreatic anastomosis stricture following pancreaticoduodenectomy: a systematic review. J Gastrointest Surg. 2018;22(11):2021–8.

Oncologic Adjuvant and Neoadjuvant Treatments in Pancreatic Adenocarcinoma

Juan José Reina Zoilo, Marta Espinosa Montaño, Francisco José Valdivia García, Rosario Carrillo de Albornoz Soto, and María Dolores Mediano Rambla

13.1 Introduction

PAC continues to be the worst prognostic gastrointestinal neoplasm, with a 5-year survival rate of 7–10% considering all stages, without a substantial improvement in the prognosis during the past decades despite therapeutic advances [1]. Based on current incidence rates, PAC is expected to be the second leading cause of cancer death in Western countries between 2020 and 2030 [2]. Surgery is the only potentially curative treatment for PAC. Unfortunately, most patients are diagnosed in the metastatic (50–60%) or locally advanced (30%) disease stage. But even in the rare 15–20% of patients performing curative-intent surgery, the probability of recurrence is 65-85% after 3 years, with a median survival of 8–12 months [3]. These data probably depict that the PCA should be considered a systemic disease, even in those cases of putative initial surgery, reinforcing the role of chemotherapy in resectable stages [4]. Pre- and/or postoperative chemotherapy in patients with PAC undergoing surgery is intended to improve these poor outcomes. Chemotherapy was traditionally given after surgery (adjuvant therapy), but recent studies have also emerged evaluating the usefulness of preoperative (neoadjuvant) treatment associated or not to the adjuvant treatment. The criteria we will use to differentiate between resectable, borderline, and locally advanced PAC (LAPAC) will be those of the *National Comprehensive Cancer Network* (NCCN) [5] and have already been explained in previous chapters.

13.2 Adjuvant Chemotherapy in PAC

The ACT is given after PAC surgery in order to prevent or delay recurrence, eliminating possible micrometastasis that may have escaped surgical procedures. For more than 10 years, ACT has become a standard for the treatment of all patients with PAC who have undergone radical surgical resection regardless of their stage, achieving a clearly significant increase in survival. As we will see, the most effective ACT regimens have been developed in the last 4 years.

J. J. Reina Zoilo (✉) · M. Espinosa Montaño
F. J. Valdivia García · R. Carrillo de Albornoz Soto ·
M. D. Mediano Rambla
Medical Oncology Department, Virgen Macarena
University Hospital, Seville, Spain

Table 13.1 The main phase III trials of adjuvant chemotherapy in PAC

Trial	Year	n	Experimental arm	Control arm	DFS (months)	OS (months)
ESPAC-1	2004	289	5-FU	OBS		20.1 vs. 15.5 HR 0.71, p: 0.009
CONKO-001	2013	354	GEM	OBS	13.4 vs. 6.7 HR 0.55, $p < 0.001$	22.8 vs. 20.2 HR 0.76, $p < 0.01$
ESPAC-3	2010	1088	GEM	5-FU	14.3 vs. 14.1 NS	23.6 vs. 23.0 NS
ESPAC-4	2017	732	GEM + capecitabine	GEM	13.9 vs. 13.1 NS	28.0 vs. 25.5 HR 0.80, p: 0.032
APACT	2019	866	GEM + nab-paclitaxel	GEM	19.4 vs. 18.8 NS	40.5 vs. 36.2 NS
CONKO-005	2017	436	GEM + erlotinib	GEM	11.4 vs. 11.4 NS	24.5 vs. 26.5 NS
PRODIGE-24	2018	493	mFOLFIRINOX	GEM	21.6 vs. 12.8 HR 0.58, $p<0.001$	54.4 vs. 35.0 HR 0.64, p: 0.003

DFS Disease-Free Survival, *OS* Overall survival, *5-FU* 5-fluorouracil, *GEM* gemcitabine, *OBS* Observation, *HR* Hazard Ratio, *NS* Not-Significant

13.2.1 ACT Indication

Most authors and clinical practice guidelines (CPG) recommend ACT in all patients, including those with pT1pN0 stage. However, a recent retrospective analysis by the US National Cancer Database (NCDB) suggests that patients with infracentimetric PAC (pT1a pN0 or pT1b pN0) may not benefit from ACT [6]. It is suggested that in these cases the indication of ACT will be assessed by a multidisciplinary committee. When the use of preoperative treatment increases, it is also possible that ACT may decrease (Table 13.1).

13.2.2 ACT Regimens

13.2.2.1 Adjuvant Monotherapy

The first study which demonstrated the benefit of ACT in OS was the ESPAC-1. With a 2 × 2 factorial design, 541 patients were assigned to two parallel studies; comparing patients receiving ACT with 5-fluorouracil (5FU) vs. those who did not receive chemotherapy. A significant benefit of ACT (median OS of 20.1 vs. 15.5 months) was observed [7]. No benefit was observed in the association of radiation therapy (RT) with chemotherapy. The multinational European study CONKO-001, compared the administration of

gemcitabine alone with the follow-up in those patients with resected PAC. As well, the results showed a significant increase in OS in the chemotherapy arm. In the most recent update, a benefit of patients receiving gemcitabine (5-year OS 21 vs. 10% and 10 years 12.2 vs. 7.7%) continues to be observed [8]. The ESPAC-3 study compared the efficacy and toxicity of 5FU vs. gemcitabine in the adjuvant setting of PAC [9]. Moreover, the OS was similar (23.6 vs. 23.0 months) but those patients who received 5FU experienced higher toxicities. With this data, gemcitabine alone was until 3–5 years ago the ACT standard in PAC. There are no studies that assess capecitabine, an oral fluoropyrimidine (FP), as a monotherapy treatment in PAC adjuvant treatment.

13.2.2.2 Combinations with Gemcitabine

The ESPAC-4 study compared the combination of gemcitabine + capecitabine vs. gemcitabine alone. The results were significantly favorable to the combination (median OS 28.0 vs. 25.5 months and 5-year OS of 28.8 vs. 16.3%). Furthermore, grade 3–4 toxicities were similar for both groups. It is important to highlight that these were poorly prognostic patients; most (60%) with microscopically resection margins (R1) and lymphadenopathy (80%) were affected [10]. Limitations of this study include the absence of postoperative computerized axial tomography (CT) for restaging and the existence of a high percentage of patients with very high Ca 19.9 levels, suggesting the presence of oligometastatic disease. The combination of gemcitabine + nab-paclitaxel has been reported to be effective in patients with metastatic PAC. The phase III APACT [11] trial evaluated ACT with that combination against gemcitabine in monotherapy. No significant differences were observed in PFS which was the primary outcome. The combination of gemcitabine with erlotinib (a tyrosine-kinase inhibitor that has been demonstrated to be effective in metastatic PAC) did not improve the results [12].

13.2.2.3 FOLFIRINOX

The FOLFIRINOX regimen (5FU + leucovorin + oxaliplatin + irinotecan) has been evaluated as an ACT in the PRODIGE-24 study, that compared it with gemcitabine alone [13]. 5FU was administered only in a continuous infusion, eliminating bolus to decrease toxicity. The main objective of the study was PFS, which was significantly higher for patients receiving ACT with FOLFIRINOX (21.6 vs. 12.8 months, HR 0.58). Significant advantage was also reported in OS (54.4 vs. 35.0 months, HR 0.64). This benefit was observed in all preplanned subgroups of patients. Besides, grade 3–4 toxicity was higher in patients treated with FOLFIRINOX, especially diarrhea (19 vs. 4%), sensory neuropathy (9 vs. 0%), asthenia (11 vs. 5%), and vomiting (5 vs. 1%). Importantly, there were no differences in neutropenia grade 3–4, but most patients (62%) who received FOLFIRINOX were associated with a granulocyte colony-stimulating factor therapy. There are no direct comparisons between ACT regimens in PAC with drug combinations (FOLFIRINOX, gemcitabine + capecitabine, and gemcitabine + nab-paclitaxel). However, in a recent meta-analysis, these chemotherapy regimens were indirectly compared [14]. The results showed that FOLFIRINOX was superior in PFS to gemcitabine + capecitabine (HR 0.69, CI 95%

0.52–0.91) and gemcitabine + nab-paclitaxel (HR 0.67, CI 95% 0.50–0.90). The advantage of FOLFIRINOX was especially significant in patients with R1 resection. Nevertheless, no differences were observed in OS. In terms of toxicity, FOLFIRINOX had an increase in grade 3–5 toxicities with respect to gemcitabine + capecitabine (except neutropenia), with no differences when compared to gemcitabine + nab-paclitaxel. Having these results in mind, the FOLFIRINOX scheme is currently considered the standard ACT in patients with resected PAC who have a good performance status (ECOG 0-1) and an adequate postoperative recovery, without significant residual sequelae.

13.2.3 Chemoradiotherapy (CT-RT)

Still, it is not clearly defined the role of CT-RT after PAC surgery, especially when using the FOLFIRINOX scheme. In the ESPAC-1 study [7] patients undergoing 5FU adjuvant CT-RT had worse results than those who were only being followed up. However, this study had significant limitations, especially with regard to the quality of RT that was far from current standards. Later, other studies with contradictory results came out. On one hand, a meta-analysis that group all together has been performed [15]. It suggests that CT-RT would benefit patients with R1 resection, although there is a high heterogeneity with R1 patients oscillating between 17 and 82%. On the other hand, the RTOG 0848 study is ongoing right now. We expect it to be able to better define the role of CT-RT in PAC therapy.

13.2.4 ACT Starting Point and Duration

Many authors and CPG recommend starting ACT within 8 weeks of surgery and that the total duration will be 6 months [16]. However, the right time after surgery to start ACT has not been certainly defined. The ESPAC-3 study [9], found no differences between initiating ACT before 8 weeks or more than 12 weeks after surgery. In line with this, other very recent retrospective studies reported that delayed administration of ACT has no influence on OS, being even effective when administered >24 weeks after surgery [17]. However, another study that uses the NCDB database claimed how OS is improved in patients who initiate ACT between 28 and 59 days after surgery, compared to those who initiate it earlier or later [18]. On the contrary, in a recent meta-analysis evaluating the optimal time for the onset of ACT in digestive neoplasms, OS was not shown to be better when postoperative treatment of patients with PAC was initiated within 6–8 weeks after surgery [19]. Based on these studies that have given the indication, the optimal duration of ACT is supposed to be 6 months, although the impact that would have a different duration is unknown.

13.2.5 Biomarkers

13.2.5.1 Ca 19.9

The Ca 19.9 tumor marker has prognostic value in all stages of the PAC. In patients with resectable PAC, preoperative Ca 19.9 levels clearly define the risk of recurrence. Several thresholds have been proposed to define prognostic values ranging from 100 to 500 IU/L [20]. Moreover, high postoperative levels have prognostic value and have been used as exclusion criteria in recent ACT studies [12, 13].

13.2.5.2 Circulating Tumoral DNA (ctDNA)

The presence of ctDNA appears to have a clear prognostic value. In an analysis of 112 patients with PAC undergoing radical resection, the presence of ctDNA before or after surgery was significantly related to PFS and OS, with very high HR between 4.0 and 5.0 [21]. One striking aspect is the value after PAC resection: 100% of patients with postoperative ctDNA showed PAC recurrence, including those who received ACT. In a meta-analysis that groups 375 patients, it is suggested that ctDNA is the most promising biomarker to assess the prognosis of resected PAC [22]. The impact that adjuvant therapy with

FOLFIRINOX would have on its detection is unknown.

13.2.5.3 BRCA Mutation

It is estimated that between 5 and 7% of patients with PAC have germline mutations in the BRCA1/2 genes. Some retrospective data suggest that treatment with cisplatin or its derivatives could improve the OS of these patients when administered perioperatively, compared to other schemes [23]. Obviously, we need confirmatory studies for this hypothesis. In the case we use the FOLFIRINOX scheme, which includes oxaliplatin, we would theoretically be using the appropriate treatment for those patients with BRCA mutated.

13.2.5.4 Predictive Gemcitabine Response Biomarkers

The so-called human equilibrative nucleoside transporter 1 (hENT1) gene, is primarily responsible for the transport of gemcitabine inside the cell. In the study ESPAC-3, the elevated expression of hENT1 was shown as a predictive biomarker of gemcitabine response for its use in ACT [24]. On the other hand, the phosphorylation of deoxycytidine kinase (dCK) is the first step in the transformation of gemcitabine into its active metabolite. High levels of dCK have been associated with increased OS in patients with PAC receiving adjuvant gemcitabine [23].

In summary, there is sufficient evidence to recommend ACT in all PAC cases with R0 or R1 surgical resection. In patients with good performance status, the FOLFIRINOX scheme is considered a standard, being able to use gemcitabine alone or in combination with capecitabine in those patients with generally poor performance status, fragility, or comorbidity. Although there is no solid evidence, ACT is preferred to last 6 months and start within the first 8 weeks after surgery. The assessment of ctDNA is considered the most promising biomarker for the prognosis of patients with resected PAC.

13.3 Neoadjuvant Chemotherapy in PAC

13.3.1 Overview

As we have previously mentioned, ACT is the standard treatment of resectable PAC. With upfront surgery, only 15–20% of patients are initially resectable [3] and the increase in this percentage of potentially resectable patients is vital to improve their prognosis. In addition, due to surgical complications, deterioration of general performance status, or early progression, only 55% of patients end up receiving ACT [25]. In the case of preoperative chemotherapy or NACT, almost all patients are able to improve the locoregional and systemic control of the PAC. Other advantages of NACT are:

- Convert in resectable those patients with irresectable locally advanced PAC.
- Increase the percentage of patients with R0 resection (free surgical resection margin >1 mm).
- Treat possible micrometastasis early.
- Avoid alterations from surgery produced during the blood infusion of the tumor.
- Decrease the rates of surgical complications such as bleeding or fistulas.
- Avoid unnecessary surgeries in patients with rapidly progressive disease.

NACT is common in other digestive neoplasms (esophagus, stomach, or rectum), but in PAC it has been struggling. On the one hand, until recent times the rate of responses to chemotherapy was very low. Another barrier is the difficulty of current radiological tests in properly assessing the response to NACT, being unreliable for predicting resectability or pathological response [26]. In addition, there is a risk of deterioration in performance status during NACT. Finally, the percentage of complete pathological responses (CR) after NACT is much lower than in other gastrointestinal tumors, ranging from 2 to 15% [27]. There are no studies comparing ACT with NACT in PAC. This comparison is difficult to make because almost all patients are eligible for NACT, while patients receiving ACT are often positively selected: they are patients with good recovery after surgery and were not found irresectable spread by laparotomy. As previously mentioned, the assessment of the NACT response is an additional difficulty. Inflammatory and fibrotic changes in the periphery of the tumor following chemotherapy with or without RT may be confused with a solid tumor mass. Therefore, during the restaging by CT after NACT no response is commonly observed. Thus, only 12–20% of patients have a radiological response after NACT, although most patients (80%) get an R0 resection. In addition, the OS of patients with CT stabilization is similar to that of responding patients. In general, anatomopathological evaluation shows complete (CR) or partial (PR) response (<50% viable tumor cells) in 56% of patients. Therefore, it is currently recommended that radiological stability is not a contraindication for surgical assessment. In short, all patients receiving NACT who do not progress locally or metastatically should undergo a surgical examination to assess the possibility of resection [28]. Other methods are being explored to evaluate the response to NACT in PAC: in a study by Tsai et al., a panel of six biomarkers was used to choose the best NACT scheme. In that study, they manage to increase the complete treatment (NACT and surgery) from 50 to 70% in borderline PAC and in 80–90% in resectable PAC. In general, there is an improvement in OS, going from a median of 38–45 months [29]. As in ACT, the absence or presence of germline or somatic mutations in genes associated with homologous recombination repair (HRR) deficiency, especially BRCA1/2, would tilt our choice of chemotherapy regimen to schemes that included platinum-based drugs such as FOLFIRINOX [23]. Probably, in the close future the assessment of the response to NACT will consist of a combination of biochemical, genetic, radiological, and pathophysiological variables. It is important to notice that PAC is currently considered a systemic disease, even in localized phases, requiring chemotherapy and not only surgery within the multimodal therapeutic strategy [28] (Fig. 13.1).

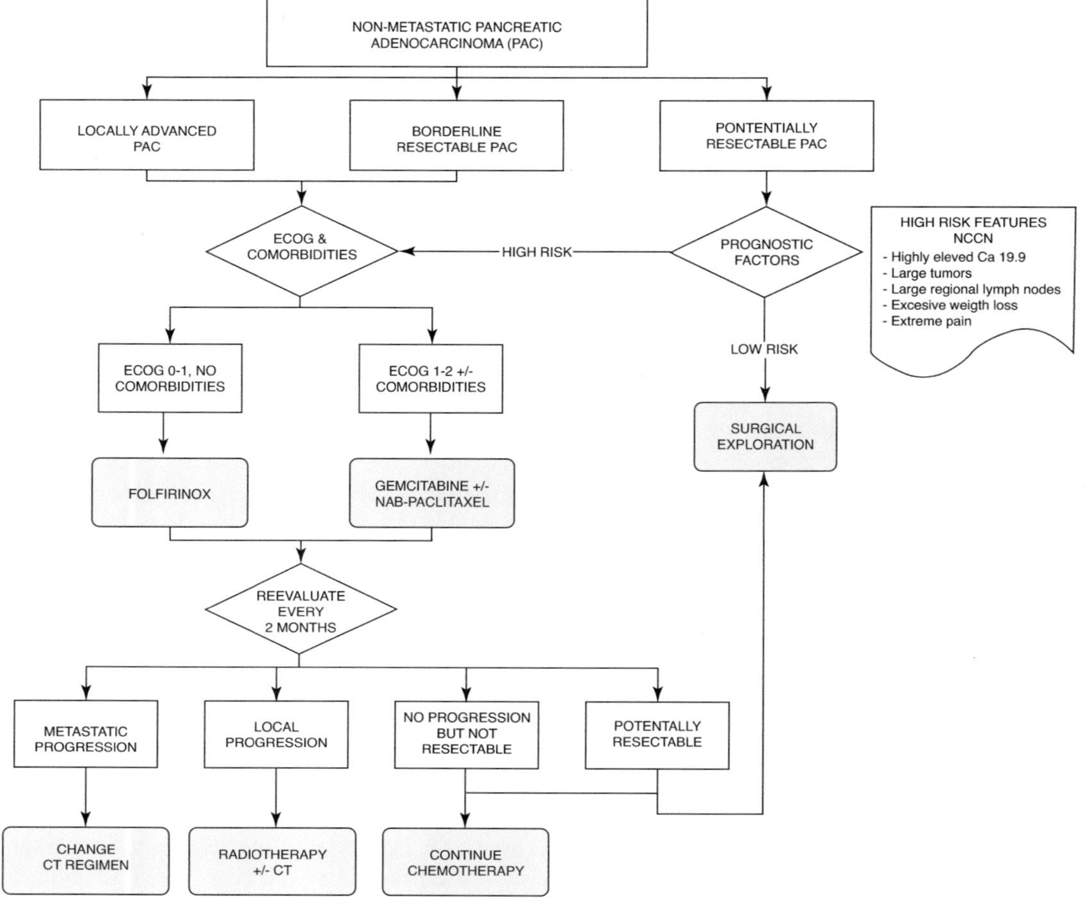

Fig. 13.1 Proposal of algorithm for the management of non-metastatic PAC

13.3.2 NACT in Locally Advanced PAC (LAPAC)

LAPAC has been defined by the NCCN [5] as the PAC that is not metastatic and for which complete resection is not possible at the time of diagnosis. 30–40% of PACs are diagnosed in this situation. Although there are multiple studies on NACT, the level of scientific evidence is low with few prospective studies. Data for resectable patient conversion are highly variable and range from 4 to 75%. The best studies are a series of cases of centers with high volume of patients. Hackert et al., from the University of Heidelberg, analyzed 575 patients (76% with LAPAC) who received NACT with various regimens. The percentage of patients who obtained surgical resec-

tion was significantly higher in those receiving FOLFIRINOX (61%) than those receiving gemcitabine + radiation therapy (46%) or other regimens. The FOLFIRINOX scheme was also associated with a better OS in multivariate analysis [30]. The Johns Hopkins's group [31] analyzed its 415 patient series, half of whom received FOLFIRINOX. One hundred sixteen patients (28%) undergone surgical examination, of which 84 (20%) achieved tumor resection and 75 (18%) R0 resection. The median OS was significantly higher in the group that achieved surgical resection (35.3 vs. 16.2 months, $p > 0.001$). Likewise, in a meta-analysis with individual data from 11 studies that included 315 patients [32], NACT in LAPAC achieved a median 24.2-month OS that is similar to that achieved in patients with borderline PAC. The first prospective study has recently been reported: the German randomized phase II NEOLAP clinical trial, in which 130 LAPAC patients were randomized to receive NACT with four cycles of gemcitabine + nab-paclitaxel or two cycles of the same scheme followed by four cycles of FOLFIRINOX, there were no significant differences between the two groups. 63.5% of patients had a surgical scan, with surgical resection reaching 35.9%. The median OS was 18.5 months in the gemcitabine + nab-paclitaxel arm and 20.7 months in the one which included FOLFIRINOX [33].

The role of RT in patients with LAPAC is uncertain. Some authors and CPG support using radiotherapy + 5FU in those LAPAC that are considered candidates for surgery following initial induction chemotherapy, but the effectiveness of this scheme has not been proven as occurred in studies such as LAP-07 [34]. The purpose of NACT in LAPAC would not be so much to decrease the tumor size in order to facilitate surgical resection, but to discover patients with early neoplastic progression indicating aggressive tumor biology contraindicating surgery. Therefore, it is important to emphasize that in the case of non-progression after NACT, the possibility of surgical examination should be evaluated to determine whether that patient should undergo resection or not. The choice of chemotherapy in LAPAC is still controversial, although it seems reasonable from the previously mentioned studies that the combinations of gemcitabine + nab-paclitaxel or FOLFIRINOX should be used.

13.3.3 NACT in Borderline PAC (BLPAC)

BLPAC has limited venous or arterial involvement [5]. Although theoretically some of these patients would be resectable with initial surgery, there is a high probability of incomplete resection (R1/R2). There is no consensus on the treatment of BLPACs. Several studies have suggested the usefulness of these patients receiving NACT. A Korean Phase II/III clinical trial [35]

compared NACT with gemcitabine + RT followed by surgery with the opposite sequence; both groups received adjuvant gemcitabine. Although only 58 of the 110 patients expected were recruited, the median OS was significantly higher in the group receiving NACT (21 vs. 12 months). Most significant is the PREOPANC study, a phase III randomized clinical trial that included patients with BLPAC and PAC resectable from the beginning. It compared three cycles of gemcitabine + RT followed by surgery with three cycles of adjuvant gemcitabine with initial surgery and six cycles of adjuvant gemcitabine. In the preplanned subgroup of BLPAC 113 patients were recruited, with a benefit observed in OS (17.6 vs. 13.2 months) for NACT. This study has limitations arising from the high rate of abandonment and the imbalance of prognostic groups impairing the initial surgery group [36]. In the recent ESPAC-5F study, 90 patients were randomized into four arms:

(i) Initial surgery
(ii) Two cycles of NACT with gemcitabine + capecitabine
(iii) NACT with FOLFIRINOX for four cycles
(iv) NACT with capecitabine + RT [37]

All patients received ACT with gemcitabine or 5FU. In the initial surgery group, 62% of patients vs. 55% were resected in those receiving NACT. Importantly, the R0 resection rate was higher in those receiving NACT (23 vs. 15%). In addition, 1-year survival was significantly higher in patients receiving NACT (77 vs. 40%, $p > 0.001$). These results served to reinforce the NCCN recommendation advising patients with BLPAC to receive NACT. A meta-analysis of 3843 patients from 38 studies that rated NACT in BLPAC found that any scheme of NACT improved OS (19 vs. 15 months). The results showed that the resection rate was higher in patients receiving initial surgery (81 vs. 66%), but R0 favored NACT (87 vs. 67%) [38]. Janssen et al. published another meta-analysis in 2019 that included 24 studies with 313 patients with BLPAC who received only neoadjuvant FOLFIRINOX [39]. The resection rate (67.8%) and R0 (83.9%) were very high. The median OS was 22.2 months and PFS was 18.0 months, although with high levels of variability among the studies. The use of RT associated with NACT varies between different studies. In one of the previously described meta-analyses [38], no differences in OS were observed between patients receiving RT and those who did not. In some studies, such as PREOPANC-1 [36], the association of RT to chemotherapy doubled the percentage of patients with R0 resection (31–65%). In the absence of randomized studies, the additional usefulness of neoadjuvant RT continues to be debated. Several clinical trials that assess NACT in BLPAC are currently ongoing, including PREOPANC-2 [40] which compares eight cycles of neoadjuvant FOLFIRINOX vs. Three cycles of gemcitabine + preoperative RT followed by surgery and four cycles of postoperative gemcitabine. In general, the CPG such as NCCN [5] and the American Society of Clinical Oncology (ASCO) [41] suggest the use of NACT in patients with BLPAC prior to surgery.

13.3.4 NACT in PAC Potentially Resectable (PACPR)

Standard treatment in patients with PACPR remains surgery. But given the benefit of NACT in patients with LAPAC and BLPAC, there is a growing interest in the use of preoperative chemotherapy also in initially resectable patients. Among other advantages it would allow almost all patients to receive chemotherapy, avoiding the high percentage of patients who do not initiate ACT due to complications of surgery or worsening their performance status. In addition, decreased accessibility of chemotherapy to the tumor, resulting from altered tumor angiogenesis caused by surgery, would be avoided. On the other hand, the high rate of R1/R2 resections and the poor long-term prognosis also support the interest in the use of NACT in these patients.

A Swiss and German study recruited 73 patients receiving preoperative chemotherapy vs. initial surgery. They did not observe any differences in R0 rection or OS [42]. The Italian study PACT-15 [43], randomized 88 patients into three arms:

(i) Initial surgery with adjuvant gemcitabine.
(ii) Initial surgery + ACT with PEXG scheme (cisplatin + epirubicin + gemcitabine + capecitabine).
(iii) NACT with 3 months of PEXG followed by surgery and another 3 months of PEXG adjuvant.

The median OS was clearly superior in the NACT arm: 38.2 months vs. 20.4 in the adjuvant gemcitabine arm and 26.2 months with postoperative PEXG. The PREOPANC study discussed above [36] included a subgroup of 133 patients with PACPR in which no differences in R0 resection, PFS, or OS were detected between patients with NACT and those receiving initial surgery. The previously commented meta-analysis [38] included the same along with 35 more phase II and retrospective studies, concluding that NACT improves OS when analyzed for treatment intent (18.8 vs. 14.8 months). A retrospective study of the NCDB conducting a *propensity score matched analysis* compared 2005 patients who received NACT for their PACPR vs. 6015 who underwent initial surgery [44]. This study claimed that patients with NACT were less likely to have ganglia impairment (48 vs. 73%), lower percentage of T3/T4 stages (73 vs. 86%), and significantly better OS (26 vs. 21 months). It is unclear what would be the best chemotherapy scheme for these patients. The recently reported SWOG S1505 study [45] compares FOLFIRINOX vs. gemcitabine + nab-paclitaxel (both administered for 12 weeks before and 12 weeks after surgery) in 102 patients with PACPR. The authors reported that R0 resections were similar in both groups, major/complete pathological responses favored the combination of gemcitabine + nab-paclitaxel (42 vs. 25%) and no differences were observed in the 2-year OS. There are currently several ongoing studies evaluating the efficacy of NACT in PACPR: the French Panache-01 (NCT02959879) evaluates NACT with FOLFIRINOX and the German NEONAX (NCT02047513) assesses the neoadjuvant with gemcitabine + nab-paclitaxel. As well as in other contexts (LAPAC and BLPAC), the question of whether patients who have received NACT or preoperative will benefit from ACT also arises in PACPR. There are no randomized clinical trials that answer this question and retrospective series data are contradictory. A retrospective analysis of 520 patients with PACPR who received neoadjuvant FOLFIRINOX suggests a benefit when associating ACT with NACT only in patients with metastatic lymph nodes [46]. Moreover, other retrospective analyses using the NCDB discussed above [44], showed benefits from ACT following NACT and surgery (HR 0.62, CI 95% 0.58–0.66). ASCO CPG [41] recommends that a total of 6 months of chemotherapy should be given in patients with dried PAC in addition to ACT and NACT periods. In summary, NACT's role in PACPR is uncertain. The most commonly used CPGs give various recommendations. ASCO [41] suggests not administering NACT in these patients, while NCCN [5] recommends its use in patients with PACPR who are very symptomatic or who have high-risk factors such as large size, very high Ca 19.9, or lymph nodes affected.

> NACT in non-metastatic PAC has theoretical advantages over ACT, but there are no randomized studies comparing these two strategies. Although the level of evidence of NACT's usefulness in initial surgery is also low, existing studies seem to suggest a consistent benefit in patients with LAPAC and BLPAC in terms of the R0 resection rate, and probably also in terms of PFS and OS. More uncertain is its benefit in PACPR, where we will probably have to wait for the results of the ongoing studies to know their usefulness.

References

1. Neuzillet C, Tijeras-Raballand A, Bourget P, Cros J, Couvelard A, Sauvanet A, et al. State of the art and future directions of pancreatic ductal adenocarcinoma therapy. Pharmacol Ther. 2015;155:80–104.
2. Ferlay J, Partensky C, Bray F. More deaths from pancreatic cancer than breast cancer in the EU by 2017. Acta Oncol. 2016;55:1158–60.
3. Groot VP, Rezaee N, Wu W, Cameron JL, Fishman EK, Hruban RH, et al. Patterns, timing, and predictors of recurrence following pancreatectomy for pancreatic ductal adenocarcinoma. Ann Surg. 2018;267:936–45.
4. Sohal DP, Walsh RM, Ramanathan RK, Khorana AA. Pancreatic adenocarcinoma: treating a systemic disease with systemic therapy. J Natl Cancer Inst. 2014;106:dju011.
5. Tempero MA, Malafa MP, Chiorean EG, Czito B, Scaife C, Narang AK, et al. Pancreatic adenocarcinoma, version 1.2019 featured updates to the NCCN guidelines. J Natl Compr Cancer Netw. 2019;17:203–10.
6. Shaib WL, Narayan AS, Switchenko JM, Kane SR, Wu C, Akce M, et al. Role of adjuvant therapy in resected stage IA subcentimeter (T1a/T1b) pancreatic cancer. Cancer. 2019;125:57–67.
7. Neoptolemos JP, Stocken DD, Friess H, Bassi C, Dunn JA, Hickey H, et al. A randomized trial of chemoradiotherapy and chemotherapy after resection of pancreatic cancer. N Engl J Med. 2004;350:1200–10.
8. Oettle H, Neuhaus P, Hochhaus A, Hartmann JT, Gellert K, Ridwelski K, et al. Adjuvant chemotherapy with gemcitabine and long-term outcomes among patients with resected pancreatic cancer: the CONKO-001 randomized trial. JAMA. 2013;310:1473–81.
9. Neoptolemos JP, Stocken DD, Bassi C, Ghaneh P, Cunningham D, Goldstein D, et al. Adjuvant chemotherapy with fluorouracil plus folinic acid vs gemcitabine following pancreatic cancer resection: a randomized controlled trial. JAMA. 2010;304:1073–81.
10. Neoptolemos JP, Palmer DH, Ghaneh P, Psarelli EE, Valle JW, Halloran CM, et al. Comparison of adjuvant gemcitabine and capecitabine with gemcitabine monotherapy in patients with resected pancreatic cancer (ESPAC-4): a multicentre, open-label, randomised, phase 3 trial. Lancet. 2017;389:1011–24.
11. Tempero MA, Reni M, Riess H, Pelzer U, Eileen M, Jordan MW, et al. APACT: phase III, multicenter, international, open-label, randomized trial of adjuvant nab-paclitaxel plus gemcitabine (nab-P/G) vs gemcitabine (G) for surgically resected pancreatic adenocarcinoma. J Clin Oncol. 2019;37(15 suppl):4000.
12. Sinn M, Bahra M, Liersch T, Gellert K, Messmann H, Bechstein W, et al. CONKO-005: adjuvant chemotherapy with gemcitabine plus erlotinib versus gemcitabine alone in patients after R0 resection of pancreatic cancer: a multicenter randomized phase III trial. J Clin Oncol. 2017;35:3330–7.
13. Conroy T, Hammel P, Hebbar M, Ben Abdelghani M, Wei AC, Raoul JL, et al. FOLFIRINOX or gemcitabine as adjuvant therapy for pancreatic cancer. N Engl J Med. 2018;379:2395–406.
14. Galvano A, Castiglia M, Rizzo S, Silvestris N, Brunetti O, Vaccaro G, et al. Moving the target on the optimal adjuvant strategy for resected pancreatic can-

cers: a systematic review with meta-analysis. Cancers (Basel). 2020;12:534.

15. Stocken DD, Buchler MW, Dervenis C, Bassi C, Jeekel H, Klinkenbijl JH, et al. Meta-analysis of randomized adjuvant therapy trials for pancreatic cancer. Br J Cancer. 2005;92:1372–81.

16. Khorana AA, Mangu PB, Berlin J, Engebretson A, Hong TS, Maitra A, et al. Potentially curable pancreatic cancer: American society of clinical oncology clinical practice guideline update. J Clin Oncol. 2017;35:2324–8.

17. Turner MC, Masoud SJ, Cerullo M, Adam MA, Shah KN, Blazer DG, et al. Improved overall survival is still observed in patients receiving delayed adjuvant chemotherapy after pancreaticoduodenectomy for pancreatic adenocarcinoma. HPB (Oxford). 2020;22:1542–8.

18. Ma SJ, Oladeru OT, Miccio JA, Iovoli AJ, Hermann GM, Singh AK. Association of timing of adjuvant therapy with survival in patients with resected stage I to II pancreatic cancer. JAMA Netw Open. 2019;2:e199126.

19. Petrelli F, Zaniboni A, Ghidini A, Ghidini M, Turati L, Pizzo C, et al. Timing of adjuvant chemotherapy and survival in colorectal, gastric, and pancreatic cancer. A systematic review and meta-analysis. Cancers (Basel). 2019;11:550.

20. Humphris JL, Chang DK, Johns AL, Scarlett CJ, Pajic M, Jones MD, et al. The prognostic and predictive value of serum CA19.9 in pancreatic cancer. Ann Oncol. 2012;23:1713–22.

21. Lee B, Lipton L, Cohen J, Tie J, Javed AA, Li L, Goldstein D, et al. Circulating tumor DNA as a potential marker of adjuvant chemotherapy benefit following surgery for localized pancreatic cancer. Ann Oncol. 2019;30:1472–8.

22. Lee JS, Rhee TM, Pietrasz D, Bachet JB, Laurent-Puig P, Kong SY, et al. Circulating tumor DNA as a prognostic indicator in resectable pancreatic ductal adenocarcinoma: a systematic review and meta-analysis. Sci Rep. 2019;9:16971.

23. Maréchal R, Bachet JB, Mackey JR, Dalban C, Demetter P, Graham K, et al. Levels of gemcitabine transport and metabolism proteins predict survival times of patients treated with gemcitabine for pancreatic adenocarcinoma. Gastroenterology. 2012;143:664–74.

24. Raffenne J, Nicolle R, Puleo F, Le Corre D, Boyez C, Marechal R, et al. hENT1 testing in pancreatic ductal adenocarcinoma: are we ready? A multimodal evaluation of hENT1 status. Cancers (Basel). 2019;11:1808.

25. Merkow RP, Bilimoria KY, Tomlinson JS, Paruch JL, Fleming JB, Talamonti MS, et al. Postoperative complications reduce adjuvant chemotherapy use in resectable pancreatic cancer. Ann Surg. 2014;260:372–7.

26. Wagner M, Antunes C, Pietrasz D, Cassinotto C, Zappa M, Sa Cunha A, et al. CT evaluation after neoadjuvant FOLFIRINOX chemotherapy for borderline and locally advanced pancreatic adenocarcinoma. Eur Radiol. 2017;27:3104–16.

27. Macedo FI, Ryon E, Maithel SK, Lee RM, Kooby DA, Fields RC, et al. Survival outcomes associated with clinical and pathological response following neoadjuvant FOLFIRINOX or gemcitabine/nab-paclitaxel chemotherapy in resected pancreatic cancer. Ann Surg. 2019;270:400–13.

28. Kaufmann B, Hartmann D, D'Haese JG, Stupakov P, Radenkovic D, Gloor B, et al. Neoadjuvant treatment for borderline resectable pancreatic ductal adenocarcinoma. Dig Surg. 2019;36:455–61.

29. Tsai S, Christians KK, George B, Ritch PS, Dua K, Khan A, et al. A phase II clinical trial of molecular profiled neoadjuvant therapy for localized pancreatic ductal adenocarcinoma. Ann Surg. 2018;268:610–9.

30. Hackert T, Sachsenmaier M, Hinz U, Schneider L, Michalski CW, Springfeld C, et al. Locally advanced pancreatic cancer: neoadjuvant therapy with Folfirinox results in resectability in 60% of the patients. Ann Surg. 2016;264:457–63.

31. Gemenetzis G, Groot VP, Blair AB, Laheru DA, Zheng L, Narang AK, et al. Survival in locally advanced pancreatic cancer after neoadjuvant therapy and surgical resection. Ann Surg. 2019;270:340–7.

32. Suker M, Beumer BR, Sadot E, Marthey L, Faris JE, Mellon EA, et al. FOLFIRINOX for locally advanced pancreatic cancer: a systematic review and patient-level meta-analysis. Lancet Oncol. 2016;17:801–10.

33. Kunzmann V, Siveke JT, Algül H, Goekkurt E, Siegler G, Martens U, et al. Nab-paclitaxel plus gemcitabine versus nab-paclitaxel plus gemcitabine followed by FOLFIRINOX induction chemotherapy in locally advanced pancreatic cancer (NEOLAP-AIO-PAK-0113): a multicentre, randomised, phase 2 trial. Lancet Gastroenterol Hepatol. 2021;6:128–38.

34. Hammel P, Huguet F, van Laethem JL, Goldstein D, Glimelius B, Artru P, et al. Effect of chemoradiotherapy vs chemotherapy on survival in patients with locally advanced pancreatic cancer controlled after 4 months of gemcitabine with or without erlotinib: the LAP07 randomized clinical trial. JAMA. 2016;315:1844–53.

35. Jang JY, Han Y, Lee H, Kim SW, Kwon W, Lee KH, et al. Oncological benefits of neoadjuvant chemoradiation with gemcitabine versus upfront surgery in patients with borderline resectable pancreatic cancer: a prospective, randomized, open-label, multicenter phase 2/3 trial. Ann Surg. 2018;268:215–22.

36. Versteijne E, Suker M, Groothuis K, Akkermans-Vogelaar JM, Besselink MG, Bonsing BA, et al. Preoperative chemoradiotherapy versus immediate surgery for resectable and borderline resectable pancreatic cancer: results of the Dutch randomized phase III PREOPANC trial. J Clin Oncol. 2020;38:1763–73.

37. Ghaneh P, Palmer DH, Cicconi S, Halloran C, Psarelli EE, Rawcliffe CL, et al. ESPAC-5F: four-arm, prospective, multicenter, international randomized phase II trial of immediate surgery compared with neoadjuvant gemcitabine plus capecitabine (GEMCAP)

or FOLFIRINOX or chemoradiotherapy (CRT) in patients with borderline resectable pancreatic cancer. J Clin Oncol. 2020;38(Suppl 1):4505.

38. Versteijne E, Vogel JA, Besselink MG, Busch ORC, Wilmink JW, Daams JG, et al. Meta-analysis comparing upfront surgery with neoadjuvant treatment in patients with resectable or borderline resectable pancreatic cancer. Br J Surg. 2018;105:946–58.

39. Janssen QP, Buettner S, Suker M, Beumer BR, Addeo P, Bachellier P, et al. Neoadjuvant FOLFIRINOX in Patients With Borderline Resectable Pancreatic Cancer: A Systematic Review and Patient-Level Meta-Analysis. J Natl Cancer Inst. 2019;111:782–94.

40. Janssen Q, Besselink MG, Wilmink JW, van Tienhoven G, Homs M, Koerkamp B, et al. The (cost) effectiveness of neoadjuvant FOLFIRINOX vs neoadjuvant gemcitabine-based chemoradiotherapy and adjuvant gemcitabine for (borderline) resectable pancreatic cancer: the PREOPANC-2 study. Available online at: https://www.trialregister.nl/trial/7094. In: 13th IHPBA World Congress. Geneva.

41. Balaban EP, Mangu PB, Khorana AA, Shah MA, Mukherjee S, Crane CH, et al. Locally advanced, unresectable pancreatic cancer: American society of clinical oncology clinical practice guideline. J Clin Oncol. 2016;34:2654–68.

42. Golcher H, Brunner TB, Witzigmann H, Marti L, Bechstein WO, Bruns C, et al. Neoadjuvant chemoradiation therapy with gemcitabine/cisplatin and surgery versus immediate surgery in resectable pancreatic cancer: results of the first prospective randomized phase II trial. Strahlenther Onkol. 2015;191:7–16.

43. Reni M, Balzano G, Zanon S, Zerbi A, Rimassa L, Castoldi R, et al. Safety and efficacy of preoperative or postoperative chemotherapy for resectable pancreatic adenocarcinoma (PACT-15): a randomised, open-label, phase 2–3 trial. Lancet Gastroenterol Hepatol. 2018;3:413–23.

44. Mokdad AA, Minter RM, Zhu H, Augustine MM, Porembka MR, Wang SC, et al. Neoadjuvant therapy followed by resection versus upfront resection for resectable pancreatic cancer: a propensity score matched analysis. J Clin Oncol. 2017;35:515–22.

45. Ahmad SA, Duong M, Sohal DPS, Gandhi NS, Beg MS, Wang-Gillam A, et al. Surgical outcome results from SWOG S1505: a randomized clinical trial of mFOLFIRINOX versus gemcitabine/nab-paclitaxel for perioperative treatment of resectable pancreatic ductal adenocarcinoma. Ann Surg. 2020;272(3):481–6. https://doi.org/10.1097/SLA.0000000000004155.

46. van Roessel S, van Veldhuisen E, Klompmaker S, Janssen QP, Abu Hilal M, Alseidi A, et al. Evaluation of adjuvant chemotherapy in patients with resected pancreatic cancer after neoadjuvant FOLFIRINOX treatment. JAMA Oncol. 2020;6:1–8.